Psychopathology

Friedel M. Reischies

Psychopathology

Characteristics of Mental Disorders and Clinical Neuroscience

Springer

Friedel M. Reischies
Arbeitsgruppe Phänomenologische
und experimentelle Psychopathologie
Charité Universitätsmedizin Berlin
Berlin, Germany

ISBN 978-3-662-70292-5 ISBN 978-3-662-70293-2 (eBook)
https://doi.org/10.1007/978-3-662-70293-2

Translation from the German language edition: "Psychopathologie" by Friedel M. Reischies, © Der/die Herausgeber bzw. der/die Autor(en), exklusiv lizenziert an Springer-Verlag GmbH, DE, ein Teil von Springer Nature 2024. Published by Springer Berlin Heidelberg. All Rights Reserved.

This book is a translation of the original German edition "Psychopathologie," Second edition, by Friedel M. Reischies, published by Springer-Verlag GmbH, DE in 2024. The translation was done with the help of an artificial intelligence machine translation tool. A subsequent human revision was done primarily in terms of content, so that the book will read stylistically differently from a conventional translation. Springer Nature works continuously to further the development of tools for the production of books and on the related technologies to support the authors.

This Springer imprint is published by the registered company Springer-Verlag GmbH, DE, part of Springer Nature.
The registered company address is: Heidelberger Platz 3, 14197 Berlin, Germany

Preface of the first edition

The special psychopathology is intended for professionals and educated laypeople who deal with individuals suffering from mental disorders—a book especially for those who work in the field of mental illnesses and have experience with psychopathological definitions. Initial impressions usually come from internships and the beginning of work with patients suffering from mental disorders; the theoretical background comes from psychiatry textbooks. In practice, however, questions or doubts arise, such as "What exactly is a hallucination, what is it related to, and how can it be explained?" The presentation of the symptoms of psychiatric disorders enables a better understanding of the various disease models in psychiatry, whether for schizophrenia, mania, or depression.

It should be a textbook for reading and a book for reference when a specific symptom or a group of symptoms needs to be considered. The book is intended to familiarize oneself with the phenomena of psychopathology and their neuroscientific foundations. It also serves to deepen already existing clinical experiences and prior knowledge.

In the symptom descriptions and introductions to the symptom groups, we see the engagement with the various traditions of psychopathology, psychology, neuropsychology, behavioral neurology, and general and cognitive neuroscience. Many disciplines are active in the field, not only psychiatrists, psychologists, and psychopathologists, but increasingly also neuroscientists with various methods. This has increased the insights. Now, the newly gained insights are to be consolidated in an attempt to further explain the symptoms of the mentally ill beyond what was possible in previous psychopathology.

Each chapter initially presents case examples, psychopathological classifications and definitions, clinical aspects, and those of diagnostics. Neuroscientific models are illustrated at the end on the one hand for the feature group, and specific neuroscientific aspects on the other hand are mentioned for the individual symptoms themselves.

I would like to thank many helpers for reviewing the chapters, Juri Katchanow, Agota Barabassy, Maria Kensche, Antonia Kersting–Reischies, Jan Holthues, Thomas Mell, and Christian Müller. Thanks are due to Springer-Verlag, especially the program planner Renate Scheddin and the project manager Renate Schulz, for the competent and prompt implementation of the work, as well as to the editor, Dr. Karen Strehlow, for the professional revision of the texts.

Berlin
January 2007

Friedel M. Reischies

Preface to the Second Edition

With the Second edition, a complete text revision is available, in which errors were corrected, inconsistencies were eliminated, and the comprehensibility of the text could be improved. The book helps the reader to understand perception and hallucination, thinking and delusion, movement and behavioral disorder, sadness and depression.

An update has been made, new research findings are presented, and new models of psychopathological features are introduced.

Thanks are due on the one hand to the publisher Springer Nature, which made the new edition possible, and on the other hand to the colleagues of the AMDP system group, especially Dr. Rainer Schaub and Dr. Sascha Augsten. Furthermore, I thank colleagues from the Department of Psychiatry at Charité, whose discussions about psychopathological diagnostics have given me many valuable suggestions, especially Dr. Martin Voss. I would also like to thank Dr. Rudolf Weiß and Dr. Antonia Kersting-Reischies for their help in editing the manuscript.

Berlin
September 2023

Friedel M. Reischies

Contents

1 Psychopathology and Neuroscience

Contents

1.1 What is Psychopathology?

Psychopathology deals with the individual signs of mental illnesses; one can speak of the smallest descriptive units of psychopathological changes, the clinical elements of syndromes and disease patterns.

Psychopathology has gone through flourishing periods when it enabled the differentiation and characterisation of the time course of various psychiatric diseases for the study of disease patterns. Just as in an early phase of language research, the study of language disorders due to localized brain lesions was important, i.e., the science of language impairment, so was psychopathology in the study of the human mind and the mental apparatus.

Now neuroscience has flourished—technical methods of imaging, biochemistry, and especially genetics are available. One goal of specific psychopathological research is now the neuroscientific explanation of, for example, delusion and hallucinations.

Psychopathology remains necessary alongside clinical diagnostics, on the one hand, to conduct good technical or laboratory investigations of mental illnesses as a research discipline, as well as to contribute to the progress of therapies. On the other hand, however, attention should be drawn to another aspect—to the models for the described symptoms: How can we explain that anxiety or delusion appear as signs of an illness? Previously, one could only ask which symptoms occur and how they are to be ordered. Nowadays, however, new questions are possible:

- What is a neuroscientific explanatory model for the elements of mental disorders?
- What are the necessary and sufficient conditions for the occurrence of the psychopathological symptom?

F. M. Reischies, *Psychopathology*, https://doi.org/10.1007/978-3-662-70293-2_1

Areas of psychopathological features such as thought disorders or ego disorders have been proposed but not accepted everywhere. For example, American psychiatry has not adopted ego disorders. In this book, the discussion of such classification problems is only mentioned in passing.

What are the psychopathological features about? In a psychopathological examination, on the one hand, the person's description of experiences and, on the other hand, events in behavior are observed. These are objective actions, both motor activity and especially speech acts. However, much that is important for the examination is not expressed by the person—they do not talk about it. This concerns very personal experiences, feelings, emotions, etc. The subjective side must be explored. For this, the person's descriptions about their experience are necessary. Only in a trusting conversation can the person be enabled to talk about it.

When the patient is better known, when much of the experience, ways of thinking, and specific feelings have been talked about, what might be considered "crazy" usually disappears. This is partly due to empathy, partly due to the appreciation of cultural differences between the person and the examiners (Heinz 2023). Another level should be added. Ramachandran (2004) emphasizes: When a patient reports something that is considered crazy by the environment, it is only because the psychiatrist fails to explain it neuroscientifically. The uncanny nature of psychopathological symptoms is partly related to this: We still understand too little about the symptoms that can develop in the human psyche. There are people who still hold magical, mystical, and supernatural influences responsible.

We have a new level of psychopathology before us: neuroscientific explanations of the abnormal actions and also the abnormal experiences of people with mental illnesses. Psychiatry is still at the beginning of the neuroscientific study of these phenomena, a psychiatric pathophysiology, but in the next few years or decades, we will be able to explain to the patient why one or another of their experiences or actions occurs. Today, patients already come to the clinic with a depressed mood and talk about a disorder in their transmitter balance. A wealth of—largely incorrect—popular explanations is circulating. This indicates the need for a scientific explanation of the symptoms on the part of the patients. In psychoeducational sessions, we talk to patients about these models.

Conclusion
The expansion of understanding symptoms to include the level of neuroscientific explanation will bring progress in the treatment of mental illness patterns.

Psychopathology enables the description of the functional state of the person concerning possible impairments of the mental or emotional realm. It uses information inferred from behavior in the examination situation or information communicated by the person. Psychopathological features are, on the one hand, objectively observable, they are to be questioned and observed in the interview, and on the other hand, they are subjective, whereby they can be spontaneously expressed, e.g., told or represented in a diary.

Objective. Experienced psychiatric examiners assess patients based on observations in the ward—this is especially true for the time course—they pay attention to psychomotor movements, emotional expression, drive, attention, etc. They rely less on the detailed interview.

Interview. In the interview, there are diverse interaction possibilities, resistances, self-presentation tendencies, simulation, etc. Additionally, there are transference phenomena, i.e., both patients transfer feelings and attitudes to the examiners and vice versa. The examiners must be aware of the possible distortions that can result from this. Furthermore, there are possibly prejudices on both sides: For example, some patients from other cultures still do not accept a female doctor as competent because they only know male doctors.

Subjective. A person can fall into despair and commit suicide due to shame, which the person do not speak about. The psychological disorder has occurred purely subjectively—up to the life-ending event. Unfortunately, this does not happen infrequently. Psychopathological diagnostics in the clinic are based on establishing contact with the patient. This includes well-trained personnel and specific framework conditions.

1.1.1 Why Special Psychopathology—Clinical Aspects

The science of psychopathology seems to have receded into the background. The symptoms are clinical everyday routine ; there is practically no research on the symptoms. Essentially, research is conducted on combinations of symptoms, on syndromes. There is the depressive syndrome, the paranoid-hallucinatory syndrome, etc.—as if we were dealing with fixed disease patterns. The syndromes are virtually fixed in their connection with the diagnoses according to the international classification systems.

This book is dedicated to the psychopathology of individual symptoms. It is organized not in syndrome groups (see below), but in psychopathological or neuroscientific groups.

The neuroscientific approach entails that the psychological explanation of symptoms is not the focus. It is not about trying to empathically trace the genesis of symptoms, to understand possible motives—why a person "freaks out," is in despair, is in a state of euphoria, or in affect committed an act.

Psychiatric Clinical Syndrome and Classification Criteria

Illnesses from the psychological domain are among the most widespread, under which many people and their relatives suffer severely. Psychological illnesses are at the top of the diseases that represent a burden to humanity.

Psychiatric illnesses are understood and diagnosed as state-time course entities What is that? A) The state is described psychopathologically: a number of psychopathological features that were observed—B) the progression is reconstructed based on the information from patients or relatives about previously occurred phases, their duration, the completeness of remission, and the acuity and circumstances of the occurrence of the current illness, etc.

Since the introduction of the international classification systems DSM and ICD, which characteristically differentiate psychiatric illnesses, the position of psychopathology in the diagnosis of psychiatry has changed. In the classification systems, much value is placed on queryable information. The classification systems emphasize information that the examined person communicates to the interviewer or that is observed by the examiner or relatives. The predominance of queryable features has led to the proposal of computer-based interviews for the diagnosis of psychiatric illnesses. Objective progression information also becomes more important than the observable and in the trained psychopathological interview elicited psychopathological symptoms. Certainly, much information about psychological illnesses can be gained through interviews—even through a computer-based interview. But by limiting to queryable features, a large part of psychopathology is excluded from the diagnostic evalutation—besides the observable features, also, for example, the sensitive and unreliably and problematically ascertainable information about symptoms of schizophrenia such as hallucination, ego disturbances, or delusion. Thus, the frequent differential diagnosis of a psychotic disorder cannot be clarified by a computer-based interview.

▶ The complete capture and diagnostic appreciation of the psychiatric illness can only be achieved through careful psychopathological examination with questioning and observation in a psychopathological interview.

An important further problem needs to be emphasized: The diagnostic criteria of the classification systems are optimized for differential diagnosis. They do not describe the entire clinical syndrome. For example, anxiety is only mentioned for anxiety disorders, as it is constitutive for the diagnosis of these illnesses. From a classificatory perspective, the symptom anxiety is therefore not valuable in other illnesses. But, for example, depressive patients, patients in a schizophrenic episode, and patients with many other psychiatric illnesses also suffer from anxiety. Anxiety is not asked for if only the diagnostic criteria are considered, for example, if the relatives have already indicated that the patient suffers from hearing voices.

The clinical reality of the health-economically streamlined diagnostic paths could enable a reduction of diagnostics to short interviews that only check the classification criteria. However, this has unfavorable consequences for the patients if they, for example, in our above examples, suffer more from anxiety than from depressed mood or ego disturbances.

Besides the approach of psychiatric illnesses as nosological units, the syndromic approach in psychiatry has been discussed (Hoche 1912, see below: Sect. 1.1.3). Psychiatric therapy is more syndrome oriented than nosologically oriented. Here, the attempt is made to make the individual symptoms, the psychopathological units themselves, the target of neuroscientific explanations. The syndromic aspect of psychiatry, however, is not at the center of psychopathology. Accordingly, syndromic references are only considered marginally.

Psychopathology is clinically indispensable, not only for its role in diagnostics but also for the observation of fine changes in the time course of an illness. These are crucial for the control and management of therapy. Currently, several psychopathological features are used in the syndrome scales for the depressive, manic, paranoid-hallucinatory, or other target syndromes.

Descriptive Psychopathology: Presentation of Mental Illness – Clinical Surface and Disturbance of Functional Systems

In a psychiatric exploration for diagnostics, a clinical "surface" of a person first becomes apparent. Various disciplines attempt to look "under" this surface: technical, for example, brain imaging, laboratory examinations such as those of body fluids, but also pychoanalytical diagnostics , behavior analysis of behavioral therapy, etc. The following will argue that the descriptive-psychopathological approach provides the basis for further investigations and therefore allows looking beneath the surface. It concerns the disturbance of neuroscientific functional systems, which are the basis of mental symptoms. The functional systems can be disturbed due to different disease processes, whether it may be emotional reactions to environmental situations or the activation of genetically determined diseases or other disease mechanisms.

An inadmissible reduction of pathological experience to coarse neuroscientific functional principles is not intended. Neuroscience does not explain and predict the complexity and diversity of individual experience. On the experience side, there are as many different syndromes as there are people who suffer from them. None is the same as the other. The investigator faces this interindividually different experience and tries to learn about it, to be empathical with the particular suffering of the person. However, the clinician must then compare the patient's experience with the coarse psychopathological categories that are supposed to classify the experience. The neuroscientific findings of psychopathology do not refer to the diversity of individual experiences but to clinically pragmatic proven dimensions and categories of describing pathological experiences.

1.1.2 Neuroscience of Psychopathology

Neuroscientists often believe that classical psychopathology cannot be made compatible with neuroscientific models . A completely new terminology must be created. In contrast, this text attempts to examine the clinically used terms with respect to their neuroscientific foundations. Some terms will be newly introduced, others will need to be changed.

In this book, the focus of interest is on the neuroscientific explanation of psychopathological symptoms. Why both: Psychopathology and Neuroscience?

Today, we know more about how the "clinical surface" of mental illness can be explained neuroscientifically. The task is to achieve a pathophysiology of mental illnesses. In the diversity of mental phenomena, features can be found that are closely related to the disturbance of the functional systems of the CNS. Neurological examples include the paralysis of the contralateral limbs after a lesion of the motor cortex. Neurologists sometimes think that if a symptom shows such dependence on neurological substrates, then this symptom becomes neurological. But that is wrong. Ultimately, many symptoms of severe mental illnesses, which, for example, are associated with genetic predisposition, will also have a neuronal substrate. An example is schizophrenia. In the coming years, genes, protein disorders, and ultimately neuronal functional disorders will be identified that produce the peculiar symptoms of schizophrenia, whether they are ego disturbances, hallucinations, or delusional perceptions. However, this does not make schizophrenia a neurological disease. Admittedly, it is still a long way to the neuroscientific explanation of mental illnesses.

▶ The disturbances of functional systems of the CNS that underlie psychiatric syndromes are not only crucial for the outbreak of the disease but also usually for the course and therapy. They are therefore not just important for diagnostics but can give us clues for the prevention, mitigation of the disease, or improvement of its course.

The example also shows another aspect of psychopathology. Research is often conducted on more sensitive techniques or laboratory chemical examination methods that may help to diagnose schizophrenia more sensitively than psychopathological features. So far, however, the most sensitive early symptoms for the first episode of the disease seem to be the psychopathological ones. This is also to be expected if we realize that the specific functions of even slight molecular changes in the functional systems of the brain can first affect the specific functions of the mental and psychological functions of the person in everyday life—long before the currently still coarse neurophysiological laboratory measurements can objectively prove this functional disorder.

From the above arguments, it can be summarized: Neuroscientific psychopathology seeks models of psychopathological symptoms, specifically models that explain the symptoms at the level of brain functional disorders.

One starting point are neuropsychological symptoms, found after brain damage. This means that the discipline of neuropsychology investigates changes found after a brain lesions or the disturbance of certain brain structures, such as symptoms of perception—agnosia, memory—amnesia, routine actions—apraxia, or language—aphasia. Classical psychopathology built on these examples and postulated that other symptoms would also be explainable neuroscientifically in the future.

Genetic Disorders with Mental Disorders

In genetic studies of psychiatric disorders, an endophenotype is sought, which is more specifically related to the genetic pathology and resulting protein disorder than the known psychopathological features. Protein disorders affect neurons and glia or their metabolic supply. Protein disorders can cause a variety of cellular or metabolic changes, such as disruption of the shape and formation of dendrites and axons of nerve cells. Furthermore, for example, the proteins involved in information transmission, such as receptors in cell membranes, can be disrupted. Or the processing of transmitters is disturbed because one of the metabolic pathways in the cell or in the surrounding glia is disrupted. When these disturbances occur in specific groups of cells, functional systems can be affected, the disruption of which causes a characteristic symptom – such as e.g. hearing voices. The impairment of certain functional systems is reflected, for example, in specific features of formal thinking or in emotional disorders. Thus, for example, the underlying disturbance important for the disruption of thought in schizophrenia seems to be that of working memory.

Not only a genetic disorder but also toxic or degenerative diseases lead to the disruption of functional systems of the CNS. The search for indicators of underlying dysfunctional CNS systems is one of the future tasks of psychopathology and modern psychiatry. What are the crucial features for the association to the disruption of certain neurophysiological functional systems?

The approach here is that psychopathology involves the damage of basic mechanisms, at least a defined number of functional systems, which are presented here. The basic mechanisms involved are explained at the beginning of each section for the symptom groups. The variety of symptoms, we suspect, arises from the complexity of the "overall apparatus" of the CNS.

It should also be considered: As clinicians, we do not see the immediate deficits caused by brain damage, but we see the organism's reaction to it. This was an important insight that Kurt Goldstein (Goldstein 1934) already pointed out, a neuropsychologist who was concerned with psychiatric symptoms. Today it is clear that there are various compensations, strategy adjustments, and cognitive-emotional reactions that make up the complexity and difficulty of psychopathological symptoms. Because not only

1. biological repair processes,
2. automatic compensation reactions in the CNS,
3. conscious efforts of the affected person to compensate, but also
4. reactions to the consequences of the change in social feedback are to be observed.

Thus, the organism reacts not only to the self-perceived dysfunction but also to the consequences in the relationship with others.

1.1.3 Psychopathology of Syndromes

Neuroscientific foundations and therapeutic principles can be found for syndromes, such as the depressive syndrome. The depressive syndrome encompasses many different areas, such as emotional, cognitive, or vegetative disease characteristics. Causes of depression apparently provoke this bundle of symptoms. The still unknown pathophysiological cause of bipolar disorder, for example, affects highly different functional systems. From this, it seems to follow that the individual symptoms have no independent significance. It seems to be the case that there are different levels of pathophysiological effects, the syndromic and the symptomatic.

The successes achieved so far in neurobiological syndromic research do not relieve us to discover the pathophysiology of individual psychopathological symptoms. If only the syndromes are examined, the individual symptoms would thereby elude neuroscientific analysis. However, this is not appropriate for many psychopathological symptoms, at least those that are already well explainable neuroscientifically. Even when considering that many symptoms occur not only in a single syndrome but in various syndromes, the explanation of the pathophysiology of psychiatric disorders must also succeed in explaining the emergence of these symptoms.

From what has been presented so far, something particularly needs to be pointed out: Behind the symptoms, there are hierarchies of causal factors:

- genetic factors,
- at the protein level: gene activators, enzymes, transmitters, receptors, etc.,
- externally metabolic factors (e.g., toxic),
- psychosocial factors, i.e., specific triggering factors that can also include complex psychological reactions.

Crucial for the concept of this book, which deals with the neurophysiology of psychopathological symptoms, is also that the criteria for psychiatric diseases vary, as can be observed in the evolution of the ICD and DSM classification criteria. Research that is oriented towards the respective classification units would have to start anew after each revision of the criteria. In contrast, the psychopathological feature diagnosis is constantly definable.

Conclusion
As long as we do not yet know the neuroscientific foundations of psychiatric disorders, it is appropriate to ask about the neuroscientific foundations of the symptoms, and it is to be expected that we will come to an understanding of the foundations of the disorders through the neuroscientific research of symptoms.

1.1.4 Research

As already stated, precise psychopathological diagnostics is, on the one hand, the basis of all neuroscientific research in psychiatry, because a precise psychopathological examination of the patients will be necessary for every study. This applies to both diagnostic criteria and the assessment of therapy response.

Research is usually oriented towards the currently valid classification criteria (Charney and Nestler 2004). The goal of this research is the therapy of etiologically homogeneous patient groups. However, this does not yet seem to be in sight. On the contrary: In clinical practice, most currently available therapies are rather syndromic or symptomatic—for example, therapy of the depressive syndrome or the symptom anxiety.

The so far limited success of nosological research in some areas may be related to the polygenic causation of many psychiatric disorders, i.e., we are rather dealing with genetic risk factors and know still far too little about the assumed causal chain:

- gene,
- protein,
- neuron function,
- functional system,
- symptom.
- In addition, there is the question of the level at which psychosocial factors exert its influence.

There has been introduced the concept of specific neurophysiological features, as endophenotypes, which come closer to the genetically caused functional disorder on the biological side than the clinical classification units. This also applies to some symptoms of psychopathology. In this sense, marker symptoms of schizophrenia such as ego disturbances could come close to the endophenotypes of schizophrenia genes in diagnostic quality, a discovery of neuroscientific foundations of ego disturbances could lead to even more specific endophenotypes of schizophrenia.

Most mental illnesses, however, cannot simply be understood as a gene-behavior causal chain, as mentioned above. In addition to protein disorders caused by altered genes, various environmental factors contribute to and partially trigger the clinical syndrome. Gene functions can be switched on or off in a specific psychological reaction to the environment. For example, a psychological reaction can lead to insomnia in a situation of stressing the person. The insomnia can, in turn, trigger gene functions that lead to the onset of a mania—in a person with a genetically disposition to bipolar affective psychosis. In other words, even if all the genes involved in a psychological clinical syndrome were known, significant variance in the manifestation of the functional disorder in psychopathology due to functional gene activation must be expected. Additionally, there are currently insufficiently inverstigated epigenetic control factors of gene activity. The described complex causality is also likely responsible for the variance of the penetrance of genetic disposition of various psychiatric diseases.

The art of psychiatry is to differentiate between psychogenic variations of the mental state and those that are based on genetic functional disorders or belong to brain damage syndromes—i.e., psychiatric research must attempt to bring this differentiation into the psychopathological phenotype of clinical diagnosis and demonstrate it in individual cases.

Most researchers agree that we must also look for the impact on the CNS in psychogenic variations of mental functions. Following the argumentation above, we assume a normal functional variance in which "normal" everyday mental life and normal mental operations take place. In psychopathological symptoms of mental illnesses, brain functions are always disturbed. However, it still requires argumentation as to what is meant by disturbed brain function. If Frege's concept of functions and arguments is applied (Kagan 2001), then we have disturbed brain "functions" before us. The current experiences or individual mental contents are to be regarded as arguments of the function. It can be left open whether the brain structure is damaged or "psychological structures" are dysfunctional; with psychological structures it is meant that, for example, experiential impacts on the brain in the development of each individual establish a corpus of functions that can, for example, have dysfunctional effects in the case of traumatically induced plastic effects.

Severity

Most readers are familiar from everyday experience that normal variance of experience and behavior and the pathological variance, caused by brain damage or brain functional disorders, overlap. An example can be the disease of the thyroid gland: In the development of hypothyroidism, there is a gradual reduction in drive and vitality. In many cases, only retrospectively, after the somatic diagnosis has been made, is the onset of psychological change revealed, i.e., retrospectively, behavioral changes are reinterpreted that had not yet given cause for concern when there was no shadow of suspicion of psychopathological symptoms. The situation is entirely different with clear psychopathological symptoms such as hallucinations.

Three gradations of features must be distinguished:

1. clearly pathological features—the proof of even slight expression of these features indicates a mental illness, for example, delusional thoughts,
2. Features with a transition into a clearly pathological area,
3. Features that, although in the normal psychological range, but
   a) in stronger expression and longer duration, and if they are not situationally explainable, must be considered pathological, such as elevated mood or
   b) can form a characteristic psychopathological syndrome together with other features.

1.1.5 Classification of Symptoms and Subdivision

Symptom List

If all terms for describing experiences and behaviors deviating from the norm were listed, many hundreds of terms would come together. These could not all be discussed here. Which terms, which symptoms are considered and which are omitted? Although there is no universally valid canon of psychopathological terms, a certain agreement is found in the list of symptoms of classical psychopathology. The basis of the symptom list was initially that of the AMDP, the Working Group for Medical Documentation in Psychiatry (2022). The AMDP symptom list has been methodically developed, i.e., the most important characteristics have been extracted from larger lists. There are meaningful solutions from factor analyses (Gebhardt et al. 1983) and scale formations for the major syndromes such as the depressive syndrome and the paranoid-hallucinatory syndrome have been successful. Some terms are added here to the AMDP-Items, which result from the basic definitions of ICD-10.

As described above, some terms are missing. Rare symptoms are not mentioned. Are symptoms dispensable, for example, because they occur too rarely or are usually closely coupled with other characteristics? Further research has to reveal this.

Certainly, additional symptoms from other psychiatric experience areas could be added, for example, those of the mentally disabled, forensic psychiatric cases, or from the observations in psychotherapy.

Classification of the Description of Symptoms and Symptom Groups
In doing so, 2 topics are presented:

1. Structure of the symptom groups,
2. Subdivision of the symptom description.

Structure of Symptom Groups
Which symptom groups should be presented first, and which last? Here, the Jaspers classification (Jaspers 1942), which distinguishes between two main groups of subjective and objective features, is not followed. The reason for this is that, for example, emotional features encompass both subjective and objective components (»Mini-syndrome« see below). For this reason, such a classification would be less meaningful.

There are a number of reasons for the chosen order, which may not seem immediately intuitive. This mainly has to do with the fact that a reader should first become familiar with certain neuroscientific contexts before dealing with features that require more complex neuroscientific explanations. Thus, the sequence of symptoms does not represent an attempt to establish a new systematics of psychopathology but follows didactically the path of a stimulus through the central nervous system:

1. How is the environment perceived, how is a stimulus perceived?
   This is the first question. Strictly speaking, it encompasses almost the entire field of neuroscience, and it will be revisited in the context of hallucinations. Nevertheless, it makes sense to begin with the principles of perception. The next step is:
2. How can an organism act independently of sensory impressions? Several aspects are addressed here, initially the ability to actively remember and the ability to focus attention on a stimulus or divert it from it.
3. How can an action be initiated? Following memory and attention, the ability for autonomous action, motor skills, and action planning is described. How can various actions be coordinated, plans made, and the realization controlled?
   How is the initiative, the drive organized?
4. How is conscious perception, conscious communication, and conscious action carried out? How is language communication and probatory action, thinking organized?
5. How does an organism emotionally respond?
6. Only at the end are the complex prototypical psychopathological features such as hallucination and delusion presented: How can imagination give rise to sensory illusions? How can a delusional explanation develop? How can a person form a judgment?

In this order, the reader first encounters the areas currently better known neuroscientifically.

This structure results in initially unfamiliar divisions at first glance: For example, neuropsychological perception disorders are separated from hallucinations, or disorders in central motor skills and disorders of drive and voluntary motor skills or dyskinesias. This seems necessary to pave a more understandable path for the reader from simpler to more complex symptoms.

1.1.6 Example: Depressed mood, Depression Syndrome, and Depression Diseases

An example of symptoms, syndromes, and specific psychopathological features is intended to illustrate the hierarchy of psychopathological features in psychiatric disease theory and psychiatric practice.

Symptom

Let us consider a situation in a psychiatric clinic: A patient is brought to a doctor on duty at the hospital at night, and the relatives say, "He wants to kill himself." What should the doctor pay attention to, what questions should he ask, and what should he examine?

The first question initially concerns the mood state, the depressed mood. This feature is a psychopathological characteristic. It is not a syndrome in the sense of the depressive syndrome, and it is also not a disease in the sense of unipolar depression or bipolar depression. Depressed mood is a low mood. One could also say low spirits. The word "sadness" means something different. This makes it clear that emotions, in most cases, cannot be precisely captured linguistically. We also do not know exactly what another person, especially a patient, understands by it. There are people who are not used to talking about emotions. So, if I ask the patient, "Are you in a depressed mood?", the patient may answer something, but I do not know exactly what to make of the answer.

In the examination situation, the doctor should trust his eyes, ears, and sense of touch: He sees the facial expressions, gestures, and posture, hears the sound of a voice and the prosody. He feels the muscle tone at the handshake. The best is to gain an impression from the totality of the behavior, not just from the emotional expressive movements or because of worry lines at the eyes (Veraguth folds), but also from the linguistic and bodily expressions as well as the muscle tone, and try to assess whether the statement "I am in a depressed mood" corresponds to one's own impression. Not only depression, but many of the psychopathological characteristics are not easily understood in colloquial language.

▶ In psychopathology, the patient's statement must be weighed against the examiner's impression. This does not mean that one does not trust the patient, but it only means that one has to pay attention to nuch more than the content of the verbal statements.

This distinguishes the psychopathological examination from having a questionnaire filled out. You can diagnose less from a transcription of an interview. But from a video recording with unintelligible verbal expression, the depression diagnosis can be largely secured psychopathologically from the gestures and the speech melody (Renfordt 1986).

depression Depression is an emotional symptom. It can be described as a mood. This distinguishes it from affects such as aggression, laughter, crying, etc. Affects are intense and usually shorter-lasting emotional expressions. But in contrast, we are usually in one of various moods, which we can describe more or less well. Some moods are also even difficult for talented people to verbalize, and it is left to the art of writers to put a certain state of mind into words. All this explains why we cannot rely solely on the patients' explanations of mood in psychopathological diagnostics.

The reader may have experienced how one feels in a depressed mood. This example could clarify some things. In the specific situation, the person would need to be asked a series of questions: Is it sadness, an anxious mood, or just tiredness and morning down? So, even for the individual psychopathological symptom, there is a differential diagnosis. Is it depressed mood or one of the other psychopathological features that can appear like depression?

Something else can be clarified with this example: there are psychopathological characteristics in various degrees—borderline, very mild, mild, moderate, severe, and extremely severe.

Conclusion

In psychopathology, it is necessary to appreciate: 1. the verbal expression, 2. the psychomotor changes or expressive movements, and 3. the integrative/overall impression of the examining person—with the differential diagnosis and the severity-judgement—this applies to each individual psychopathological feature.

Symptom, syndrome, psychiatric clinical syndrome

In the second step, it must be distinguished whether a symptom, a syndrome, or a disease can be diagnosed. Depressed mood can be part of a depressive syndrome, which also includes other features such as vegetative disturbances, cognitive features like certain ways of thinking, motor symptoms, and sometimes additional affective features. The frequency of personal experiences of depressed mood makes it clear that the presence of a psychopathological feature is not necessarily equivalent to the presence of a psychiatric illness. Conversely, many people consider depressed mood from their own experience to be normal, given the circumstances, and react with incomprehension when this feature needs to be treated within the framework of a psychiatric illness.

What constitutes the depressive syndrome? First of all, the depressive mood; in addition, there is the affect of anxiety or an anxious mood. Furthermore, there is a reduction in drive. The persons cannot motivate themselves, they can no longer manage their daily tasks. Specific ways of thinking are also symptoms of the depressive syndrome, they are called depressive cognitions. The patient has for example, feelings of guilt ideas of guilt and their self-esteem is significantly reduced. Furthermore, vegetative disturbances are of great importance. This includes disturbances of sleep, appetite, and sexuality. The individuals can not focuss attention for a longer period and have difficulty making decisions. Finally, psychomotor disturbances also occur. The patients often experiences their limbs as heavy or are retarded in performing movements.

The hospital doctor does not have to fill out a depression scale. But in the psychiatric clinic, the documentation of the syndrome on scales is gaining influence. On the scales in circulation, a feature is asked about and 1–4 points are given for the severity of the feature, for example, for sleep disturbance, depressed mood, drive, anxiety, suicidality, etc. The rater arrives at a sum score based on the number and severity of the depression symptoms (see above). However, based on observation, the experienced observer will also have an independent subjective weighting of the severity of the depression. The observational assessment and the sum score of the rating often contradict each other, for example, when a severely depressed patient with suicidality receives only a few additional points on a scale. But based on observation, they exhibit a large number of depression features that the scale does not ask about, such as pronounced fatigue, a quiet monotone voice, lack of *emotional resonance*, and lack of strength in the handshake, etc.

▶ Observation during a careful interview is usually more valid than the sum score of a depression scale.

Clinical Pictures

In the third step, after securing the symptoms and identifying the syndrome, the criteria of the classification systems must be checked for a diagnosis of a psychiatric disease.

The US-American DSM-V classification system essentially lists symptoms in its criteria list for a depressive episode. Additionally, the threshold for diagnosing a depressive episode—a major depression—is set such that more than 4 of these symptoms must be present for the disease to be diagnosed. Studies have found that there is a significant difference between a depressive syndrome with 2 or 3 symptoms and one with 6 or 7 symptoms: it has different genetic, familial, course, and therapy response characteristics.

There are also additional criteria: on the one hand, the syndrome must be differentiated from other syndromes. An acute grief reaction is often cited as an example here. Another criterion is the significance of the syndrome for everyday life. A disease is only diagnosed if the person suffers from the syndrome and is significantly impaired in their daily functions or professional life.

In the next step, differential diagnostic considerations become necessary.

The depressive syndrome occurs, with minor differences, as part of various psychiatric depression diseases. The most important are: the depressive episode or major depression, which belongs to unipolar depression, bipolar affective psychosis, where manias have also occurred in the course, dysthymia, and depressive adjustment disorder. Clinically, the need for treatment is important in this context. Its criteria are recorded in the psychopathological examination. Here, the severity, for example, the number of symptoms, the burden of the syndrome in everyday life, but also delusion or suicidality must be mentioned. Suicidality is a feature that must be examined with the aspect of acute self-harm, i.e., whether the patient needs to be treated in a protected ward (see above).

▶ For certain psychopathological symptoms, there is often a reduced or absent willingness to undergo treatment. This reduction in insight into the need for treatment is itself a psychopathological feature. A lack of insight into the illness and a lack of willingness to undergo treatment play a prominent role in psychiatry.

With the more modern imaging brain examinations, it has been discovered that in depression, particularly the amygdala and the medial orbitofrontal cortex are disturbed. What do these neuroscientific findings mean for the psychopathological examination? Currently, the neuroscientific imaging findings in patient groups mean very little for an individual patient. Not much can be said neuroscientifically about the nature of the depressive syndrome. It is still unclear what ultimately causes this dysfunction in parts of the brain.

It is also still unclear why the various symptoms of a psychiatric disease occur together in a syndrome. The disturbance of an element of the central nervous system (CNS) can have multiple consequences. Genetic factors with changes in proteins, gene activation, disturbances in transmitter metabolism, or neuroendocrinological disturbances affecting many functional domains are discussed. There can also be connections of processes, for example, neuroanatomical and neurophysiological connections between brain function systems, which cause the spread of pathological functions to other functional systems.

In general, the view prevails that the criteria for diagnosis have improved the quality of psychiatric diagnostics. But the current criteria are far from convincing and will be revised over time.

Example Suicidality

How is the psychopathology of suicidality—as an example—to be assessed? One of the most important differential diagnostic steps is already successful after the above-mentioned examination steps: It can be clarified whether it is a severe depressive disorder, then a possibly life-threatening suicidality must be taken particularly seriously. If suicidality is found in the context of a delusional depression, the danger is even more severe and inpatient psychiatric treatment is often necessary. The affected person must be protected – because after treatment, these patients regularly state that they would have killed themselves and are now grateful that they were saved. They describe that during the illness phase, they could not come to a clear, correct judgment about their situation. If it is a temporary despair of a person without a psychiatric disorder, a short crisis intervention may already be sufficient to de-escalate.

In the case of suicidality, it has proven useful to distinguish between imminent, prepared actions that are very likely to lead to suicide, and suicide attempts that can also have the character of help seeking behavior. A psychopathological feature that has been observed more frequently in recent years is self-harm. This has usually less to do with suicidality.

The prognosis of the type of suicidality and the likelihood of suicide is one of the main tasks of psychopathology and succeeds all the better the more precisely the examiner gets to know the patient in his life course, his goals, and hopes, and how precisely he examines him psychopathologically. Features of acute suicidality are, for example, besides the presence of a severe depressive disorder, the patient sees no values anymore, his previously existing value system is changed, everything that previously meant something to him seems lost; and if he has concrete plans to kill himself and he is caught up in fantasies about it.

1.2 Introduction to the Chapter Structure

First, an overview of the structure and features of the individual sections will be given. The chapter structure applies to all chapters from Chap. 2 onwards. In the descriptions of the feature groups, examples are first given and then an outlook on the disturbances in the features is provided. This is followed by diagnostics and then the neuroscientific explanation of the psychopathological features and their disruptability, as far as this currently seems possible.

Individual Symptoms
The features are described in categories, whereby the following 15 categories are not fully considered for each feature but are omitted if there are no comments for a category.

Subdivision of Symptom Description
Definition. The psychopathological symptom is first presented with a clinically manageable description, with a definition and explanation.

Example. If possible, several short examples are given. The examples should be illustrative and already show the possible diversity of the clinical manifestations of the feature.

Position in Psychopathology. The concept and use of features have changed for some symptoms over the course of the development of psychopathology. In such cases, important concepts and terms from the development are presented. The AMDP feature number is given. In some cases, the feature is new, varied, or changed.

Related Terms. There are often synonymous terms for a feature, sometimes only semantically related terms or old terms that should be mentioned.

Psychopathological Interactions
The independence of psychopathological features has often been demanded for assessment (e.g., in the AMDP system). This is also to be supported in order to document the most valid individual observations possible. However, many features are complexly interrelated. For example, thought pressure and increased drive interact—and these, in turn, with incoherence, i.e., disconnected thoughts. The principle dependence or interaction is easy to imagine in extreme cases, because if a person is mute, speaks very little or not at all, a disturbance in formal thinking cannot be diagnosed—this also applies to all features that require a statement from the patient. The levels at which the interaction of the features is effected are not easy to determine. The interaction can be sought at the core of what constitutes a psychiatric syndrome. In this sense, e.g. the question of the relationship between sleep disturbances and depressed mood touches the foundations of the depressive syndrome.

Interactions can also arise only at the diagnostic level: Features can only be diagnosed if another feature is present or absent.

Another reason for interactions is that features have common constraints. Such constraints do not belong to the narrow concept but influence the feature, such as vigilance/fatigue—an example is the functions of thinking, which are dependent on alertness or fatigue. This specific constraint may not apply to other features, such as emotional symptoms.

An interaction between two psychopathological features can reduce the reliability of the diagnosis, the reliability, both for psychopathological features and for clinical neuropsychological examination procedures such as tests of memory functions.

From a neuroscientific perspective, an interaction between two symptoms arises on the one hand from the dependence of the two underlying disturbed brain functions on each other. The attention system, for example, influences the system of memory encoding, so that the encoding of memory items is more successful when attention is undisturbed. On the other hand, the activity of one functional system may affect many others. For example, the many vegetative, cognitive, motor manifestations of an anxiety reaction, in turn, affect other brain functions, which then trigger further psychopathological features. The dysfunction of one functional system triggers many others. A syndromal connection arises.

There are often unavoidable overlaps of two symptoms with differential diagnostic aspects: Are there two features, or is one feature simply an expression or variant of the other? For the documentation of the psychopathological findings, noting both features is important. For the analysis of an individual case, an attempt can be made to differentiate diagnostically whether only one influencing factor is present, i.e., whether this factor fully explains the observed or reported phenomenon. Otherwise, it must be asked whether, for example, one feature is only a variant of the other (see above) or whether the interaction is rather based on the diagnostic level.

Differential Diagnostic Distinctions

Is there the differential diagnosis of a psychopathological feature? Differential diagnosis is commonly conceived as excluding alternative diseases. For precise psychiatric diagnostics and if one aims to identify underlying functional disorders causing the symptoms, the question must be answered whether the psychopathological features actually apply in the specific case or whether another psychopathological feature is present that modifies the clinical syndrome at this point.

To emphasize the importance of this point in special psychopathology, two examples should be given. An important differential diagnosis arises in schizophrenia: There are patients who believe that other people can read their thoughts, simply because these other people speak about content that only the patientsy have thought. They have wondered where the people they hear got this information and concluded that the people can read their thoughts. This is a different feature than the experience of thought broadcasting or the experience of a kind of mystical unity of two people with the telepathic exchange of feelings and thoughts. The second example of attention disorder has already been presented. An attention disorder that leads to a memory disorder is pathophysiologically different from a memory disorder without the attention disorder, which is found in "true" amnestic syndromes, also as part of an Alzheimer's-type dementia syndrome.

The psychopathological dimension of differential diagnosis is often not considered. However, it cannot be overlooked that differential diagnostic problems exist with individual features and in certain situations. The need for differential diagnostic clarification also applies to individual psychopathological features in the criteria of classification systems. The individual features must be carefully examined to determine whether other disease signs not mentioned in the criteria determine the feature in question.

There is an overlap with the previous category "psychopathological interactions." In differential diagnosis, it is a matter of weighing whether the other feature better describes the experience or behavior of the patient. It builds on the knowledge of interaction possibilities.

Further Characterization

What is additionally important in the appreciation of the feature beyond the definition – what are further critical properties, what is central for diagnostics and psychopathology?

- Not important for definition, but useful to mention for the characterization of the feature,
- clinically significant, but not observable in all cases.

Self-evaluation vs. observation by another person-/other persons's judgment

This and the following sections of the presentation of a psychopathological symptom are dedicated to diagnostics. First, a fundamental distinction must be addressed, which is between the self-evaluation, where it is documented whether the patient says e.g. they hear voices, feel depressed or happy, etc., and another persons's judgment, where the clinician, companions, or nursing staff document observations about a symptom. Obviously, different factors play a role in self-evaluation than in other persons's judgment. Nevertheless, there are overlaps, as some information about a feature comes from the patient, and some additional information comes from observation. For example, it can be observed that the patient who says they hear voices gazes thoughtfully into a corner of the room and then talks to an absent person. Or in statements about emotions, the entire behavior, but especially the affective expressive motor skills, matches the statement that the person is depressed or happy.

Attempts have been made to indicate self-evaluation and other persons's judgment in proportions (see AMDP system). The question of what percentage the self-evaluation contributes to the diagnosis is often unanswerable. Therefore, only the indication self- and/or other persons's judgment is given here.

The documentation of external and self-evaluation should be done separately whenever possible. This is the preferred approach in documenting therapeutic success. In depression remission, for example, there are regularly differences in the judgement of mood improvement. Relatives or visitors may already report that the person is significantly less depressed and has better drive. However, the patient maintains that the signs of depression are maximal. Not only for documenting this frequently observed delay of subjective in contrast to objective mood improvement in the resolution of depressive symptoms is it useful to separate self- and other persons's judgment; but also for the perception of suicide risk, which is particularly high during this time when objective drive improvement and subjective persistence of severe depression coexist.

Even though the statements of the person are decisive for many features, "the patient does not dictate the psychopathological status"; ultimately, the examining person must reach to an independent assessment of whether the feature is present or not.

Interview for Psychopathological Rating
In the case of a self-assessment characteristic, a person must be asked, for example, how they experience their mood or whether they feel retarded. A wording of the question that has proven effective should be used.

a) The person should explain an introspection. Much criticism has been directed at the scientific base of introspection. But in psychopathology, it must be asked whether a patient feels severe pain, grief or shame, whether they ruminate or experience obsessive thoughts. Of course the information based on this introspection statements are characterized by diagnostic uncertainty. The interviewer must learn to what extent they can trust the information in the specific case for psychopathological assessment.
b) In some cases, a history taken from other persons must be used because it is expected that the patient has not made the observation, does not want to talk about it, or has forgotten it. Examples are the occurrence of failures in every day actions in apraxia, which is usually forgotten by a person with a dementia syndrome, and the aggressive action, about which the person would prefer to remain shamefully silent.
c) The characteristic can be observed in behavior and during the course of the interview. Behavior can also be observed in a ward or an emergency unit.

Neuropsychology/objectification
Some features cannot be queried or reliably observed, such as disorientation; a task must be given, for example, to name the current date or the current location. In psychopathological testing, for example, remembering 3 words for 5 minutes or performing a serial subtraction (100 minus 7, 93 minus 7, etc., see below), we observe behavior and can document errors and compare them with normative data. Patients generally do not like to be tested; this circumstance means that they usually answer such questions reluctantly and perform the tasks unwillingly. In other cases, it happens that they

do not invest sufficient effort during testing. For this reason, testing must be introduced with particular care. For example, by announcing that a short test of concentration is to be carried out, which is necessary for all patients, and that the data will be treated confidentially, etc.

There are not only examination procedures for cognitive features—but also, for example, for examining emotional reactions. For this, the interview topic should be directed to positive or even cheerful content, paying attention to the expected emotional reaction.

The question for the many different psychopathological features is, therefore, whether there are appropriate examination procedures. If an examination procedure exists, the examiner must be trained in its execution and interpretation: A) Which behavior must be observed in the patient? B) What influencing factors are to be expected?

Is an objectification of a feature possible? A test result does not necessarily provide objective information, as a tendency towards response distortion also affects performance in the testing situation, for example, in reducing the effort during testing. The objectification of psychopathological findings has so far remained in a dormant state and is a subject of future research.

Currently, it is relevant primarily in court expert reports. But that may change. For long-term care insurance, the low objectifiability of the psychological and cognitive impairments of demented patients play a role. A test result is to some extent valid and reliable regarding high performance; low performance can always be related to a bias, for example, in order to reach a higher severity rating for long-term care insurance, a retirement request or financial compensation after accidents.

For the somatic investigation the question of whether there is a dissociative or a neurological disorder is often discussed, for example, with respect of a questionable psychogenic epileptiform seizure. But psychogenic loss of consciousness also occurs in the psychiatric clinic. Here, with all clinical knowledge and as much information as possible about the person's history, the consistency or inconsistency of the clinical picture must be clarified.

In the USA, after the first edition of this book, the initiative to establish the neuroscientifically foundation of psychiatric diagnostics was launched (Research Domain Criteria, RDoC, Review Morris et al. 2022). In 5 basic dimensions, neuroscientific findings are being investigated, which are to form the basis for the objectification of psychiatric diagnoses: arousal and arousal regulation, positive and negative valence, sensorimotor, cognitive, and social processes. Considerable research activity has been stimulated—in various parts of this 2nd edition, we will address new research results. However, at the present time, we unfortunately cannot yet state, that there is already a neuroscientific foundation of the psychiatric diagnoses. The concept of this book has the—somewhat more modest—goal of explaining the neuroscience not immediately of diagnoses, but the neuroscience of individual symptoms in the context of disturbed functional systems.

Regarding the credibility of psychopathological findings, the internal consistency of all diagnostic informations is crucial. If inconsistencies are found—for example, in the performance profile, where the relative difficulty of the tests is well known—then the finding is no longer to be considered trustworthy. In the AMDP system, it is emphazised that the psychopathological finding always remains judgment of the investigator and in case of doubts about the consistency of the findings, the critical feature should be rated as "not assessable."

Severity of the psychopathological symptom

What findings are there for the severity of a psychopathological symptom, i.e., a mild or severe manifestation of the psychopathological feature, and how can this be correctly assessed?

Assessing the severity requires experience in the variance of the manifestation of the psychopathological feature. Someone who has never seen a severe depressive illness will consider a person who is currently sad and crying to be severely depressed. But usually, patients with a lack of emotional responsiveness, who can no longer cry, suffer from the most severe manifestation of depressed despair. If an examiner only knows mildly depressive and anxious outpatient patients, he cannot assess the severity of delusional depression or acute severe schizophrenic psychosis.

How should one be able to compare the severity levels of different features? It is tempting to apply external criteria. In some approaches, purely subjective feature manifestations were classified as mild, and those that disturb the environment were classified as severe. But this does not always lead to satisfactory results because many features remain predominantly subjective.

When presenting the features, the variance of the symptom will be indicated to give the reader initial hints about the range of severity of the phenomenon.

The severity of a syndrome, for example, the depressive syndrome, is often estimated in clinical practice using rating scales. In part, a respective severity assessment of the relevant individual symptoms is summed up—in part, only the number of symptoms are counted. Everyone will immediately agree that the latter is a problematic procedure. However, the reason for this approach is, among other things, that the severity assessment in training for psychopathological scales always appears to be the least reliable, while there is more agreement on the presence or absence of a feature. A trained and reliable assessment exclusively of the feature "depressed mood" is much closer to the core of the syndrome and could thus provide a more appropriate assessment of the severity of depression.

Pathognomonic—the symptom is pathognomonic for a psychiatric clinical syndrome

Some features are diagnostically decisive for one of the psychiatric disorders. In other words, there is practically no differential diagnosis, but the identification of this feature diagnostically reliably indicates the presence of the specific disorder. These symptoms have a prominent position in nosology: for example, ego disturbances in the form of experiences of external influence and phonemes in the form of dialoguing voices have a high value in identifying schizophrenic disorders.

Specifications

Are there specific groups of individuals in whom a feature is found? If a separate smptoms were coined for each specification, we would be dealing with drastically more psychopathological symptoms. When is an observation to be considered a psychopathological symptom, and when as a specification of another symptom? One could only speak of psychopathological domains and document everything else in specifications. For example, many specifications are listed for delusional thoughts, such as delusion of guilt, paranoia, or megalomania, which in other psychopathological schools are considered additional symptoms. On the other hand, summarizing the features into very large groups results in too coarse a psychopathological classification. For example, it does not help to speak only of content-related thought disorders without further subdivision.

For these reasons, a compromise has been attempted below. The goal is to make pragmatic, valid distinctions in the abundance of psychiatric observations, i.e., those that have proven to be useful in achieving a characterization of more homogeneous groups of psychological/physiological states.

One factor that has been used for the classification of psychiatric observations is the terminological distinctiveness, as in the case of illusion, hallucination or pseudohallucination. In the early days of psychopathology, symptoms could not be explained, but distinctions could be made that were related to the logical structure and especially the psychological-philosophical definability. In delusional thoughts, the different delusional contents can involve different mechanisms. A depressive delusion is certainly based on different pathophysiological mechanisms than a theft delusion of a demented person. In the early days of psychiatry, they were discussed as different diseases.

For the specification of a feature, in the sense of a further subdivision, the first important question is whether there are distinguishable classes of the feature. Future research may find that only a limited number of features and specifications are associated with the disorder of neuroscientifically identifiable brain dysfunctions, which will enable a sufficient description of the mental suffering - for therapy. It is therefore possible that some global features can be identified that are centrally closely associated with genetic-pathophysiological factors of psychiatric diseases.

Personality Influences
Variance in the manifestation of psychiatric disorders mentioned above is significantly related to characteristics of the personality. For instance, grief expresses itself differently in an anxiously avoidant person compared with a narcissistic histrionic person. The influence of the processes responsible for personality traits on the manifestation of psychopathological symptoms should not be underestimated. This means, however, that diagnostics in psychiatry is already a difficult art, as on the one hand, the beginner must already know the personality types to assess their influences on the modification of psychopathological features, and on the other hand, these personality-forming processes themselves can be deformed by the pathological factors of the disease process.

Personality influences should indeed represent a kind of "error variance" for most features, which must be considered in diagnostics. Beyond that, however, pathophysiological interactions are possible or likely for some features. This is evident in the case of compulsions: In the symptoms, personality characterization, and the disease of compulsive phenomena, the interaction of psychopathological symptoms and personality characteristics becomes clear. However, differences in the syndromes between compulsive personality and compulsive disorder must be pointed out here; that is, it is not simply a matter of a different degree of dysfuntion that determines whether it is a compulsive personality or a compulsive disorder. There can be a mild compulsive disorder with a severe compulsive personality disorder. The same applies to the schizotypal personality, which has a content-related kinship to schizophrenic illness, and of course to anxiety and anxiety disorders.

Thus, on the one hand, we have specific symptoms that belong to the corresponding personality forms and also specific mental illness patterns, and on the other hand, personality forms that generally color the above-mentioned manifestation of psychological features—such as narcissistic or avoidant personality types.

Conceptual Problems of the Feature
Finally, the conceptual problems associated with all the above-mentioned influences will be addressed for each feature.

An example is the distinction between thought broadcasting as an ego disturbance and delusional explanation of commenting voices.

For the specific psychopathological feature, there may be conceptual doubts regarding the definition; or controversial models of the philosophy of mind may refer to the specific symptom.

These problems of the individual psychopathological symptom affect the diagnostic relevance of the feature, the reliability of a diagnosis made with it, or a possible close association with other features.

Neuroscientific/Cognitive Neuroscientific Models
In addition to the general neuroscientific introduction to the feature group, both neuroscientific and specifically cognitive-neuroscientific models are mentioned for each symptom. These cannot be explained in detail for each feature. Therefore, at the beginning of a chapter, the neuroscientific introduction attempts to illustrate the most important basic mechanisms. The neuroscientific factors mentioned for each symptom often represent no more than hypotheses and model drafts. In part, there is a plethora of hypotheses, so not all can be mentioned.

References

AMDP, Arbeitsgemeinschaft für Methodik und Dokumentation in der Psychiatrie (2022) Das AMDP-System, 11 edn. Hogrefe, Göttingen. Engl. translation: W Guy, TA Ban 2012, Springer Berlin

Charney DS, Nestler EJ (2004) Neurobiology of mental illness, 2. edn. Oxford Univ Press, Oxford

Gebhardt R, Pietzcker A, Strauss A et al (1983) Skalenbildung im AMDP System. Arch Psychiatr Nervenkr 233:223–245

Goldstein K (1934) Der Aufbau des Organismus. Einführung in die Biologie unter besonderer Berücksichtigung der Erfahrungen am kranken Menschen. Martinus Nijhoff, Haag

Heinz A (2023) Das kolonialisierte Gehirn und die Wege der Revolte. Suhrkamp Verlag, Frankfurt

Hoche AE (1912) Die Bedeutung der Symptomenkomplexe in der Psychiatrie. Z Ges Neurol Psychiatr 12:540–551

Jaspers K (1942) Allgemeine Psychopathologie, 4. edn. Springer, Berlin

Kagan J (2001) Biological constraint, cultural variety and psychological structures. In: Damasio AR, Harrington A, Kagan J et al (Eds) Unitiy of knowledge. The convergence of natural and human science. Ann N Y Acad Sci 935:177–190

Morris SE, Sanislow CA, Pacheco J, Vaidyanathan U, Gordon JA, Cuthbert BN (2022) Revisiting the seven pillars of RDoC. BMC Med 20:220

Ramachandran VS (2004) A brief tour of human consciousness. Pi Press, New York

Renfordt E (1986) Quantitative analysis of speech behavior of depressed patients under a drug therapy. Psychiatr Dev 4:135–146

Perception—Neuropsychological Disorders

2

Contents

On the path of a stimulus through the brain, we consider the first step, perception. How do we perceive what is happening around us? Which people or animals are there, which houses, which streets, etc.? How does understanding the mechanisms of elementary perception help us understand complex perceptual disorders such as hallucinations?

Elementary perception is impaired in focal brain injuries and degenerative brain diseases. Since disorders of primary perception have little significance in psychopathology, the disorders are only briefly presented. The complex perceptual illusions, the much more common hallucinations, are described in Chap. 12.

Example

An almost 90-year-old man complains of poor vision. The optician could no longer fit a better pair of glasses. Sometimes he tries an old pair of glasses or both on top of each other. But he can no longer read the newspaper. He has to be accompanied on every walk. Only in his house does he know his way well enough to move alone. The examination

F. M. Reischies, *Psychopathology*, https://doi.org/10.1007/978-3-662-70293-2_2

showed sufficient visual acuity and ruled out visual field restrictions. When trying to trace overlapping figures with his finger, it became apparent that he could no longer distinguish the individual figures from each other and could not name which figures were hidden in the tangle of lines. ◀

Is the elementary perceptual disorder dispensable as a psychopathological symptom area? Many psychiatrists have seen agnosia or other elementary perceptual disorder rarely or not at all. But they occur in the syndromes of dementia, delirium, or as hallucinations with sensory impairment (Förstl et al. 1991).

In older depressed patients, a sense of insufficiency is common, especially affecting vision, and help-seeking behavior can contribute to this. So the question of perceptual ability must be examined. In young people with anxious histrionic syndromes, tunnel vision and so-called hysterical blindness are described.

2.1 Perceptual Elements

The first group of perceptual disorders includes those involving elements of the objects to be perceived. In this type of disorder, edges, corners, or colored surfaces are incorrectly perceived. In the auditory modality, sound properties are no longer reliably perceived—for example, speech, especially when multiple speakers are speaking simultaneously. In the following, we will primarily illustrate agnosias using the example of visual perception.

The elements of perceptual objects are not perceived individually in everyday perception, but only as complete objects. This becomes clear to anyone who tries to draw more complex figures, such as the image of a person. Perceptual elements do not stand out to a person in everyday life, but only when, for example, they cannot identify an object they have never seen before in poor lighting. However, once it is identified, the meaning is clear to the person, and the perception of the elements of the visual form completely recedes into the background. We can focus on seeing the figure elements through the control of attention.

The disturbance of information processing at the level of elementary perceptual features leads to problems with the delineation of objects, i.e., the question of what belongs to one object and what to another (see below Poppelreuter figures, Fig. 2.1). Other problems exist with the identification of the same objects in different views, from different perspectives and distances.

The perception of a class of elementary perceptual features can be disturbed. An example is color blindness, which can be genetically determined—however, brain damage in the occipitotemporal area may also lead to achromatopsia, the inability to perceive the colors of objects, e.g., in a quadrant of the visual field. In depression, the subjective experience of colors can be diminished, with people feeling that colors are faded or everything seems to be "gray in gray." The perception of the movement of objects can also be disturbed. Patients may not be able to reliably distinguish different objects because they cannot see whether two shapes are the same or different (Milner and Goodale 1995;

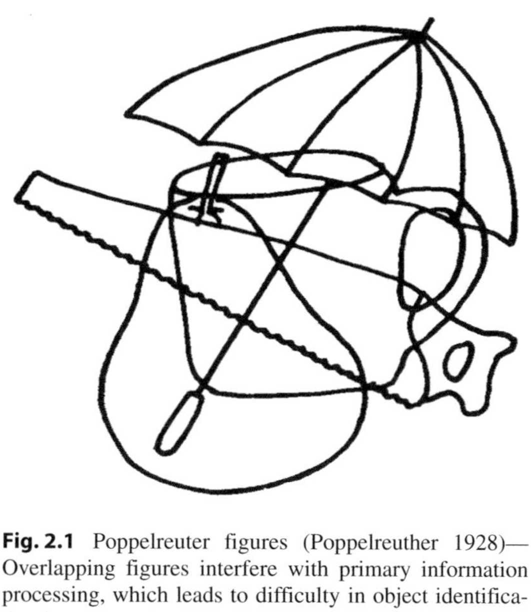

Fig. 2.1 Poppelreuter figures (Poppelreuther 1928)—Overlapping figures interfere with primary information processing, which leads to difficulty in object identification in apperceptive agnosia. A patient with speech problems should be asked to trace the outlines of the figures, as this can distinguish between naming disorders and agnostic disorders.

Hildebrandt et al. 2004). When elements of the objects to be recognized cannot be correctly identified, the disorder is referred to as apperceptive agnosia.

The distinction between two levels of perception, that of elementary perceptual features and that of object recognition, is evidenced by a "double dissociation," which is essential for neuropsychological proof of distinguishable brain functions: After damage to one brain region, elements of perception such as shapes, edges, corners, or even colors cannot be recognized—after damage to another brain region, objects cannot be recognized—but these individuals can describe or draw the elementary perceptual features. This demonstrates the specific vulnerability of the levels of feature and object recognition.

2.2 Object Perception

The second group of elementary perceptual disorders deals with object perception, the recognition of, for example, a house, a pair of scissors, or a face. In object agnosia, the person finds no access to the meaning, although the edges, corners, and curves, i.e., the elements of the perceived objects, are correctly identified (see, for example, Hécaen and Albert 1978). The person can draw the figure but does not know what he has drawn; he cannot describe what can be done with the object. A patient managed to copy a delicately drawn beach crab but did not know what the picture was supposed to represent and guessed helplessly.

The described subdivision leads to the assumption that there must be at least 2 levels of neural representation of objects in the brain:

1. Psychophysical level of the elementary perception of sensory elements such as edges and corners, as well as surfaces with their visual properties:
   - visual, somatosensory,
   - spatial, sensorimotor,
2. Object meaning, semantic level of object recognition.

Specific qualities of the object can indeed be available to the person (color, form elements, etc.), but the level of meaning, the semantic and thus also linguistic level, is not reached—"perception stripped off its meaning" (Teuber 1968). If a patient cannot name an object, it must be differentiated diagnostically whether it is due to 1. an agnostic disorder or 2. an aphasic disorder (see Chap. 9), a word-finding disorder. Object agnosia is described further below in Sect. 2.4.3.

Early on, there was a concept of a disconnection, which refers to the disruption of the information flow from the level of object perception to the level of word finding, the lexicon (Humphreys et al. 1999). For these logically clearly delineable stages of information processing, there is again a spectrum of cases that rather belong to a disturbed analysis of the perception elements or conversely to a disorder of object naming, which has been referred to as optical aphasia or modality-specific visual misnaming.

Conscious Perception

Another subdivision of the processes of perception can be made according to the degree of consciousness: conscious perception in contrast to unconscious, implicit perception and reaction (Farah and Feinberg 1997, Chap. 8 consciousness). Unconscious perception can lead to reflexive movements, such as in traffic when quickly reacting to a vehicle coming from the side. We have learned to react before we have clearly seen and consciously perceived the object. In everyday life, adults perceive most objects in their environment unconsciously and react more or less reflexively to them.

Definition

1. apperception is understood as the conscious perception of objects.
2. perception is understood as the process of perception; for example, in reaction time experiments, one can react to perception to elements of an object before the entire object is consciously perceived.

For the quality of consciousness of perception, refer to Chap. 8 consciousness.

2.3 Clinic

Agnostic disorders are noticed e.g. due to naming difficulties and problems with recognizing people. Observing clumsiness in everyday life can also, upon closer inspection, indicate whether a person has "visual problems." For agnosia, for example, it is valuable to have reports from others that objects and people are no longer consistently and reliably recognized or named (Grüsser and Landis 1991, Sachs 1985).

Example

It is often the case with gerontopsychiatric patients that they say they can no longer properly recognize their environment, that they are blind in one eye, or that they need increasingly brighter lamps, stronger magnifying glasses, and newly adjusting their glasses for reading. Then often they buy new glasses or use multiple pairs of glasses ("multiple spectacle syndrome"). Upon examination, it turns out that they have a form of agnosia. ◀

2.3.1 Apperceptive agnosia

In apperceptive agnosia, the elementary sensory features of the objects no longer help in recognizing the objects (see above). In diagnostics, the worsening of perception is examined using, for example, interference lines. In the case of apperceptive agnosia, such a variation in perception conditions makes perception difficult. For example, crossing out objects or letters leads to them no longer being recognized, or the overlapping Poppelreuter figures see Fig. 2.1. A patient with apperceptive agnosia will not be able to name the outlines of all figures despite intact point perception and an intact visual field.

Example

A patient with a right occipital infarction and a left temporal middle cerebral artery infarction could only partially recognize large overlapping objects in the Poppelreuter figures: He said "bell or sack" for the bell but could not identify and name the comb and hammer. The identification of the object in the Poppelreuter figures was also unsuccessful when they were traced by the examiner's hand. ◀

Agnostic symptoms occur after states of oxygen deprivation in the brain, after herpes simplex encephalitis of the temporal lobe, etc. Agnostic symptoms also occur in advanced Alzheimer's dementia. In posterior atrophy, agnostic symptoms occur, with apperceptive agnosia predominating (Schmidtke et al. 2005). There is a test with drawings whose lines are more or less interrupted or only rudimentarily depicted. It investigates at what degree of completeness of the figure the person can recognize the object (Kessler et al. 1993).

2.3.2 Simultanagnosia

In clinical observation of this form of agnosia, it is noticeable that a patient looks around perplexed. For example, he may correctly name some individual parts in a complex picture—but he "cannot make sense" of the whole. The integration of the correctly perceived objects into an overall view of the scene is disturbed (Allison et al. 2000). This form of agnostic disorder is found in older patients in the course of dementia development.

2.3.3 Disturbance of spatial exploration

Cortical visual disturbances often also lead to a disturbance in the perception of the spatial relationships of objects and their surroundings (De Renzi 1982). This may become evident in grasping. A form of apraxia relates to the lack of information for the adjustment of grasping movements (Sect. 5.1.4 errors in routine motor skills).

The visual-spatial disturbances are also evident, among other things, in trail making tests. A test was developed for visual exploration using arrows, whose direction must be followed with the eyes (Reischies et al. 1989; Reischies and Berghöfer 1995).

2.4 Neuroscience

The elementary perceptual functions are—at least in principle— during evolution already developed in the animal kingdom, as with almost all functions of the first chapters of this book. This means that significant insights could be gained from the neuroscience of animal research. We can investigate many of these functions independently of consciousness and language.

2.4.1 Object Identification—"what pathway"

How does the brain manage to reliably identify the multitude of different objects, even when they are shaped differently or seen from unusual perspectives? Essential steps of information processing in the various modalities are now explainable (see Karnath and Thier 2003 for neuropsychology).

Neuroscience describes two separate information processing pathways, one for object identification and one for the localization of objects. The pathway for object identification runs through the temporal lobe, for visual objects through the inferotemporal cortex. Visual object identification occurs there after the perseptual elements of the visual object have been processed in the primary visual areas.

The other information processing pathway, the "Where Pathway," runs to the parietal lobe and concerns, among other things, the spatial aspects of action preparation, e.g., when an object needs to be grasped or avoided (Milner and Goodale 1995, see above and Chap. 5).

When comparing neurons in the primary brain areas and the inferotemporal cortex, characteristics of higher information processing become apparent. The visual neurons of the primary sensory areas have narrowly limited receptive fields, i.e., they "see" a point of light, edges and corners only in a specific small section of the visual field. On the way to the inferotemporal cortex, researchers find neurons with increasingly larger receptive fields that include the fixation point. In other words, the recognition of perception elements becomes increasingly independent of the visual field position, which changes with each eye movement. Additionally, neurons are found in the inferotemporal cortex that encode complex shape elements or objects such as hands or faces.

2.4.2 Ensemble Coding

A principle of the organization of information processing in perception is ensemble coding. Neurons are grouped in overlapping ensembles, i.e., they can belong to many object ensembles. This is easy to understand: an edge can belong to a house, a book, or a cube.

How do the ensembles come together? The process of bonding of binding the elementary feature neurons into an ensemble assigned to an object is currently being intensively researched. It can be assumed that during the phase of imprinting visual discrimination of visual objects according to the model of neural networks (see below), the identification of objects and faces is trained. The bonding to object ensembles is plastic and changeable over the course of life, i.e., a person can still train new ensembles for new objects (see, for example, Karnath and Thier 2003).

2.4.3 Object Identification

bottom-up

The physiological process of object identification can be explained as an activation of ensembles of neurons found in the inferotemporal cortex for visual perception. On the one hand, the primary identification of visual elements in specific orientation and relative localization in neuronal networks, like in artificial intelligence (see below) will automatically result in an activation of the object-coding ensemble neurons.

This automatic recognition from the perception elements can be characterized as "bottom-up", i.e., progressing from basic to higher information processing (Riesenhuber and Poggio 2000). Apparently, this involves characteristic high-frequency rhythmic potentials. For the automatically occurring, not necessarily conscious recognition of objects, which is achieved in about 150 ms (Thorpe et al. 1996), bottom-up information processing is more important than top-down processes (Fig. 2.2).

Sensory information enables the sensory representation of the object. One speaks of the representation of an object in the cortex when neurons become specifically active when this object is presented. The term representation is to be understood in this narrow sense in neuroscience and psychopathology.

2.4.4 Constructivist Position of Perception

top down

The physiologist Helmholtz formulated early on that perception should be based on unconscious inferences. How is this to be understood: Optical illusions or ambiguous images are usually shown to demonstrate mechanisms of visual perception. In neuropsychology, incomplete figures are shown, where the person being examined has to guess what the completed figure means.

The identification of difficult-to-recognize objects, for example, those depicted incompletely, can be explained as follows: Imagine a soldier who has to identify a figure on the horizon at dusk and in fog. In this situation, a preselection of objects is possible. As a result, one or another perceptual unit is repeatedly triggered as a tial, but the complete explanation of the elements does not succeed. In everyday psychological terms, an attempt is made to explain the object visually. Over time, a group of neurons can be activated that contributes to a coherent explanation of the figure. Such a process of figure identification is due to the testing of stored object schemata - one speaks of top-down identification, i.e., the already higher organized information processing helps the more elementary object perception.

An example can illustrate the principle: A drawing of a wire cube can always be seen in two ways. Either the top square is in front or the bottom square. The perceptual interpretations switch after some time (Necker cube). This indicates that the sensory data are interpreted by the

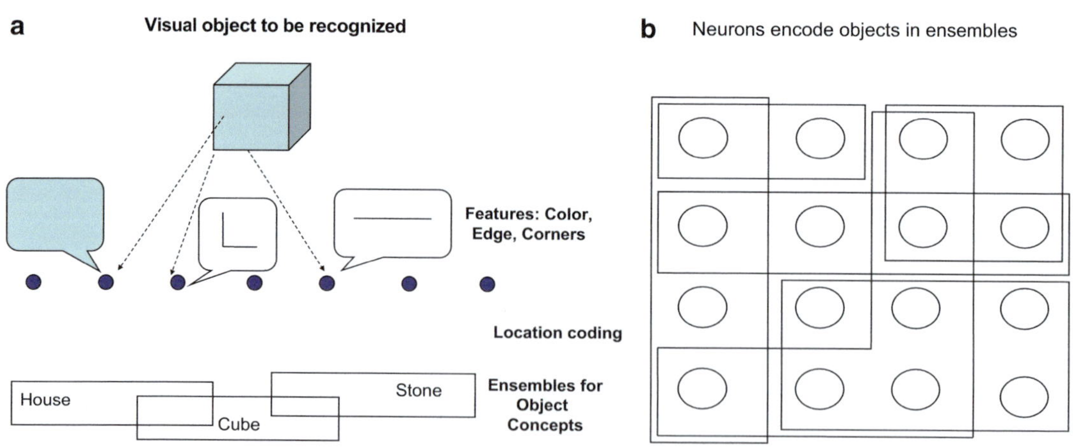

Fig. 2.2 Perception elements. A) Each object is represented separately by different neurons in terms of its sensory elements—a visual object, for example, by neurons that encode color, edges, and corners. Each neuron that encodes an element has a spatial coding through its receptive field. For object recognition and differentiation from similar objects, the information is reassembled. B) Nerve cells of the sensory systems are activated in ensembles by an object, apparently in a transient process, where the activated cells assume a high-frequency synchronized activity. Each neuron can belong to several overlapping ensembles

brain in different ways, whereby this happens by alternately activating different object models after a certain time.

Many neurophysiologists assume a constructivist concept of perception. Already the above-mentioned imagination that for the elements of the objects represented in the cortex, models that could explain them are "tried" until one is found that sufficiently explains the sensory data, points to an active, constructivist concept of perception. In human perception, we are not dealing solely with a passive imaging process.

This aspect becomes particularly clear in the construction of a stable visual environment. We experience the eye movements as wandering around in a constant environmental image. But this image is obtained from the information in the eye, which is upside down and also jumps with every fast eye movement. From the jumping images on the retina, the stable image of the resting environment must first be constructed so that the eye movements can be experienced as an exploration in a stable environment.

The plasticity of this constructed environmental stability has been investigated using inversion goggles. These experiments have shown that after a period of adaptation, people see the environment upright again. The constructivist nature of human perception is important for explaining psychotic perceptual disorders and hallucinations (Sect. 12.1.2).

2.4.5 Specialized Neurons in Perception

The question of whether there is a neuron specialized for the image of well known objects, like the respective grandmother has been discussed in the neurophysiology of perception for decades. The first answer to this question was the finding of hand- and face-specific neurons. They encode, for example, the particularly important information about faces for humans and monkeys (Perrett et al. 1982). Prosopagnosia, the disorder of face perception, had already been described clinically early on.

Generally speaking, the representation of classes of objects in the cortex apparently arranges itself in groups, i.e., closer to each other than to other object classes. There are cortical areas where neurons representing certain object groups are more likely to be found, while in other cortical areas, other object groups are more likely to be identified sensorily.

2.4.6 Memory, knowledge, or perception

However, the "grandmother neuron" has not been found. Presumably, there is no grandmother neuron, but rather ensembles of neurons that first identify a specific face as familiar and then specify that it is the grandmother. It is unclear to what extent the imprinting and early training of the mother's image lead to a more specific representation.

The recognition of objects is already related to visual memory (De Renzi 2000). The classification of objects as "familiar" or "known" is also processed in temporal brain areas. Furthermore, there is a concept that the episodic memories of objects is consolidated into a visual knowledge base—in the sense of a visual lexicon.

2.4.7 Imagination

The visual imagination of perceived objects can be very vivid and plastic. The models for this assume that the top-down information from higher organized brain areas to the primary brain areas is a prerequisite for this. Kosslyn et al. (2002) have attempted to demonstrate that visual imagination activates the primary sensory areas top-down and that imagination can be disrupted by temporary inactivation of the primary sensory areas (see also Ganis et al. 1999). These aspects of elementary perception are valuable for an explanation of hallucinations (see below).

2.4.8 Attention Effects

What we perceive is complexly connected with attention (Chap. 4 attention and Chap. 8 consciousness). Stable points in a cloud of moving points are no longer perceived after a short time. They remain represented in primary visual areas. But we only see these stationary points if they represent something that is consciously perceivable, e.g. a known shape. Another instructive phenomenon is masking an object by immediately following images. As a result, objects are not perceived, virtually erased. For these masked objects, traces are present in the primary visual information processing, but they are not further processed. Attention also plays a role here (Fig. 2.3). Only about 4–5 different objects can be perceived simultaneously in a short time interval. Apparently, they require something like attention resources, which seem to be exhausted with 4–5 objects. It is known that attention to an object or a feature significantly modifies the neuronal response in the cortex (Desimone and Duncan 1995; Maunsell and McAdams 2000) and that different objects in a neuron's receptive field compete for attention resources. The object can be suppressed for perception. Due to the attention dependency of perception, there are numerous top-down influences on perception, which are presented in perceptual psychology and neuropsychology. These attention effects can also be used to explain complex psychiatric perceptual disorders (Sect. 12.1).

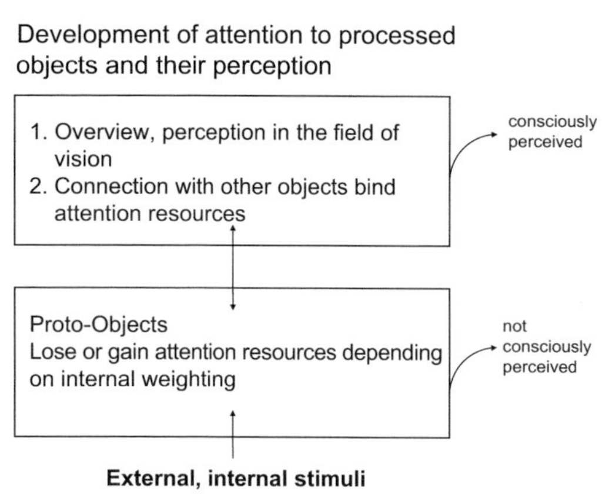

Fig. 2.3 An object that is not primarily focused on by attention can bind attention resources during processing. In this process, it is decided whether it can attract enough attention and reach consciousness

2.4.9 Forwarding of Object Information

After the identification of the object in the inferotemporal cortex, the information is forwarded from there—on the one hand, primarily to the hippocampus and the parahippocampal region, where, for example, familiarity is checked and possibly memories of the object are activated (Chap. 3 Episodic Memory; Fig. 2.4). Furthermore, the information is forwarded to the language areas, where, for example, names are found, and to the brain areas that perform emotional evaluation, to e.g. the amygdala and the orbitofrontal cortex.

The recognition of an object, for example, a house, has both general semantic, linguistic aspects and individual memory aspects that go back to episodes of experience with this house. Even in healthy individuals, an error can occur, whereby an object is mistakenly regarded as familiar, mistakenly recognized (Chap. 3 Episodic Memory). This déjà vu feeling is described by Scharfetter (2002) as perception disorders. The false feeling of familiarity in a perception is more related to the quality of the personal experience with the object than to the cognitive, semantic aspects of perception.

2.4.10 Effects of Disturbances in Elementary Information Processing Steps

Can errors in the initial, elementary information processing have consequences in further processing steps at a higher hierarchical level? For example, does disturbed primary sensory information lead to delayed and uncertain object identification, which in turn causes a disturbance in semantic processing? This has been discussed as the "Weak Input" Model. The concept

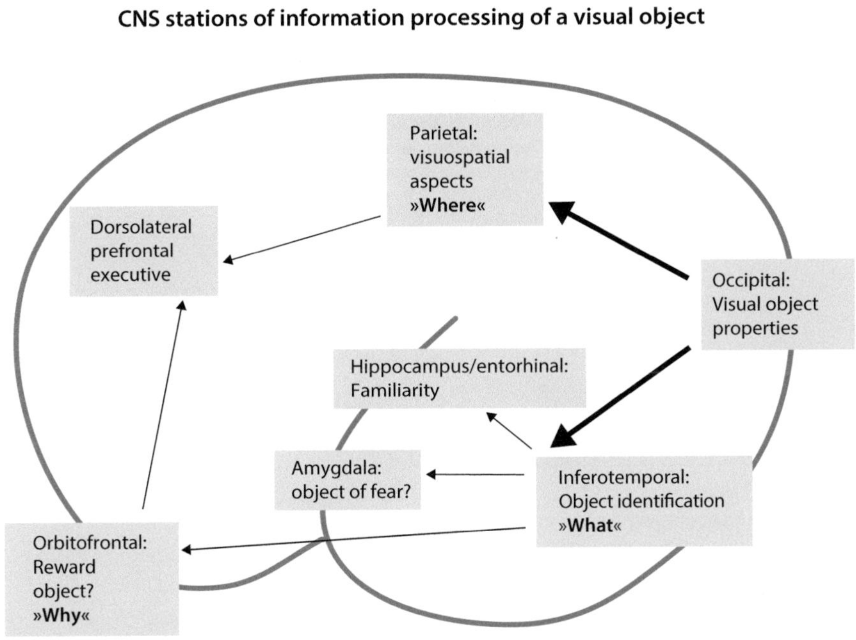

Fig. 2.4 Two information processing streams have been roughly characterized for visual perception: A ventral stream for object identification and a dorsal stream for visual-spatial information processing. In the ventral stream, in the inferotemporal cortex, an object is recognized and the information is further processed in the entorhinal cortex and hippocampus with regard to possible memories (Chap. 3). In the amygdala system and orbitofrontal cortex, the object information can activate emotional aspects, such as anxiety, negative or positive valence or reward sensations (Chap. 11 emotion/affect). In the dorsolateral prefrontal cortex, both streams of information processing can then be integrated, for example, for action preparation

of hierarchical information processing would assume that no further disturbances result. Because once an object is recognized, further processing can proceed undisturbed: retrieving episodic information about the object, monitoring in working memory where it was just found, analyzing the context and possible meaning the object might have, etc. All of this should proceed undisturbed once object identification is achieved.

According to a more holistic conception of cerebral information processing, however, a disturbance in the initial information processing could result in a propagated disturbance in the subsequent steps. This would be the case if the object representation, which is eventually achieved with difficulty, is disturbed, i.e., the neural activity is sufficient for a person to say: “That is a boot” when shown one. But the object representation, the activity of the neuron ensembles that encode the object, is in some way abnormal. Neurons that would otherwise be activated might be missing, or the temporal or rhythmic activity of the neurons might be altered. All of this would lead to the activation of incorrect further nodes in the semantic network during further processing. Then, primary information processing problems result in difficulties at the hierarchically higher levels of cognitive processes.

Today, there are technical object recognition systems with high performance—they can recognize objects quickly and efficiently. The training of neural networks is used in this process. As an indication that understanding elementary perception can facilitate the understanding of complex disturbances, it should be mentioned that in the so-called deep learning layers (hidden layers), categories of objects, elements, but also incorrect solutions can be found, which should later be deleted in the neural network processing. These incorrect “intermediate results” can

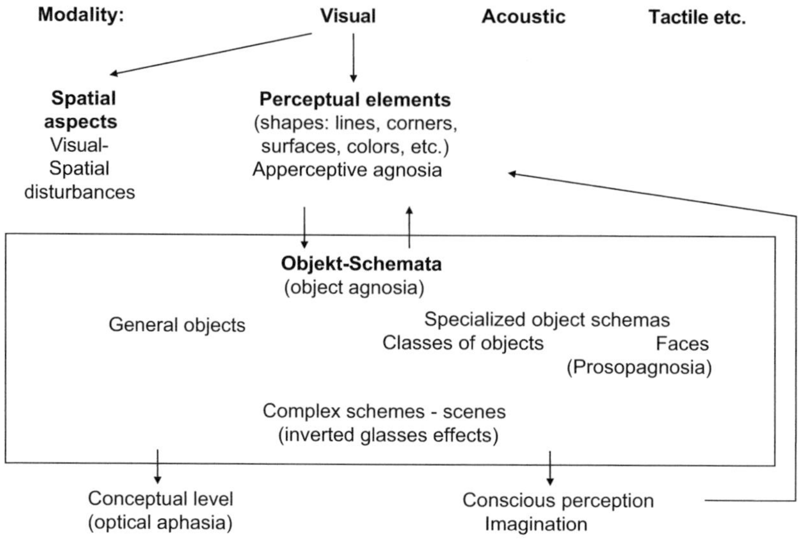

Fig. 2.5 Taxonomy of object agnosia using the example of the visual modality

further help to explain the hallucinatory errors of mentally ill persons (see Chap. 12) (Fig. 2.5).

2.5 Psychopathological Symptoms of Elementary Perception

Agnostic Disorder
Definition: Perception is disturbed despite unimpaired functions of the sensory organs (e.g. in the visual, auditory, or somatosensory modality).

Example. A patient no longer recognizes things seen in his environment. He tries to recognize these objects better, e.g. with several pairs of glasses, but often fails.

Position in Psychopathology. Not in AMDP (AMDP-system 2023), but in the AGP-system, as a symptom of dementia.

Differential Diagnostic Distinctions

- Peripheral or central disease of the sensory organs (or the visual pathway),
- Disturbance of consciousness, disturbance of eye motility or attention,
- Disturbance of language, through which perceptions are to be expressed (e.g., optical aphasia—specifically visually perceived objects cannot be named, e.g., sounds, however, are unaffected).

Further Characterization

a) Disturbance of the differentiation of percepts,
b) Disturbance of the activation of the meaning of percepts, object recognition.

self-/other persons' judgment. Usually only vague subjective complaints, other persons' judgment.

Neuropsychology/objectification. Exact description of the percepts by the patient, in case of suspected visual agnosia let the patient draw objects (which then may not be able to name),

- show incompletely drawn figures (neuropsychological tests are available for this),
- let the patient trace Poppelreuter's overlapping figures.

Severity. Individual perceptual errors up to the inability to find one's way in the environment.

Specifications

1. Modality:
   - visual,
   - sound agnosia,
   - tactile
   - concerning other sensory modalities.
2. Type of agnosia:
   a) Disturbance of the elements of object perception, disturbance of the differentiation of perception elements, (apperceptive agnosia)
   b) Disturbance of the activation of the meaning of the identified perception elements, e.g., the identification of objects (object agnosia),
      - Subtype: prosopagnosia—Visual agnosia for faces.
3. Contexts: simultanagnosia—Integration of percepts disturbed (e.g., of the visual field as a visual scene—the complexity of a diverse image can no longer be comprehended).

Conceptual problems of the feature. Belongs to the so-called brain tool disorders, i.e., disturbance of information processing, which affects one of the "modules" of the mind (Fodor 1983)—in which there is automatic information processing.

Neuroscientific/cognitive-neuroscientific models

a) In the case of apperceptive agnosia forms a complication of the perception conditions (crossing out, overlapping different figures, but also brightness, etc.) prevents the perception of objects/letters, etc.: The object elements that can be perceived,
   - no longer differentially activate the neuron ensembles that encode the objects, i.e., the ensemble that could pass the information in the What-Pathway, for example, to linguistic processing can no longer be activated,
   - it is also a complication of visual "figure-ground differentiation"
     (problems of figure-ground differentiation exist not only for visual perception but generally for semantic units, declarative units of perception, i.e., elements that can be identified by the person and of memory-items).

b) In the case of object agnosia the person does not realize what objects are involved—they cannot explain what properties the object has.

In the case of optical aphasia, it is assumed that it is one of the many possible cases of disconnection due to a brain lesion: Specifically, the disconnection of the pathway from object identification to the neurons that process the lexical unit of the word.

References

AMDP-System (2023) Manual zur Dokumentation des psychischen Befundes in Psychiatrie Psychotherapie und Psychosomatik, 11. edn. Hogrefe, Göttingen. Engl. translation: W Guy, TA Ban 2012, Springer Berlin

De Renzi E (1982) Disorders of space exploration and cognition. Wiley, Chichester

De Renzi E (2000) Disorders of visual recognition. Semin Neurol 20:479–485

Desimone R, Duncan J (1995) Neural mechanisms of selective visual attention. Ann Rev Neurosci 18:193–222

Farah MJ, Feinberg TE (1997) Consciousness of perception after brain damage. Semin Neurol 17:145–152

Fodor JA (1983) The modularity of mind. MIT Press, Cambridge

Ganis G, Sukel KE, Alpert NM (1999) The role of area 17 in visual imagery: convergent evidence from PET and rTMS. Science 284:167–170

Grüsser OJ, Landis T (1991) Visual agnosias and other disturbances of visual perception and cognition. Vision and visual dysfunction, Vol 12. MacMillan, Basingstoke

Hécean A, Albert ML (1978) Human neuropsychology. Wiley, New York

Hildebrandt H, Schütze C, Ebke M, Spang K (2004) Differential impact of parvocellular and magnocellular pathways on visual impairment in apperceptive agnosia? Neurocase 10:207–214

Humphreys GW, Price CJ, Riddoch MJ (1999) From objects to names: a cognitive neuroscience approach. Psychol Res 62:118–130

Karnath H-O, Thier P (2003) Neuropsychologie. Springer, Berlin Heidelberg New York Tokio

Kessler J, Schaaf A, Mielke R (1993) Der fragmentierte Bildertest—Handanweisung. Hogrefe, Göttingen

Kosslyn SM, Pascual-Leone A, Felician O et al (2002) Single-neuron correlates of subjective vision in the human medial temporal lobe. Proc Natl Acad Sci U S A 99:8378–8383

Maunsell JHR, McAdams CJ (2000) Effects of attention on neuronal response properties in visual cerebral cortex. In: Gazzaniga M (Ed) The new cognitive neurosciences, 2. edn. MIT Press, Cambridge, MA, pp 315–324

Milner AD, Goodale MA (1995) The visual brain in action. Oxford Univ Press, Oxford

Perrett DI, Rolls ET, Caan W (1982) Visual neurones responsive to faces in the monkey temporal cortex. Exp Brain Res 47:329–342

Poppelreuther W (1928) Die psychischen Schädigungen durch Kopfschuß im Kriege 1914–1918; Vol 1 Die Störungen der niederen und höheren Sehleistungen durch Verletzungen des Okzipitalhirns. Voss, Leipzig, p 1918

Reischies FM, Berghöfer A (1995) Saccadic tracking test—normal data and reliability. J Clin Psychol 51:262–267

Reischies FM, Stieglitz R-D, Mielewczyk A, Vogel A (1989) Impairments in a saccadic tracking task in schizophrenic patients. Eur Arch Psychiatry Neurol Sci 239:58–61

Riesenhuber M, Poggio T (2000) Models of object recognition. Nat Neurosci 3(Suppl):1199–1204

Scharfetter C (2002) Allgemeine Psychopathologie. Thieme, Stuttgart

Schmidtke K, Hüll M, Talazko J (2005) Posterior cortical atrophy: variant of Alzheimer's disease? A case series with PET findings. J Neurol 252:27–35

Teuber HL (1968) Alteration of perception and memory in man. In: Weiskrantz L (Ed) Analysis of behavior change. Harper & Row, New York

Thorpe S, Fize D, Marlot C (1996) Speed of processing in the human visual system. Nature 381:520–522

Further Reading

Allison T, Puce A, McCarthy G (2000) Social perception from visual cues: role of the STS region. Trends Cogn Sci 4:267–278

Förstl H, Almeida OP, Owen AM et al (1991) Psychiatric, neurological and medical aspects of misidentification syndromes: a review of 260 cases. Psychol Med 21:905–910

Sachs O (1985) The man who mistook his wife for a hat. Duckworth, London. Deutsch: Der Mann der seine Frau mit einem Hut verwechselte (1990). Rowohlt, Reinbek

3 Episodic Memory

Contents

3.1 Introduction

A loss of episodic memory, an amnesia, is currently depicted a lot in novels and films, probably because of the somewhat eerie, frightening clinical picture. What does it mean to lose the memory of situations, episodes of one's life? This section addresses that. First, to illustrate, the memory of the last family dinner should be evoked. We remember the spatial situation, the seating arrangement, the sequence of courses, and the conversations. After an event that led to amnesia, patients with a severe amnestic syndrome always live in the present and the very distant past. In the case of Sacks (1994), the patient experienced a shock every morning when he looked in the mirror. Because he remembered himself only as a young man, which he was many years ago. He had forgotten all impressions since that time after a short delay. This example characterizes a patient with an amnestic syndrome and can answer the question of why

F. M. Reischies, *Psychopathology*, https://doi.org/10.1007/978-3-662-70293-2_3

practically all cases of severe amnestic syndrome need to be closely supervised, usually even in a sheltered home.

We know several memory systems: Episodic memory must be distinguished from other forms of human memory. Other memory functions that play a role in psychopathology are:

1. Working memory see Chap. 6
2. conditioning of behaviour see Chap. 11
3. Learning of manual skills or motor abilities such as riding a bicycle

(see Neuropsychology of Memory, Markowitsch 1992, 1998; Baddeley 1976; Baddeley et al. 1997).

The disturbance of episodic memory is an integral part of psychopathology, as distortions in the process of encoding and retrieval from episodic and autobiographical memory are significant for a patient's self-image. In the diagnostic process they affect every life history. Amnestic patients must be tested regarding the functions of episodic memory. Autobiographical memory, i.e., the episodes that are stored enduringly, are lost, for example, in Alzheimer's dementia.

Example

In the amnestic syndrome, only episodic memory is impaired, i.e., the other forms of memory remain intact. An amnestic patient in his apartment forgets everything within a very short time, for example, to turn off the stove; he forgets whether he has already taken his medication, how much money he has available, and similar things. However, he can argue cleverly. Since he can retain something in his mind for a short time, for example, repeat a short phone number or a short series of words, the fundamental deficit may be not immediately noticeable. However, he forgets after a few seconds that he has repeated the phone number or the words. In the diagnostic examination, it becomes apparent in the anamnesis interview that he has forgotten the part of his biography that occurred after the onset of the amnestic syndrome. ◀

In the amnestic syndrome, intelligence is not affected. Here we can demonstrate a double dissociation: Severely amnestic patients can have high intelligence. However, the reverse pattern is found in patients with severe intellectual disability: These individuals can show a surprisingly good memory. The double dissociation is important for neuropsychology to show the independence of two functional areas. Indeed, episodic memory can fail while other brain functions remain intact.

Why is the name episodic memory correct, in what way is the storage of episodic information impaired? The amnestic patient has forgotten personal experiences, i.e., episodes that he experienced where, when, with whom, how, etc. These are his personal memories of the episodes, memories of how he experienced them. These memories can usually be described. One therefore speaks of declarative memory. The diversity of personal experiences of a situation can be well illustrated by disputes between two witnesses about an event, where each person experienced the event differently and thus stored it differently in episodic memory.

3.2 Autobiographical Memory

The autobiographical memory has been characterized as a highly revised episodic memory that is therefore more firmly stored in the brain and is stable for years and decades. It is affected in retrograde amnesia, which can occur in forms of degenerative dementia. Works by Rubin et al. 1986 have illustrated the extent of forgetting that normally takes place. Practically all unimportant details of the day's experiences are forgotten in the following weeks. In his study, only a few entries from the diary from 2 years ago could be actively recalled.

Not all features of autobiographical memory are determined by processes of episodic memory itself. For the processing and storage of life events, complex reinterpretation and repression processes become effective. For example, persons avoid remembering events that are unpleasant for them. Over time, a person may forget the unpleasant event because it is not consolidated, as we will see further below. Thus, many different, complex mental processes, both conscious and unconscious are effectively shaping autobiographical memory.

Before the clinical manifestations and the neuroscience of episodic memory can be described, the distinctions of various processes that have been elaborated in memory psychology must first be addressed (see also Parker et al. 2002).

Episodic memory can be discussed based on

a) processes,
b) modalities—such as visual, verbal, olfactory, etc.—or
c) the methods of investigation.

Here, the division of the processes of episodic memory into encoding, consolidating, storing, and retrieving will first be explained.

3.3 Memory Processes

3.3.1 Encoding

Information must be processed in a certain way so that it can be retrieved later. In the first phase, the hippocampus is critically involved. The neuroscientific findings about storage in the hippocampus are reported in detail below. The function of the hippocampus can be metaphorically compared to that of a librarian:

- The hippocampus registers all incoming objects,
- assigns them an identifier,
- when a request comes, it issues a message whether it is present, whether it is known (recognition),
- it issues the identifier with which the object can be found and retrieved from storage (recall from memory, retrieval, comparable to the address in a computer by which stored information can be read out),
- if the customer has searched for the book more frequently, they go directly to the correct place on the bookshelves without the help of the librarian (automated recall from memory).

We can remember images that we have seen superficially only once. Apparently, no further storage work beyond perceptual processing is necessary for this. Visual memory has a special status. For remembering names, we often have to make an effort. For memorizing phone numbers or the credit card PIN, a storage routine is recommended, as they are otherwise frequently forgotten.

Deficits of encoding functions are common. On the one hand, insufficient processes are activated; on the other hand, the function of the hippocampus and the parahippocampal region, which is activated during encoding, is disturbed—as in Alzheimer's dementia.

The "depth of processing" is an important variable for storage. If the information was only processed superficially, it will be less well retrievable. This can be demonstrated by comparing the retrieval performance of words that were processed only as words—in contrast to nonsense words—and words with which sentences were formed. The words with which sentences had to be formed are better retained.

Encoding Strategies

A long series of suggestions for improving storage has been made. Words that have been visualized can be reproduced better (Reischies et al. 2000). One of the best storage methods is the method of places: for instance a shopping list is to be memorized. The person visualizes the objects to be remembered, for example, on a path through their own house, a) at the front door, b) in the hallway, c) at a coat rack, d) in the bathroom, e) in the kitchen, f) in the living room, g) on the balcony, h) in the bedroom. They can also be visualized at different places on the body. In antiquity, it was suggested that speakers should remember the sequence of their arguments by wandering through their house and visualizing a keyword for the next argument in each room. This storage strategy is particularly advantageous as it is also suitable for recall in the correct sequence.

One can distinguish between trained efforts and automatic processes for storage. An untrained person will probably process the information to be remembered more attentively, with more mental energy, and engage in a "rehearsal", i.e., silently repeating the items to be remembered internally. Nowadays it happens, that patients come to the memory clinic after memory training and distort the test results by applying efficient storage strategies.

3.3.2 Consolidation

After encoding, the memory content is available for a transitional period through the mediation of the hippocampus, i.e., for a period of weeks to months, there is a dependency of the stored information on the hippocampus until the information is permanently stored.

Since early memory research, it has been assumed that there must be a consolidation phase for newly imprinted memories. The consolidation processes are, for example, responsible for the observation of a gradient of retrograde amnesia after a traumatic brain injury: the events immediately before the brain injury are completely forgotten, while the episodes experienced weeks before the event are partially remembered, and the events that occurred years ago are normally available.

3.3.3 Storage

Where is the information about the experienced episodes stored? Today, it is assumed that there is widely distributed storage in the hippocampus, the parahippocampal region, and especially the cortical association areas. In the hippocampal phase, the hippocampus mediates the memory processes (Sect. 3.3.2).

3.3.4 Recall

As complex as the storage is, so is the recall of the stored memories of episodes. The recall begins with a hint of the storage episode—as a cue. Compared to a computer, one can speak of an "address" that is necessary to read out information stored in the computer.

Example

As an example, let us consider the situation: Someone meets another person whom the person has seen before. Everyone has experienced gradations of recognition and remembering people they do not know well. The process of recalling the episode, in which one saw the person first, breaks off. Initially, the other person just seems "familiar" (Fig. 3.1). ◀

Process of Recall

a) "seems familiar" or "I have seen this before, but I don't know in which situation",
b) recall of the episode in which they met the person, but not specifically, "I know her from work" or from a party—an initial performance of "recollection", "reminiscence" "recollection" of further details from the episode—but still insufficient, because, for example, the name cannot be remembered, e.g., "that's Mrs. …",
c) conscious remembering of the episode of the personal encounter, "Remembering",
d) "reminiscence" "recollection" of further details, e.g., "that was at the dinner at the sports club after the club tournament" and recall of the name,
   "Retrieval" refers to the process of recall from memory, in this case the recall of the name,
e) Routine recall: model of neural networks, e.g., when meeting a colleague whom one sees every day, "oh look, he looks tired today, he must have had a party yesterday."

In the example of searching for the name, we first consider the recall from episodic memory before the Consolidation, i.e., in the phase in which hippocampal function is still necessary (Fig. 3.2).

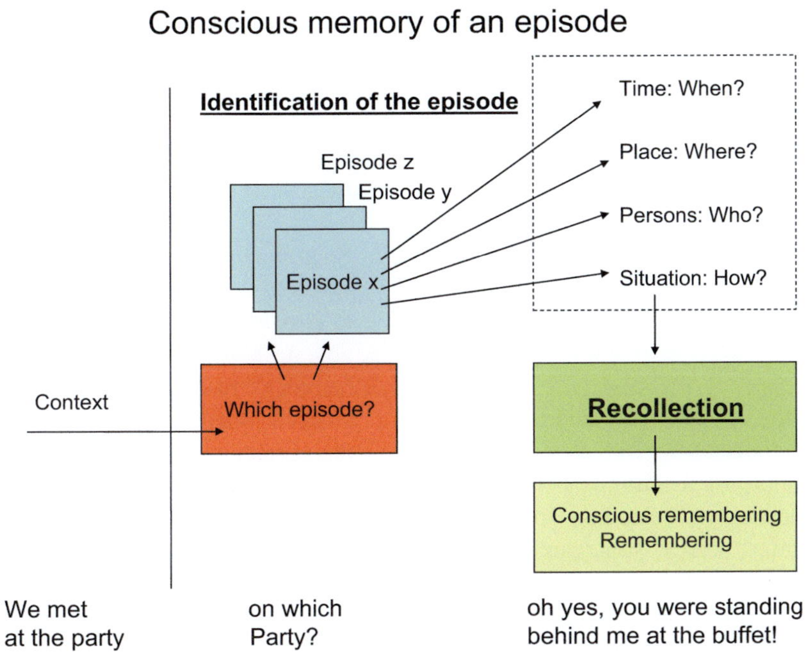

Fig. 3.1 Memory 1. of the episode as context and 2. of details from the episode. Usually, a detail is only remembered when the context of the storage episode has been remembered

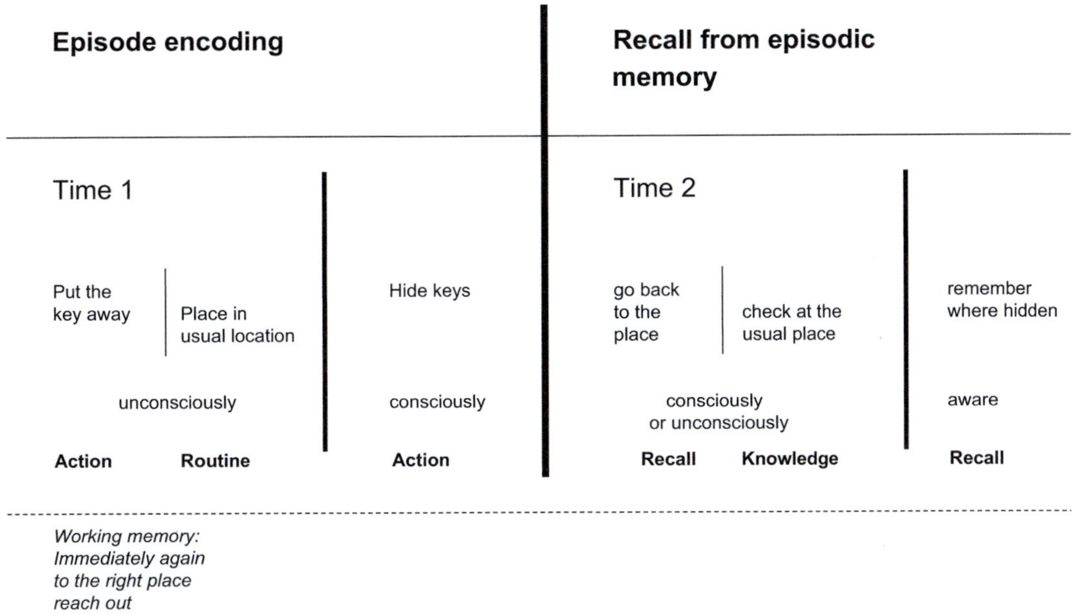

Fig. 3.2 Memory processes using the example of putting away and finding keys again. A storage episode (Episode 1) can occur consciously or unconsciously. Without intermediate distraction, the information about the location of the keys is available in working memory. After a distraction, the storage location must be recalled from memory (Episode 2). This can occur in the knowledge system (if, for example, the keys, as always, hang next to the front door). The recall from episodic memory can occur consciously and unconsciously

From the aforementioned gradation of the recall of episodic information, a gradation in the certainty of consolidated memory contents, especially knowledge, is to be differentiated: For example, one meets a famous person whom one knows from newspapers, television, or movies and says to oneself: "I know who the person is." Here, the focus is not on the memory of an episode, but on the knowledge about a person, which usually originates from many different episodic sources, such as movies, news broadcasts, or newspapers.

Remembering episodes is linked to the function of the hippocampus. But as can be seen from the example of meeting a person whom one knows fleetingly, "searching in memory" occurs. For this, search strategies are used, which are under executive control (see below). In patients with frontal lobe disorders and disturbances of the frontal cortico-subcortical projection loops (Frontal Loops), there occur dysfunctions in the recall from memory. These are evident in free recall, where strategies must be used to search for the mnemonic words. However, if the mnemonic words are offered and only need to be recognized, the memory performance of the individuals is unremarkable.

3.4 Modalities

Visual memory differs from acoustic verbal memory, for example, in its seemingly almost unlimited ability to recognize images that have been seen once. Recently, many studies have also been conducted on olfactory memory, which cannot be discussed here due to space constraints; they apparently play a role in Alzheimer's dementia.

3.5 Methods of Investigation

If a detail from an episode is to be reproduced, for example, a conversation from the last family dinner, this is sometimes difficult. However, if it is only to be recognized whether topic x was discussed at the last family dinner, the decision is easier. Memory psychology has shown that reproduction requires the involvement of different processes than recognition.

Using the example of the task of remembering a list of words, the most important types of memory tests can be demonstrated:

1. Reproduction after mentioning the encoding episode: "a short time ago I gave you words to remember, try to recall them, because now your task is to reproduce these words from memory." In reproduction, it is to be distinguished whether it should be reproduced in the correct sequence or freely—i.e., without regard to the order.
2. Reproduction with a cue: In a second group of query methods, assistance is provided. This can involve
   - a restriction of the solution set: For example, the semantic category is mentioned.
     In the special form of paired association learning, one word of a word pair that was learned is given and the associated word is requested from memory: learning word pairs, e.g., book-fish. Query: "What was paired with book?"
   - Another class of tasks arises when the word to be learned is given among alternatives for recognition: identical stimulus as a cue ("identity cue").

People can recognize those objects well that they have seen in a specific episode. If a person is shown words to learn and later presented again mixed with alternatives, the evoked potentials in the brain differ in the electroencephalogram depending on whether a word shown during the learning period or a word not shown is presented. This recognition performance and the differences in evoked potentials are impaired in cases of brain damage with amnesia (Mecklinger et al. 1998).

3.6 Clinic

Of central importance in the clinical field is the distinction between anterograde and retrograde amnesia.

3.6.1 Anterograde amnesia

A disturbance in the formation of new memory traces in episodic memory is referred to as anterograde memory impairment. From a certain severity of impairment of episodic memory functions, it is no longer possible to encode into episodic memory. New information can no longer be reproduced after a short distraction, and thus in severe cases of anterograde amnesia, nothing new can be learned. An exception is learning in other memory systems, such as learning motor skills and emotional associations.

3.6.2 Retrograde amnesia

In contrast to this, in retrograde amnesia, information stored in episodes from a time ago, which was previously available, can no longer be recalled or recognized. An motorcyclist who suffered a traumatic brain injury during his first test ride, for example, no longer remembers the birthday party where he received the motorcycle as a gift. Information that was encoded before the brain injury or any other dysfunction of the memory systems and was retrievable before this point is forgotten. For example, a face of a famous person from the media or politics, which was certainly known to the person before, is not recognized. In delirium, the availability of recent memories, which was just given before, is suddenly lost; the patients no longer know what year it is or where they are. In delirium, there is thus a temporary retrograde amnesia—temporary because the memories become practically all available again after the delirium subsides (Fig. 3.3).

3.6.3 Course of the Development of Anterograde and Retrograde Amnesia

In retrograde amnesia following a sudden head trauma, there is usually a gradient from recently experienced events to episodes experienced many years earlier. This is because, while recent events are forgotten, already consolidated information from long-term memory remains available, i.e., information from decades before the damaging event.

However, amnesia often develops slowly, e.g., the amnesia of Alzheimer's disease; or in alcoholics, the encoding was already disturbed during phases of high alcohol consumption before the onset of Wernicke-Korsakoff syndrome. Then, anterograde and retrograde amnesia combine for longer periods. In Alzheimer's disease, retrograde amnesia expands over the course of the disease, so that in the later stages, only memories of youth remain.

A special form of retrograde amnesia occurs without the characteristic gradient in memory. It is suspected that this involves a disturbance in recall from long-term memory, i.e., a disturbance in the mechanisms that provide the addresses for retrieving specific memories from autobiographical memory. Therefore, patients cannot recall otherwise readily available information, e.g., about school years, marriage many years ago, etc.

The slow development of anterograde and retrograde amnesia must be distinguished from the temporary loss of availability of memories of recently past times. This is observed in delirium and transient global amnesia (Sander and Sander 2005). Retrograde amnesia develops suddenly, and the person can no longer recall episodes from the recent past.

Error types of episodic memory that occur in psychopathology are shown in Table 3.1. Recognition and recall of information from episode "x". First, the situation is considered in which the event was forgotten, then that memories of the episode are incorrectly activated.

3.7 Diagnostics

In the clinic and especially in the outpatient psychopathological examination, a disturbance of episodic memory can go unnoticed if the patient is not specifically examined for it. This is particularly true if the person confabulates, i.e., fills memory gaps with spontaneously invented

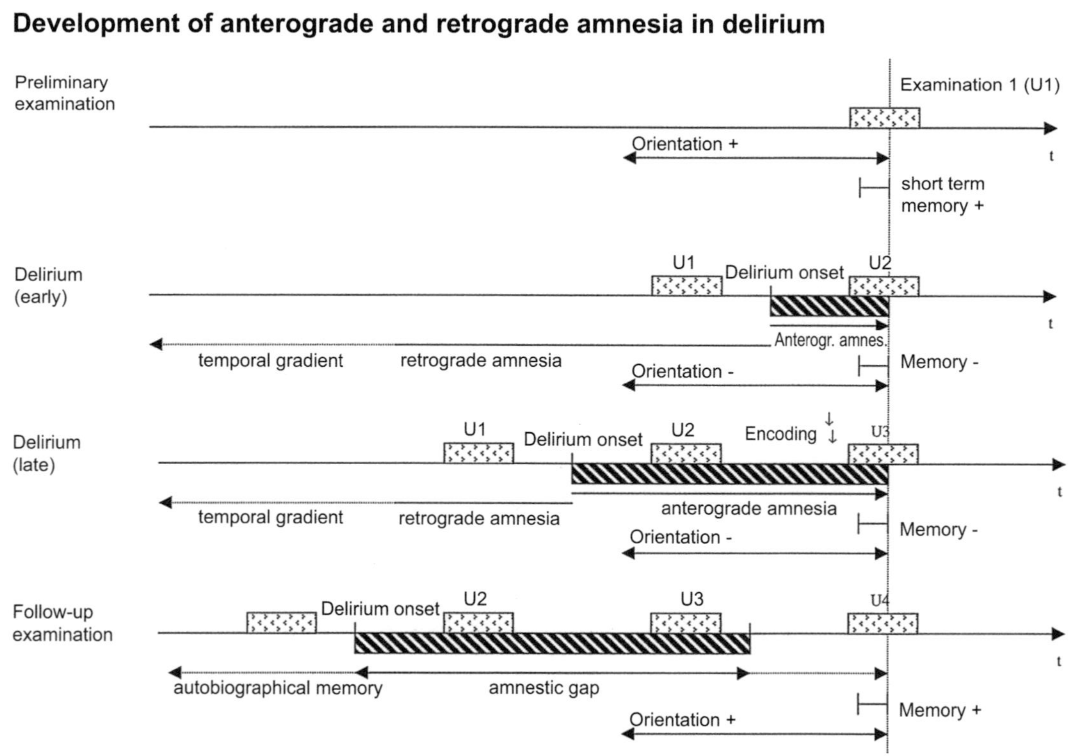

Fig. 3.3 Temporal sequence of anterograde and retrograde amnesia at the onset and after the end of delirium. Initially, a patient can store and recall words. He is oriented and remembers recently past episodes. However, after the onset of delirium, he can no longer store and recall words and has forgotten recently past episodes. He is also disoriented. Finally, after the end of delirium, the ability to remember is no longer disturbed, and the patient is oriented. He remembers the events of the recent past but not the events during the delirium (amnesic gap). (According to Reischies et al. 2000)

Table 3.1 Episodic Memory: Error Types

		Recognition	Recall
Event occurred in episode x	False negative (this event forgotten)	Anterograde: Amnestic error Psychogenic amnesia	Anterograde amnestic errors Psychogenic amnesia
		Retrograde: Jamais vu	Retrograde amnestic error
	False positive (incorrectly recalling another event)	Amnestic error (intrusion)	Correct positive but: dysfunctional retrieval dysfunctional implicit memory, flashback, traumatic memory, obsessive memory, etc.
			Confabulation (filling gaps)
No event	False positive (incorrectly remembered)	Déjà vu	False memory Delusion memory

information. An important interview technique for this is to ask for detailed information again, where in the case of a confabulation, other details are then reported.

How can disturbances of episodic memory be inferred from the course of the conversation?

- Information is told multiple times
- Vague information about the way to the examination room ("how did you get here, or to the clinic"—route, means of transport, brought by whom)
- Vague or no information about events of the last weeks/months (city, politics, world events)
- A piece of news (news of the last few days) is not recognized as such by the person
- When asked about everyday life using the example of the previous day: details about getting up with breakfast, morning activities, lunch, afternoon activities, evening with dinner, TV/radio, news, going to bed?—consistency and richness of detail are assessed
- When asked: "Did I already tell you…?" the repetition is not recognized
- Temporal relation of information about recent events shows disorder (the events could not have occurred in this sequence): time grid of the last few days
- "How old are you?" with information about the date of birth
- After the examination: does the person suggest the wrong way at the examiner's door—or get lost in the practice or clinic?

If relatives who care for the patient should be questioned and can verify the patient's information, for example, the information about the activities of the previous day (as well as observations about forgotten episodes), this is of utmost value:

- does the person get lost (first in unfamiliar surroundings, later in the development of dementia also in familiar surroundings),
- does the person misplace things and forget the place where the things are located,
- are important appointments forgotten,
- are entire episodes of the last few days, which the patient has certainly experienced with full attention, forgotten (visit of the children, etc.)—or details thereof.

Testing the memory and especially the orientation implies a break in the course of the conversation of a psychopathological examination. This break should be made explicit, and with introductory, explanatory words, the special situation must be announced, for example, "I would now like to test the memory, as we have to do with all patients." Otherwise, the testing of orientation is often perceived as insulting—as an "idiot test".

3.7.1 Anterograde amnesia

Neuropsychological Examination Procedures
Frequently learning tasks are applied (see Lachner et al. 1994). A word list is to be learned and reproduced after a period of distraction, or the words are presented among distractors and are to be recognized. In the non-verbal domain, figures are to be drawn and reconstructed after a delay. Why is such a task a test of episodic memory, what can be considered an episode in this context? The repetition of the words or even just reading them aloud for encoding functions as a encoding episode, i.e., as an event that the person should be able to remember. During the recall, reference is made to this process in the encoding episode: "I had just given you words to remember." In severe amnestic syndromes, the storage episode itself is forgotten, and the patients are confused and do not know what the request to recall the learned words refers to.

The better the task is stored, the more valid an omission error in the recall test is for diagnostics. Because if a person did not attentively perceive the memory words, a disturbance of episodic memory could be mistakenly diagnosed. First, it must be ensured whether the memory objects were processed more than superficially by the person being examined, whether the person perceived them attentively. This cannot be assumed as certain in clinical situations of anxiety, resistance, thought disorders or perception disorders. When reading aloud, people can be thinking about something else, considering something else—therefore, a single reading of learning words alone is probably not sufficient to ensure information encoding. For this reason, repetition of reading in several rounds is often chosen. Conversely, it should also be considered today that some patients have participated in memory training and perform inexplicably well because they use encoding strategies.

The repetition of the memory objects, which is the procedure in the frequently used Mini Mental State Examination (MMSE), proves to be a good control of information intake. However, with this method, 10 or 12 words cannot be stored, as people can generally only repeat about 7 words. Most patients to be examined, however, can only reproduce about 4 or 5 words from the sensory register (an immediate memory system) with sufficient certainty.

The duration of the distraction period in word list learning tasks is clinically highly variable. Certainly, the primary effect of clearing the working memory is particularly important. This occurs after a short engagement with another task. The further duration of the distraction, whether it lasts 1 minute or 10 minutes, seems less crucial for clearing the memory objects from the working memory. Longer intervals, such as an hour or more, are not clinically practical and have not proven necessary when episodic memory is to be clinically tested.

In the MMSE, the 3 words are asked again after 1-2 minutes. In another clinical neuropsychological test battery, the CERAD-NP, the recall of the learning list and the reconstruction of geometric figures occur after about 10 minutes. The AMDP requires the same latency. For some tasks, a delay of one or half an hour is required.

However, if immediate recall is tested, it should be noted that by omitting the distraction, both working memory and episodic memory are tested. This results in a contamination, which is mostly not neuropsychologically meaningful. But in more severe dementia syndromes, both working memory and episodic memory are impaired, so such a test result at least has diagnostic value for this syndrome.

Testing Recall from Memory
How is recall from episodic memory tested? Mostly the reproduction of the memorized objects is used, naming the memorized words after referring to the encoding episode "I

recently introduced you to a series of words" etc. Reproduction is usually tested as free recall—recall without regard to the correct sequence of items in the learning lists. In this case, it shold be said that the order of reproduction of the memorized items does not matter.

In many clinical memory tests, encoding and retrieval are examined in several trials in order to measure learning success. However, it should be noted that learning success may be influenced by other factors that are not directly related to episodic memory. For example, the age effect on learning, in contrast to other parameters of episodic memory, is small or non-existent (Reischies and Lindenberger 1996).

When reproducing word lists, not only episodic memory is tested, but other functions also play a role.

1. Aphasic disorders in dementia can interfere. Apraxic disorders can interfere with the reconstruction of non-verbal-figural information.
2. Searching for the memorized words in memory is referred to as retrieval. In this process, search strategies are used. Some patients may show a premature cessation of searching. In other words, other processes needed for searching the items in memory, which are not directly related to the processes of episodic memory, can be affected in certain brain diseases, such as those of the frontal lobe, leading to a reduction in the reproduction of memorized words.

In the clinic, for some diagnoses, memory disorders must be confirmed or ruled out during the initial examination.

Clinical Testing—Bedside Tests of Episodic Memory

3-word list—Repetition:
Query after 5-10 minutes of distraction (MMSE after about 1–2 minutes, Folstein et al. 1975).

10-word list with imagination encoding aid:
(Patient should imagine the objects and compare the size of the memorized object with a table—"larger or smaller than a table").
Words: potato, letter, sea, clock, armchair, photo, forest, policeman, infant, cat
Immediate free reproduction—threshold 4/5 (Reischies et al. 2000; Strotzka 2021).

3.7.2 Orientation Disorders

The temporal Disorientation in time is closely correlated with episodic memory disorders. For disorientation in time, some additional influencing factors come into play, particularly the availability of information about daily events and dates. Even patients who, in pronounced social withdrawal, show no interest in their environment can easily appear temporally disoriented.

It is not yet known which mechanisms become effective for temporal orientation. On the one hand, an updating of a time monitoring could occur. On the other hand, time monitoring could be related to remembering time markers. An example would be the memory of changing the calendar page, a significant birthday date in recent days, etc. This could explain why temporal orientation is closely linked to episodic memory and why the disorder of orientation is highly correlated with the disorder of episodic memory performance.

In the clinical examination, the person should name the current date and location. If they do not know the date, they should be asked to guess it. Numbers can be offered for the estimation of retrograde amnesia, such as 1990, 1995, 2000, 2005, etc for the year. Thus, an estimation of the extent of the orientation disorder in time should be carried out. For this purpose, the Benton Score has been developed, for example.

Benton orientation test (Benton 1983)

5 answers regarding orientation in time:

- Time—1 point/error (unit half an hour); max. 5 points.
- Day of the week—1 point/error; max. 3 points.
- Day of the month—1 point/error; max. 15 points.
- Month—5 points/error; max. 30 points.
- Year—10 points/error; max. 60 points.

Patients with moderate dementia score approximately 40-50 points (Solomon et al. 1998). Delirious patients score approximately 50 points. There are no data for early or mild delirium. In the normalization sample by Solomon, no healthy individuals scored more than 6 error points, which corresponds to the clinicians' assessment that disorientation by more than about 1 week is generally considered pathological and needs further investigation (Reischies 2005).

Spatial orientation is better understood. It can already be quite reliably associated with the place cells of the hippocampus and the grid cells in the entorhinal cortex (Moser et al. 2015). The information from the (1) place cells combined with that from the (2) grid cells provides information about the (1) current position of the organism (2) on a map of the environment. This can enable orientation. These neurons play a central role in spatial orientation, which is discussed in Sect. 3.8 Neuroscience. The early loss of spatial orientation in Alzheimer's dementia due to hippocampal and entorhinal damage is consistent with this model. Patients initially get lost in unfamiliar environments, later also in familiar surroundings.

Some researchers state that orientation disorders should be strictly distinguished from episodic memory disorders. This applies to disorientation for the situation, which will be addressed in the chapter about consciousness disorders (Sect. 8.3.1). However, the disorder of episodic memory certainly contributes at least to some extent to situational disorientation in consciousness disorders.

3.7.3 Retrograde amnesia

Clinically the current chancellor, president, or mayor is asked about in many diagnostic protocols, whereby mentioning, for example, the last officeholder instead of the current one can be taken as a symptom of retrograde amnesia, at least for the examination of acutely amnestic patients who are known to have followed daily events with sufficient interest, listened to or watched the news, and read the newspaper. One can also ask about recent news and thus try to determine the extent of the retrograde disorientation in time (Fig. 3.4).

If it is known that the person's episodic memory was good until recently, the question about temporal orientation captures the retrograde amnesia. In delirium and transient global amnesia (TGA), temporal orientation is suddenly disturbed, and the memory of the last few days is lost.

In formalized tests, the recognition of names or pictures from the last year, decade, several decades ago, etc., are tested (Schmidtke and Vollmer 1997). Unfortunately, these tests have to be revised every few years, which means that no current test is on the market

3.8 Neuroscience

In almost all neural structures, plasticity phenomena can be observed, which are attributed to memory phenomena. Using the example of afterimages with bright light stimuli, one can demonstrate one of the many enduring phenomena of information processing in the CNS. Neurons continue to provide information about a light stimulus for a certain period, even though it has already disappeared. This chapter is limited to a specific memory system—that of episodic memory. What does neuroscience know about this memory system? How can it be explained that it is possible to store and retrieve an experience

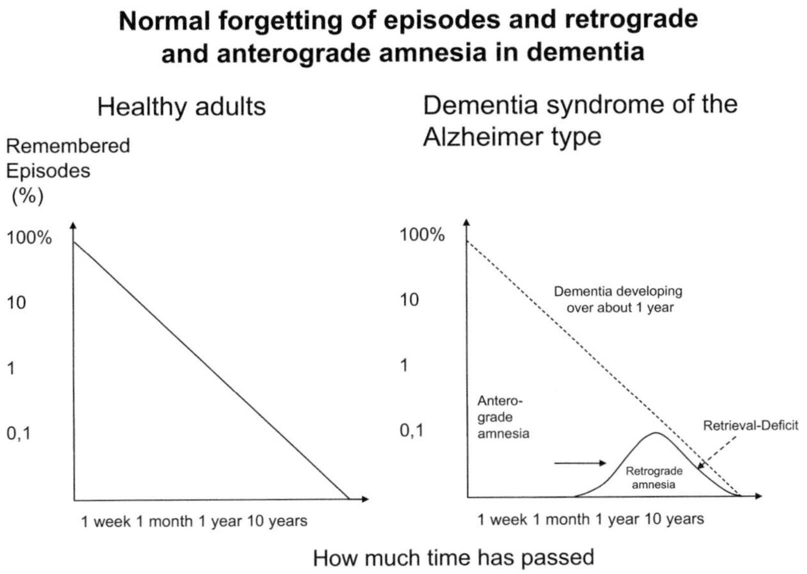

Fig. 3.4 Forgetting episodic information over time In amnestic disorders in dementia, new data are not stored (anterograde amnesia) and increasingly autobiographical data that had already been consolidated is forgotten (retrograde amnesia). Additionally, some patients experience a specific retrieval disorder, making all autobiographical data less accessible without a temporal gradient (Based on data on the availability of diary information, Rubin et al. 1986)

in the brain? When we recall episodes, we usually imagine the visual-spatial conditions, sound experiences, or even the smell, etc. The initial example in this chapter was remembering the last family dinner. Who sat next to you, what was talked about, what was eaten, and many other pieces of information become available again, including the one sought after. For this, the functions of the hippocampus are to be explained.

Hippocampal Phase

The question of how the hippocampus works has been addressed with great energy over the past decades and has already been clarified in some aspects. Three important mechanisms must first be presented:

1. the cellular principle of enhancing synaptic efficiency, “long term potentiation” (LTP),
2. properties of hippocampal neurons and their connections,
3. and the problem of restructuring neuronal networks when training new associative connections, which comes into play especially during consolidation.

Before cellular mechanisms are presented, it should first be explained what kind of information the hippocampus receives. The answer to this question can be inferred from the anatomical connection of the neurons of the hippocampus. The type of neuronal information processing in different regions of the cortex is now known. Of course, it would be inefficient if the brain stored information about all the individual edges and corners of a figure or , e.g., elementary acoustic properties of a word. The principle is that the hippocampus receives information about objects, i.e., information about sensory impressions that, after stimulus identification in the temporal cortex, is already preprocessed at a high level and now exists as information about objects (Chap. 2 Perception; Fig. 3.5).

The hippocampus receives information from various brain areas and sends the processed information back to the same brain areas. What this processing consists of will be roughly outlined in the following, insofar as functional models of neuroscience have already been tested.

Incidentally, it should be mentioned here that the hippocampus is additionally closely connected to the diencephalon. This second afferent of the

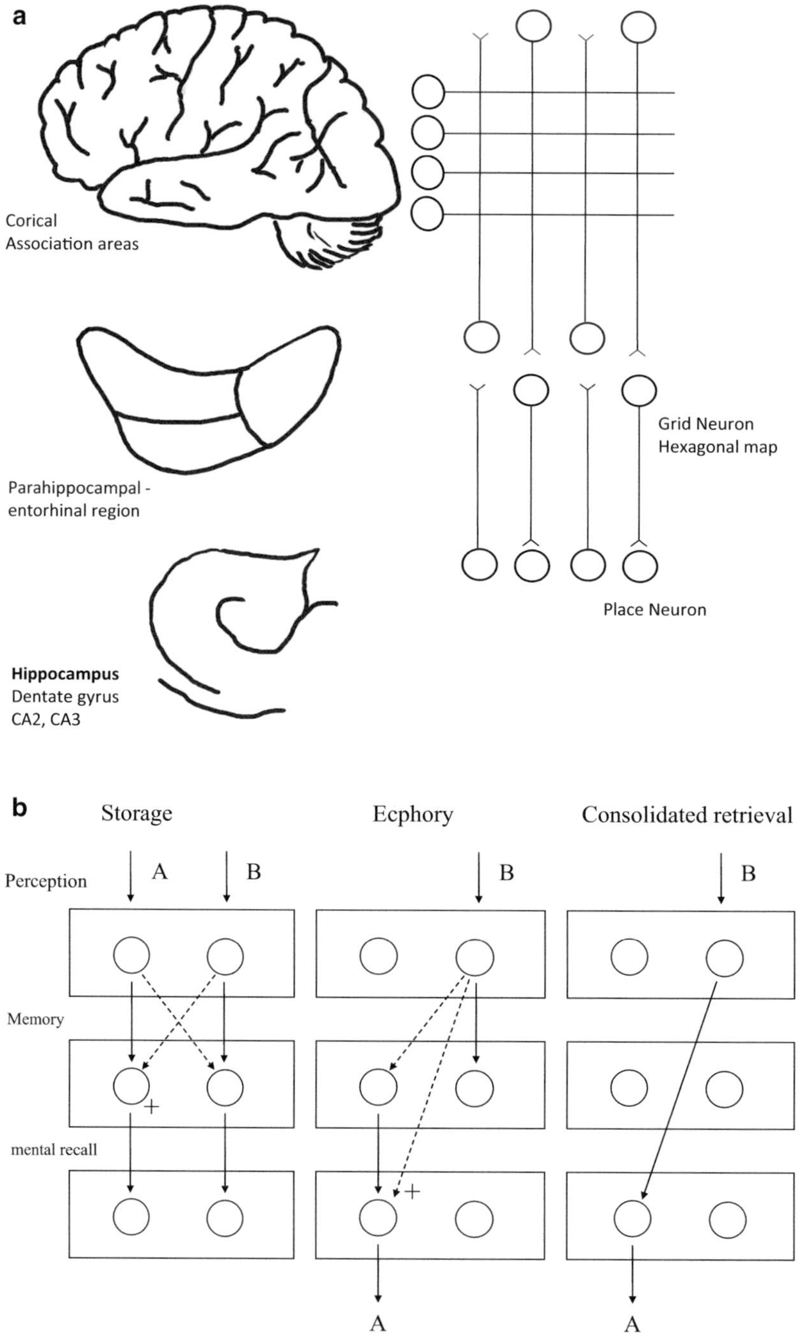

Fig. 3.5 a, b. Mechanisms of episodic memory and retrieval through context stimulation. a) Several cortical networks send neuronal information to the entorhinal cortex. There, the "grid" neurons (Moser et al. 2015), which represent a kind of map grid function, were found. From there, the information about the memory content and the context is fed into the hippocampal network and mediated back from the hippocampal network to the entorhinal cortex. The context information can in retrieval reactivate the activity of the neurons representing the information to be remembered in the cortical networks (see Squire and Zola-Morgan 1991), b) Stimulus A is to be remembered. Stimulus B, which was associated in the storage situation, is given as context for this (in the test, e.g., "You were just supposed to remember a series of words"). The networking of the innervation enables the recall of Stimulus A through activation of the perceptual units of Stimulus B. After final consolidation, the memory is independent of the hippocampal system, and a purely cortical-cortical connection is sufficient for the activation of Stimulus A upon the presentation of Stimulus B

hippocampus from the septo-hippocampal system is critical for hippocampal functions. If the cholinergic neurons of the septal system are damaged, the hippocampus loses its rhythmic activity, and a loss of function, as observed after hippocampal damage, can be observed. This afferent is disrupted in an anticholinergic delirium.

3.8.1 Neuronal Memory Phenomena—Changes at the Synapses

Neurons exhibit various memory or plasticity phenomena. After a plastic change, the neuronal response is facilitated (enhanced) or habituated (diminished).

In this process, the presynaptic, synaptic, or postsynaptic processing can be altered:

- presynaptic: from the action potential to the release of synaptic vesicles as well as the provision of the transmitter in the presynaptic vesicles,
- synaptic: the metabolism of the released molecules, their inactivation, or the re-uptake into the presynaptic vesicles,
- postsynaptic: the number of receptors, their reaction, the intracellular processing, etc.

Through a single or several different changes in the mentioned synaptic mechanisms, the enhancement (or reduction) of the effect of the same neuronal information, which was transmitted as an action potential propagates along the axon, is achieved.

Long Term Potentiation and Long Term Depression

Cellular and molecular mechanisms of specific associative memory have been elucidated. This was possible because a plasticity phenomenon had been discovered that can be studied in laboratory investigations (Lynch 2004), namely Long Term Potentiation (LTP).

The principle of Long Term Potentiation is initially simple: A neuronal response to a weak stimulus x alone does not lead to a neuronal response. However, if it is paired with a strong stimulus y, the response is enhanced upon repetition that later the weak stimulus x alone leads to a neuronal response.

In LTP, an essential principle of associativity is realized: A stimulus-response is only enhanced if it occurs temporally associated with others at the neuron or synapse. Since a hippocampal neuron only fires when more than about 100 synapses on the dendrites are activated (Eichenbaum and Cohen 2001), strong afferents must first be active to enhance a new weak stimulus over a certain period.

Neurophysiologists have uncovered the biochemistry and metabolism of this phenomenon. Only the basics of molecular physiology will be presented here. In the first part of LTP, two types of receptors of the transmitter glutamate play a key role:

1. AMPA receptors respond to an initial stimulation with sodium influx and potassium efflux, causing depolarization.
2. A second group of glutamate receptors, the NMDA receptors, is only involved in the response to the second stimulus. Normally, the NMDA channel is blocked by a magnesium ion. The initial AMPA activation has now triggered a membrane depolarization, and this membrane depolarization causes the NMDA receptors to release the magnesium ion that blocks the channel for calcium ions. Only then can the docking of the glutamate molecule of the second afferent at the NMDA receptor open the channel for calcium. Thus, an initial membrane depolarization and a second transmitter action work together.

In the second part of LTP, the reaction to the docking of the transmitter glutamate at the receptor is sustainably enhanced. In LTP, the processes after the docking of the transmitter change. An increase in the concentration of calcium in the neuron is responsible on the one hand for gene activation and protein synthesis, which are necessary for the maintenance of LTP. There is also an activation of AMPA receptors. The end effect is a potentiation of the cellular response to a stimulation that lasts for a long time. LTP can last for many hours and days. For further explanations of the details, refer to presentations of molecular neuroscience of LTP and LTD (Kandel 1991, 2001).

With the described molecular machinery, an association of synaptic information from a weak stimulus with the practically simultaneous, i.e., only milliseconds preceding, neuronal depolarization by other stimuli is achieved. Additionally, the response of the cells to precisely this weak input is enhanced. Subsequently, the weak stimulus is sufficient to activate the hippocampal neuron. This molecular mechanism can explain how the processing of stimuli changes neuronal activity in the CNS for a certain period.

Recently, it has been questioned whether LTP is indispensable for episodic memory. However, the answer to this question depends on what is considered the measure of episodic memory. Apparently, the functions of the parahippocampal region are sufficient for simple recognition tasks. In the recognition of seen objects, the hippocampus does not need to be active. Thus, certain memory phenomena can be preserved in the case of experimental damage to the LTP mechanisms. A wealth of genetic studies and the association of age-related impaired LTP phenomena with memory changes in old age suggest a role for LTP in the complex mechanisms of episodic memory (Rosenzweig and Barnes 2003).

Properties of Hippocampal Cells

The hippocampus is activated by almost all newly arriving stimuli. What does this activation do for the storage of the stimulus? As mentioned above, the hippocampus represents the spatial or, more generally, the situational context according to animal studies (Eichenbaum and Cohen 2001). It provides the orientation map on which the incoming stimuli are related to the respective place and other contexts of the situation. Interestingly, the method of loci (see above) is, in accordance to the above, one of the best memory aids.

For each situation, the hippocampus has to capture the relation of ,e.g., objects in a room, such as where the door is, where the radio is, who is in the room. These are familiar relations and people have an independent long-term representation of it linguistically and semantically. It is about the ad-hoc situation, the current arrangement of familiar things in the present situation that is being experienced. This constitutes the episode that one can remember later.

The hippocampus must therefore fulfill two tasks: on the one hand, to update the spatial map when something has changed, and on the other hand, to associate stimuli with places, i.e., to register them in terms of their location (or in terms of another context).

What do the neurons of the hippocampus respond to, what do they represent, as far as can be shown in electrophysiological studies? A finding has been known for decades is: the cells respond to the position of the animal in relation to spatial markers of the environment. This has been referred to as a "cognitive map". This consists of the set of cells that each represent the relationship of one's position to a feature of the environment, or the spatial relationship between two objects in the environment. A memory space in the hippocampus has been discussed, which is realized in individual relational representations (Eichenbaum and Cohen 2001). The animal studies mainly refer to rodents, and it has been speculated that in humans, not only spatial but also more complex relations of situations are processed in the hippocampus.

It is not certain whether animals have episodic memory, that is, specifically, whether they can remember episodes of their lives with any form of awareness (see Hampton and Schwartz 2004). Most likely, an analogy to human episodic memory can be assumed in great apes. This is mainly related to the awareness of remembering and—related to this—the communicability of conscious remembering. Likewise, we do not know whether an animal can perceive consciously. Although it would make sense to present the concept of consciousness at the beginning of the book to better explain these aspects, components necessary for understanding the elements of consciousness are to be introduced in the following sections.

How can the findings of place neurons be reconciled with those of Long Term Potentiation? At present, one can only make model considerations about this, since the LTP phenomenon is a laboratory phenomenon and could not be studied in animals in their natural environment. According to such model considerations, the place of an object can serve as a situational context for episodic memory. An example of a memory of an episode should make the concept clearer. When a place is mentioned, a person remembers an episode with a person he experienced there. In the episode during encoding, in the past, the environmental stimuli activated the hippocampus. The spatial map was established, i.e., the neurons of the hippocampus encoded the place. The perception of the person then triggered an LTP, which associated the new stimulus information with the place information. The stimulus of the person was then neurally associated with the pre-stimulation of the place. During retrieval, the information about the place is transmitted to the hippocampus, for example, triggered by the question: What happened at place x? The hippocampal neurons for the specific place can now activate the cortical ensemble for the stimulus representation of the person. Thus, the experience of the person is remembered for the place. The example is very specific. In general, it is apparent that the hippocampus can separately associate the relation of stimuli of an episode, which are represented, for example, in the temporal lobe.

Computer scientists have been able to model the possibility of retrieving words from memory, for example in paired-associatiates learning. A better performance in recognition could be demonstratd by transmitting information from the neurons of the entorhinal cortex with input from the other association areas via the dentate gyrus to the CA3 region of the hippocampus. It is particularly relevant there that the synaptic connection is supposed to be plastically changed via LTP mechanisms. This leads to a reciprocal activation of the memory item (e.g., a word) by the context (e.g., a situation) during retrieval from memory; or, on the other hand, during recognition, the presentation and processing of the memory item leads to the activation of the situation-coding neurons (Hasselmo and McClelland 1999; Fig. 3.6). While the neurons in the hippocampus are activated by the situational context, a characteristic rhythmic theta activity has been shown.

3.8.2 Hippocampus and the Storage in Neuronal Networks

How can memory information be read out from the hippocampus? If one wants to explain how the brain can retrieve episodes, one must trace the path of the information back to the storage episode. Let us consider an episode again: A person sees a hat they recognize in a place, i.e., in a specific spatial context. The neuronal representation of the hat is activated, and simultaneously with this neuronal activation of the object's representation, the spatial coding, or context coding, from the hippocampus arrives—the conditions for long-term potentiation are met. The recall can thus be explained by the fact that the hippocampal place cells are specifically addressed when the situation is named or described again for the recall: There in space x, what did you see there? During retrieval, the memory space of the place is now activated, and thus the cortical representation of the hat, i.e., the probability increases that the person will come up with "the hat" when asked, "what did you see there?" The recall from episodic memory involves two pieces of information, a cue, the address, and a targeted memory content, the remembered object. Normally, the recall starts from an episode and asks for details, such as the words learned in the episode. But one can also remember the place where an experience occurred in reverse. For example, many people still remember the place and situation where they learned that a terrible event had occurred, a terrifying terrorist attack, a declaration of war, or a personal event, such as the news of a family member's death. In this case, the information about the event, "NN has died," reaches the

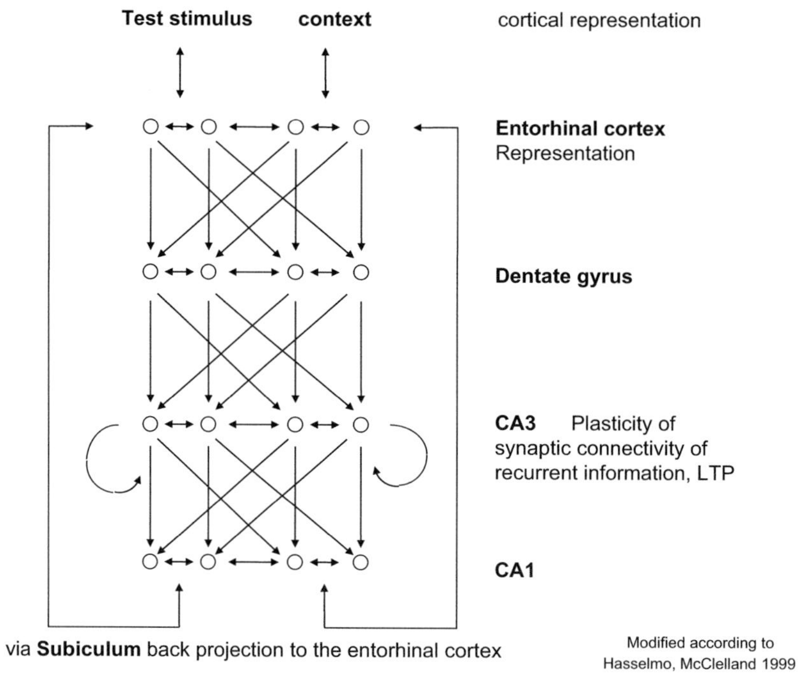

Fig. 3.6 Hippocampal network. Information about the stimulus to be remembered and the context stimulus is transmitted from the entorhinal cortex to the first station of the hippocampus, the nerve cells of the dentate gyrus. There is close networking at every level of the hippocampus. The phenomenon of long-term potentiation is particularly observed in the CA3 neurons. The activation of the context can thus enhance the initially weak reactivation of the representation of the stimulus to be remembered. (Mod. after Hasselmo and McClelland 1999)

hippocampus. This stimulus can then reactivate the spatial map that applied to this event. Many remember that they knew the place in a school book where a vocabulary word was located but no longer the meaning of the English or Latin word. Later, the spatial information of the vocabulary is lost, and the semantic information is automatically available. This will be discussed further below in the consolidation.

For the regular case in which information about an episode is given, the recall is more complicated to imagine. A stimulus x has been associatively coupled with a place, or more generally with the situational context, through hippocampal activation. If a question now arises in which the place or situation is given as the address for the recall of the memory content, the corresponding place cells or codings for the situation in the hippocampus are activated in the first step. In the second step, these neurons must now amplify the neuronal trace of the stimulus x so that the neuronal representation of the stimulus x is reactivated. How can they achieve this? It is known that hippocampal activity is connected via the entorhinal region with the association areas of the entire cortex, where the various aspects of objects are represented (Fig. 3.5a). This information is very specific.

How do we search our memory when the memory does not immediately set in automatically? How is the retrieval , the ecphoria ecphory organized? If the memory does not automatically succeed effortlessly, i.e., when trying to remember, a context stimulus is sought. If the correct context is activated, the queried stimulus can in turn be reactivated.

When the context is sought, it involves partial goal patterns that can be understood as "addresses" like in a computer. In doing so, search strategies are applied. Search strategies can be dysfunctional and lead to a reduction in retrieval performance. For the effortful memory, search strategies are needed that involve executive functions. For this reason, frontal lobe functions play a significant role in the usual recall tests, such as the recall of learned words.

3.8.3 Post-Hippocampal Phase

Cortical storage occurs in cortical neuronal networks. How can storage in the neuronal networks in the cortex occur after the specific cortical activation by hippocampal neurons? The transfer to or incorporation into cortical neuronal networks occurs in the consolidation phase.

First, it must be explained how neuronal networks can fulfill memory functions. They operate according to the principle of Gestalt completion. A part of the pattern to which the neuronal network is trained is sufficient as input to obtain the entire pattern as output. This principle also plays a central role in perceptual physiology. It has been recognized many years ago (Rosenblatt 1961; Steinbuch 1961; Marr 1971). The episode serves as context, as a partial pattern from which the entire pattern of the information to be remembered, i.e., the memory of details from the episode, is worked out. In the memory domain, the principle of completion of stimulus patterns is applied to the completion of situation-context patterns. This principle can explain that the brain can reconstruct target patterns learned in the past with neuronal network structures. The context is perceived as a stimulus or can also be generated internally. The detail experienced in the episode is then remembered as described above.

Rummelhart et al. have presented a parallel-distributed-processing model for this purpose (Rummelhart et al. 1986a, b; Spitzer 1996; Chap. 9 Language). During the training of a neural network, the activation thresholds in the connection from one input neuron to the next neuron change. This corresponds molecularly to the change in synaptic transmission at the nerve endings (see 3.8.1). In the example in Chap. 9, it is about the recall from a linguistic memory. The language model serves to illustrate how people can retrieve words for speech production from semantic memory.

The training follows a principle of specific feedback: If the network has produced the correct stimulus during a training round, all connections that were active in this round are strengthened. The system of the neural network must therefore be able to plastically change the currently active synaptic connections. Over the course of training through many hundreds of learning rounds, a specific constellation of connectivity is formed in the neural network, so that the sought item is always activated when the context is the input. These neural networks have been successfully trained in many studies and technical applications up to today's AI large language model.

New Information in Trained Neuronal Networks

For neuronal networks, there is a significant complication: When a trained network is supposed to store new information, the connectivities at all nodes, the neurons, change. However, if the connectivity has been changed for the new stimulus, the retrieval performance of the previously trained memory contents collapses. The term "catastrophic interference" has been coined for this. For this reason, it is assumed that the hippocampus lies in a kind of bypass to the cortical networks. This ensures that not every new stimulus that arrives and is stored at any moment disrupts the previously consolidated stored contents. But how does the later integration of the information to be stored into the cortical networks occur?

Neural networks are good models for explaining the retrieval of information. They play a crucial role in long-term consolidated memory contents that needs to be retrieved automatically and quickly. We have a neural network function before us that should ideally not be changed, because a change in the weights of the neuron connections would cause the retrieval performance to collapse (see above). The modules for language comprehension, for example, remain essentially unchanged in a person's later life. The retrieval processes of word meanings in semantic memory are to be imagined as automatic rapid processes in semantic neuronal networks.

Neuronal networks are initially not good models for changing repeatedly newly stored information about the environment. Here, the specific context-memory object associations that the hippocampal system can work out function better. They can explain the high memory performance of humans in monitoring what happened over the course of the day or the last few days.

The solution to the consolidation problem starts from a phase of transfer of information from hippocampal storage to storage in cortical networks. In the consolidation phase, according to McClelland's ideas, a retraining of the new and old stimuli should proceed together (McClelland et al. 1995). Through new training of the old and new information, a gentle new representation of the added information and a preservation or correction of the damaged representation of the old information can occur.

The hypothesis has been investigated that in sleep phases, a replay of past information is realized, in which ultimately over months an integration of the new and old memory contents in the neural networks of the cortex is achieved. The question of how the integrating retraining occurs is still unresolved.

After a long time, usually after months, the information that can be remembered is no longer dependent on the integrity of the hippocampus. However, after months, many episodes have already been forgotten. Only a small part of the total information, that is available, for example, about the previous day, can be recalled 3 months later (Fig. 3.4).

The described mechanisms of neuronal networks apply to cortical plasticity and retrieval processes. In contrast to the neuronal networks, another principle was presented above, that of specific targeted neuronal activation. Because in learning in the hippocampal system, there is apparently the strengthening of specific connections that can attach to and activate already trained cortical representations. So we have 2 principles before us:

- that of distributed parallel processing in neuronal networks and
- that of specific strengthening of neuronal representations.

Long-term Storage

Where in the brain are a person's biographical data stored? Certainly, almost all cortical areas are involved in the storage of consolidated information. However, from a series of recent studies, it has been concluded that the prefrontal areas, especially of the non-language-dominant hemisphere, hold a large part of the autobiographical long-term information. Damage to the cortical representation or the recall or activation mechanisms for these brain regions results in retrograde amnesia, which also encompasses the more distant time periods, as observed in degenerative dementia diseases.

Age Effect on Episodic Memory

Old people generally have memory problems. This is particularly striking in the "Memory" game, where two identical object cards lying randomly among others on the table are repeatedly turned over, and the goal is to find as many pairs as possible. Children can effortlessly remember where a particular card was previously uncovered when the second, matching one for the pair is turned over. Older people usually still know that an object has been uncovered before, but not where.

The effortless encoding of children is likely related to an undisturbed hippocampal representation of all stimuli in their context, i.e., all stimuli with all relations to each other, of the entire relational memory space (Eichenbaum and Cohen 2001). This is no longer possible for older people because physiological changes in the hippocampus reduce synaptic connectivity and may have shifted the LTP mechanisms in favor of LTD processes, which can have dysfunctional effects (Rosenzweig and Barnes 2003).

> Diagnostically, the physiological reduction of memory functions with age must be distinguished from that in incipient dementia (Heden et al. 2004). Benign age-related forgetfulness is characterized by the fact that unimportant details are forgotten, but important information can still be retained in episodic memory by the elderly through selection and compensatory efforts (see, e.g., Reischies and Lindenberger 1996).

Déjà vu

When a new environment seems familiar to us or an event that we encounter for the first time appears to have been experienced before, it is called déjà vu (Table 3.1, Brown 2003). The cause can be seen as a pathological activation of neurons in the parahippocampal region or the hippocampus, which signal "This is familiar" even in an unfamiliar environment. This is supported by déjà vu experiences in the aura of patients with an epileptic focus in the mediotemporal region.

A second explanation refers to false recognition, which selectively relates to elements of the new environment. These elements are indeed present in the experience from earlier contexts—however, the entire new environment has not yet been experienced. The recognition of the elements now leads to the impression of having somehow seen the new environment before (Brown 2003).

It is assumed that there is a two-part memory. The simpler first step is recognition. Neurons of the temporal lobe are engaged with various classes of recognition phenomena (Desimone et al. 1995). As already indicated, the activation of the hippocampus is not necessary. It involves a changed activation of neurons when the stimulus that was shown has already been shown once before. This corresponds to the fact that in the electroencephalogram, the neuronal response is altered when an object is shown a second time, compared to the neuronal response when the object is shown for the first time.

Besides elementary recognition, the experience of familiarity is important here. It apparently accompanies our daily life and immediately signals to us if something new has occurred. In certain psychopathological situations - such as the delusional mood - this familiarity is lost.

Everything new must be specially evaluated. It usually triggers curiosity. However, the new can also triggers anxiety. It is assumed that the unrecognized, i.e., new objects are evaluated in the amygdala. Other emotional reactions can also be triggered. Thus, a collaboration of specific brain areas, such as the amygdala with the hippocampus, can be observed for the characteristics of emotion (see there).

3.9 Psychopathological Symptoms of Episodic Memory

Impairment of short term retention

Definition. Facts or information about an episode cannot be retained or recalled by the patient after distraction, i.e., over a period of engagement with other content.

Specifically: If features of the encoding episode, in which the contents to be remembered were communicated, are given as cues, this does not help to recall the contents.

Example

- An older patient cannot recall 3 items (e.g., tree, soap, and airplane) after a distraction of 10 minutes, although he was able to repeat them immediately after they were mentioned, indicating he understood them.
- A patient cannot say what he had for lunch the previous day.
- A woman cannot remember having met the interviewer before at the second interview.

Position in Psychopathology. Term introduced by Wernicke, AMDP 11.

Related Terms. Neuropsychological and experimental psychological terms that partly contradict each other (e.g., different usage of "short-term" and "long-term memory"),

- postdistractional short term memory ,
- secondary memory,
- episodic memory.

Psychopathological Interactions. attention, motivation, consciousness disorder, aphasia, diagnostic cooperation.

Differential Diagnostic Distinctions
Afference: aphasia, comprehension disorder in encoding:

- Task not understood,
- Motivational problem,
- After memory training: encoding strategies applied,
- Wrong strategy (e.g., encoding with rhymes in aphasia) etc.

Recall:

- Disorganized—frontal lobe disorder,
- From intermediate storage ("primary memory"),
- Simulation; appropriate pattern of performance in memory tasks of varying difficulty must be recognizable,
- Pseudodementia as a depressive feature with immediate "I don't know" answers, where upon further questioning the correct recall can still be provided.

Efference: aphasia, apraxia, decision-making disorder.

Further Characterization. Anterograde false negative errors; loss of the ability to remember the elements of the encoding situation.

Self-/Other Person's Judgment. self-evaluation usually not valid—tendency for minimalization.

Interview for Rating. History taken from other persons about the forgetting of episodes in everyday life, especially forgetting appointments, disturbance in recognizing facts, things, and people.

Neuropsychology/Objectification. Some patients retain the information in memory but cannot recall it. For them, a recognition task must be given, e.g. for the 3 word test: Was the word "bicycle (car, or airplane)" included? More severe Severe memory impairment if items cannot be recognized (excluding aphasic disorders).

- Problem with demented, echolalic patients who repeat but do not understand the information.
- Problem with aphasic patients for whom non-verbal memory items must be used, which are not comparable in difficulty (the patient redraws three symbols (e.g., a "*", a "#", and an "upward arrow") after distraction or recognize faces of staff, etc.),
- Today, older individuals come for examination who have learned mnemonic techniques in memory training,
- For these problems, a uniform encoding routine such as imagination (see above 10-word test with imagination encoding aid).

Severity. A mild disturbance corresponds to forgetting 1 out of 3 items in young adulthood, and about 2 in old age. A severe disturbance is present when no word can be reproduced or recognized, or it is no longer remembered that words were given to be remembered at all.

Specifications. dissociation of reproduction and recognition:

- pronounced reproduction disorder with minor recognition disorder

Neuroscientific/cognitive neuroscientific models

1. The cue mentioning the encoding episode can no longer fully activate the specific hippocampal activity after distraction, or the activation of hippocampal activity cannot promote the ecphoria of the memory items,

- therefore, the episode is no longer remembered and the reactivation of those items processed in the episode does not occur.

2. Recognition is impaired because mentioning the memory word does not trigger recognition potential in the medial temporal brain region,

- recognition is apparently processed in the parahippocampal region,

Anterograde amnesia
Patients with amnesia developing over years or decades are also impaired in recalling events from the more distant past, which they could no longer efficiently encode due to the already existing amnestic disorder.

Retrograde amnesia
Definition. Contents of episodic memory that were available to the person before the time of a damaging event are not recallable, e.g., familiar facts cannot be reproduced or recognized.

Example

- Memories of days before head trauma are not available, although the person consciously experienced them and can usually remember daily events in detail,
- delirious patient, who according to relatives showed no memory impairment, can no longer say where he was yesterday, what he experienced in recent months, and does not recognize names (or photos) of people from current events.

Position in psychopathology. In AMDP (Item 12) memory disorder – no distinction between anterograde or retrograde disorder. However, this is not always clearly determinable—e.g., in alcoholics or long-lasting dementia development.

Differential diagnostic distinctions

- Distinction from normal forgetting,
- "Psychogenic amnesia": Memory contents originating from strongly emotionally tinted episodes may be subject to disorder of retrieval,
- Overlap with and transition to simulation phenomena (spectrum of conscious and unconscious blocking of retrieval).

Further characterization. Episodes no longer retrievable that could previously be reliably remembered.

Self-/other persons's judgment. other persons's judgment and self-evaluation.

Neuropsychology/objectification

- Situation descriptions, history taken from other persons,
- Tasks such as listing the order of politicians (chancellors/presidents),
- relating episodes to be recalled with respect to the time of brain damage,
- Showing pictures of famous people from a contemporary history book.

Severity. In head trauma, the duration of the retrograde disorder is prognostically useful,

Period of time of retrograde amnesia in a delirium is the duration of the period from which information is not available (months, years—question about chancellors, presidents).

Specifications
a) temporarily e.g. in delirium, or permanently (e.g. in dementia),
b) the temporal order of events is disturbed in the reproduction from memory.

Conceptual problems of the feature. Awareness of retrieval blocking in denial, simulation and highly emotional episodes is only vaguely detectable: spectrum from clearly conscious feigning of memory disorders to not subjectively noticeable avoidance of stimuli that are emotionally stressful (also as self-protection).

Neuroscientific/cognitive neuroscientific models

- Lack of retrievability in the stage of dependency of episodic memory on the integrity of the hippocampus, i.e., before the consolidation of memory contents, thereafter retrievability without mediation of the hippocampus (over time, however, also "revision" into highly overlearned autobiographical texts),
- Lack of retrievability after damage to cortical structures and pathways associated with effortful retrieval from consolidated memory. For example, lesions in frontal brain areas - especially right/language subdominant,

> **Disorder of autobiographical memory**
> **Definition.** Autobiographical information can no longer be remembered or can no longer be remembered in detail.

Example
- A patient cannot describe details of past significant family events, such as weddings, children's baptisms, although he tries, and he no longer remembers his profession, the stages of his professional life.

Position in psychopathology. Not specified in the AMDP, but listed as an orientation disorder to the person. Quantitative transition of the disorder of autobiographical memory contents to orientation disorder to the person.

Related terms. Orientation disorder about one's own person.

Psychopathological interaction. Memory impairment and retrograde memory disorder.

Differential diagnostic distinctions

- normal forgetting of events long past,
- delusional reinterpretation of life situation, delusional identity falsification.

Further characterization. Retrograde disorder of reproduction (less of recognition).

Interview for rating. Anamnestic questioning, history taken from other persons.

Neuropsychology/objectification. In addition to the standard data on biography, address details of some situations (such as last day of school, marriage, start of the professional career, etc.) - with external anamnestic verification,

- if diaries are available, more detailed diagnosis can be made.

Severity. Range of the disorder of the availability of autobiographical information from details (e.g., at the wedding) to essential information about one's own person, such as the date of birth.

Pathognomonic for: Not only, for example, in dementias, but also difficult access to autobiographical data as a mild disorder of autobiographical memory in the depressive episode.

Conceptual problems of the feature. At the beginning of psychopathology, in the 19th century, research was conducted on memory disorders in states such as fugue. If they are genuine memory disorders, they include retrograde disorders of autobiographical memory and orientation. This symptoms also occurs in transient global amnesia.

Neuroscientific/cognitive neuroscientific models
1. special form of retrograde amnesia, especially in severe dementia syndromes of the Alzheimer type,

- special susceptibility of autobiographical memories has been shown in research (dissociation from other memory areas); however, the influence of psychogenic retrieval disorders is difficult to exclude,
- normal forgetting rate (see Rubin et al. 1986).

2. Affective processes interfere with or distract from the recall and processing of autobiographical material - possibly to be characterized as avoidance behavior or resistance Chap. 11.
3. Storage of autobiographical information undergoes a transformation into cortical associations after the stage of episodic memory in the process of consolidation, in which one's own interpretation of the personal life story distorts the actual facts and relationships, resulting in the storage of an edited and censored autobiographical information, which has often also been trained in narratives.

False memory
Definition. Misinterpretation of a perception or a thought as a memory, although the episode did not actually occur. Supposed recognition.

Example

- A man thinks he has already experienced something, believes the situation is familiar to him, which, however, cannot be the case (Déjà-vu),
- someone claims to have had a terrible experience, which, however, did not occur.

Position in psychopathology. In AMDP paramnesia as a collective term, which, however, encompasses more, e.g., also hypermnesia included.

Related terms. Also involved in confabulation—a patient is supposed to remember an episode and fills memory gaps with false content, believing to remember it (confabulatory tendency).

Psychopathological interaction. derealization (see self-disorders, Chap. 13): A situation is experienced as altered – in the sense of false familiarity.

Differential diagnostic distinctions: Simulation, paralogy (lying), e.g., in witness statements; delusional memory falsification.

Further characterization. False positive errors of episodic memory, where no event to remember—the encoding episode—has taken place.

Interview for rating. Inquire if a memory might be false, external validation through third party anamnesis.

Severity. Range: Isolated vs. important statements falsified and thus unreliable in communication.

Specifications

- false familiarity, Déjà vu,
- delusional memory falsification,
- emotional experiences are falsely remembered, especially from childhood.

Conceptual problems of the feature
- Disturbance of memory in the sense of non-recognition not included here (likewise not the hypermnesia, which can be described as such)

Neuroscientific/cognitive neuroscientific models
1. Faulty reconnaissance signal false familiarity signal in the mediotemporal cortex,
2. fantasized experience, which is highly emotional (feared or desired), is perceived as a memory, for example, in the course of repeated fantasies over time,
3. source of information is not correctly categorized: fantasy or imagination is identified as a memory.

Confabulation
Definition. Filling memory gaps with false content.

Example

- A man with memory impairment reports false events from the past few days, i.e., events that did not happen, and believes he is remembering.
- A woman mentions an unusually high number of false positive items (intrusions) in a memory list task—and upon repetition, she bring up other false words (confabulatory tendency).

Position in psychopathology. AMDP 13

Related terms. paramnesia, disinhibition.

Psychopathological interaction. General disinhibition, phantasy, euphoria.

Differential diagnostic distinctions. Lying (pseudologia)—examination of the possible intention to the presentation of false content.

Further characterization. The patients know that they are supposed to report on elements of a situation to be remembered, filling in gaps.

Interview for rating. Repetition of a request to remember. History taken from other persons when reporting recent events.

Neuropsychology/objectification. Memory tasks with counting and evaluation of false positive errors.

Severity. Range from individual false positive errors up to general unreliability of statements in communication situations.

Specifications

- many false positive recall errorsin learning list tests,
- simple confabulation in gaps of recall,
- fantastic confabulation with embellishments that are not necessary.

Personality influences. An ambitious person faces a conflict between leaving omission errors, which the person notices, and filling in gaps that may not be checked by the examiner (e.g., when asked about daily events).

Conceptual problems of the feature

- Problem of awareness that false information is being provided,
- relationship to false memory, for example, when a memory gap is not admitted in court testimonies but is filled with false information.

Neuroscientific/cognitive neuroscientific models
1. Threshold of acceptance of mental contents, which are activated during the attempt of retrieval of the episode, as memories is lowered,
2. Part of a personality change in frontal lobe lesions,
    - especially fantastic, spontaneous confabulations (Schnider et al. 1996)

Model: Anxiety relief through disruption of afferents from the amygdala (see also euphoria model).

Flashback

Involuntary remembering mostly of a negative experience or a catastrophic episode. It is recurrently remembered without the person having consciously recalled the memory content.

- There are different types of forced retrievals of contents that are unpleasant or frightening to the person,
- relationship to obsessive thoughts should be investigated.

Disorientation in time
Definition. The current time cannot be correctly stated or identified.

Example:
- The patient does not know the current date and cannot recognize it from alternatives offered to him. He also cannot indicate the time range the current date lies in.

Position in psychopathology. AMDP 5—there defined as the knowledge of the date that is disturbed.

Psychopathological interaction. Memory impairment, retrograde memory disorder, attention to the environment, hospitalization.

Differential diagnostic distinction

- Prolonged state of disturbance of attention to the surroundings, in which no environmental information was grasped,
- aphasia—the person does not understand the task and cannot find the words,
- hasty "don't know" answer especially in depression—then it should be calmly asked whether the date could be estimated and the time range further narrowed down.

Self-/other person's judgment. Other person's judgment, possibly metacognition (knowledge about one's own memory and orientation disorder).

Interview for rating. Interview about current events.

Neuropsychology/objectification

- Name or guess the current date (recognition from alternatives 1990, 2000, 2010, 2020, 2030 etc.),
- Quantitative estimation of the extent of temporal disorientation, e.g., Benton score (see above) or asking the sequence of heads of state, etc.

Severity: According to the distance of the mentioned date from the current date, e.g., Benton score, mild—only a few days, weekdays wrong, severe—many years or decades wrong.

Specifications

- Suddenly out of full orientation—retrograde amnesia,
- Slowly progressive disorientation—mixing of anterograde amnesia (since the onset of dementia) and retrograde amnesia.

Neuroscientific/cognitive neuroscientific models
1. Time markers are not stored or cannot be retrieved,
2. anterograde amnesia—in amnestic syndrome and Alzheimer's dementia,
3. retrograde amnesia— e.g. in delirium,
4. Failure in the updating of time data, or it cannot be stored, see also above.

Disorientation in space
Definition. The current location of the person cannot be identified or cannot be spatially correctly classified.

Example

- A man gets lost in a city he is visiting for the first time, although he otherwise knew his way around after a single glance at a map.
- A patient does not have the many detailed pieces of information about the local conditions of his own city available, which he previously knew for sure.
- A patient gets lost in the surrounding of the house in which he has lived for a long time.

Position in psychopathology. AMDP 6—there, getting lost in familiar environments is referred to as a visuospatial memory disorder.

Psychopathological interaction

- declining visuospatial perception,

- declining interest in the spatial conditions of a foreign city,
- in severe disorders like in dementia also recognition problems and visual perceptual problems.

Differential diagnostic distinctions. People who have always had difficulty finding their way in unfamiliar environments.

Further characterization. Disorder of the automatic identification of one's own position in a spatial environment.

Neuropsychology/objectification

- Behavioral observation and history taken from other persons about "getting lost",
- let the person describe the current location,
- let the patient describe the way to the examination room (also memory impairment involved) or observe behavior.

Severity. From temporary problems in unfamiliar surroundings to the inability to find rooms in one's own house.

Neuroscientific/cognitive neuroscientific models

1. Disorder of place cells in the hippocampus, relation to spatial markers provided by the grid neurons,
2. The process of converting a traveled path onto an external "map" has either never been mastered, or is no longer possible after brain damage, see also above.

Reduplicative paramnesia

A patient knows, for example, that he is in the clinic. But he believes his location is also at home—or at his work.

- Distinction from spatial disorientation
- correctable, otherwise see also Delusion

References

Baddeley AD (1976) The psychology of memory. Harper, New York

Baddeley AD, Wilson BA, Watts FN (1997) Handbook of memory disorders. Wiley, Chichester

Benton AL (1983) Contributions to neurospychological assessment. Oxford Univ Press, Oxford

Brown AS (2003) A review of déjà vu experience. Psychol Bull 129:394–413

Desimone R, Miller EK, Chelazzi L, Lüschow A (1995) Multiple memory systems in the visual cortex. In: Gazzaniga MS (Ed) The cognitive neurosciences. Bradford, Cambridge, pp 475–486

Eichenbaum H, Cohen NJ (2001) From conditioning to conscious recollection—memory systems of the brain. Oxford Univ Press, Oxford

Folstein MF, Folstein SE, McHugh PR (1975) »Mini-mental state«. A practical method for grading the cognitive state of patients for the clinician. J Psychiatr Res 12:189–198

Hampton RR, Schwartz BL (2004) Episodic memory in nonhumans: what, and where, is when? Curr Opin Neurobiol 14:192–197

Hasselmo ME, McClelland JL (1999) Neural models of memory. Curr Opin Neurobiol 9:184–188

Kandel ER (1991) Cellular mechanisms of learning and the biological basis of individuality. In: Kandel ER, Schwartz JH, Jessell TM (Eds) Principles of neural science. Elsevier, New York, pp 1009–1031

Kandel ER (2001) The molecular biology of memory storage. A dialogue between genes and synapses. Science 294:1030–1038

Lachner G, Satzger W, Engel RR (1994) Verbal memory tests in the differential diagnosis of depression and dementia: discriminative power of seven test variations. Arch Clin Neuropsychol 9:1–13

Lynch MA (2004) Long term potentiation and memory. Physiol Rev 84:87–136

Markowitsch HJ (1992) Neuropsychologie des Gedächtnisses. Hogrefe, Göttingen

Markowitsch HJ (1998) Gedächtnisstörungen. Kohlhammer, Stuttgart

Marr D (1971) Simple memory: a theory for archecortex. Philos Trans R Soc Lond Biol Sci 262:23–81

McClelland JL, McNaughton BL, O'Reilly RC (1995) Why there are complementary learning systems in the hippocampus and neocortex: insight from the successes and failures of connectionist models of learning and memory. Psychol Rev 102:419–457

Mecklinger A, von Cramon DY, Matthes-von Cramon G (1998) Event-related potential evidence for a specific recognition memory deficit in adult survivors of cerebral hypoxia. Brain 121:1919–1935

Moser M-B, Rowland DC, Moser EI (2015) Place cells, grid cells, and memory. Cold Spring Harbor Perspectives in Biology 7(2): a 021808

Parker AE, Wilding EL, Bussey T (2002) The cognitive neuroscience of memory encoding and retrieval. Psychology Press, New York

Reischies FM (2005) Die Stellung von Screeninguntersuchungen und neuropsychologischen Markertests in der Demenzdiagnostik—allgemeine Aspekte. Zeitschrift für Gerontopsychologie & -psychiatrie 18:105–114

Reischies FM, Lindenberger U (1996) Grenzen und Potentiale kognitiver Leistungen im hohen Alter. In: Mayer KU, Baltes PB (Eds) Die Berliner Altersstudie. Akademie Verlag, Berlin, pp 351–377

Reischies FM, Kühl KP, Krebs M (2000) Zehn-Wort-Merkliste mit Imaginations-Einspeicherhilfe. Erste Ergebnisse mit einem neuen Instrument zur klinischen Gedächtnisprüfung. Zeitschrift für Gerontopsychologie & -psychiatrie 13:30–37

Rosenblatt F (1961) Principles of neurodynamics. Spartan Books, Washington

Rosenzweig ES, Barnes CA (2003) Impact of aging on hippocampal function: plasticity, network dynamics, and cognition. Prog Neurobiol 69:143–179

Rubin DC, Wetzler SE, Nebes RD (1986) Autobiographical memory across the adult lifespan. In: Rubin DC (Ed) Autobiographical memory. Cambridge Univ Press, Cambridge, pp 202–221

Rumelhart D, Hinton G, Williams R (1986a) Learning representations by back-propagating errors. Nature 323:533–536

Rummelhart DE, McClelland JL, PDP-Research Group (1986b) Parallel distributed processing: Explorations in the microstructure of cognition. MIT Press, Cambridge

Sacks O (1994) Der Mann der seine Frau mit einem Hut verwechselte. Rowohlt, Reinbek

Sander K, Sander D (2005) New insights into transient global amnesia: recent imaging and clinical findings. Lancet Neurol 4:437–444

Schmidtke K, Vollmer H (1997) Retrograde amnesia: a study of its relation to anterograde amnesia and semantic memory deficits. Neuropsychologia 35:505–518

Schnider A, von Däniken C, Gutbrod K (1996) The mechanisms of spontaneous and provoked confabulations. Brain 119:1365–1375

Solomon PR, Hirschoff A, Kelly B et al (1998) A 7 minute Neurocognitive screening battery highly sensitive to Alzheimer's disease. Arch Neurol 55:349–355

Squire LR, Zola-Morgan S (1991) The medial temporal lobe memory system. Science 253:1380–1386

Spitzer M (1996) Der Geist im Netz. Spektrum, Heidelberg

Steinbuch K (1961) Die Lernmatrix. Kybernetik 1:36–45

Strotzka S (2021) 20 Jahre Zehn-Wort-Merkliste mit Imaginations-Einspeicherhilfe. Psycho-Neuropraxis 24:110–115

Further Reading

Hedden T, Gabrieli JD (2004) Insights into the ageing mind: a view from cognitive neuroscience. Nat Rev Neurosci 5:87–96

Attention

4

Contents

4.1 Introduction

Attention is a little-understood sister of consciousness. We speak of "wakefulness" and the image of the spotlight of attention when we illustrate consciousness as a stage. Intentional consciousness makes use of attentional functions. We are dealing with a variety of attentional functions. At the beginning, the wide range of phenomena concerning attention in psychopathology will be shown using the example of undirected and directed attention.

Undirected attention

Example

A man dozes on the sofa in his apartment after work—on the upper floors of a high-rise building. Suddenly, the doorbell rings. He starts up and presses the door opener, looking through the "peephole" in the apartment door and seeing that no one is standing in front of it. Apparently, someone is coming up using the elevator. The man is now suddenly "awake"—compared to the previous state on the sofa. ◄

F. M. Reischies, *Psychopathology*, https://doi.org/10.1007/978-3-662-70293-2_4

In the example, the state of attention is reactively triggered. After the doorbell rings, there is a phase of startle—an alarm state—and then a longer-lasting phase of attentive wakefulness. However, attention may not yet be directed at an object that can be seen or heard. Mental search processes are taking place, such as: "Who could that be?".

In psychiatric conditions such as acute paranoid disorder, there is a change in the level of undirected attention. For example, a high level of attention is observed—the patient is hyperalert and pays attention to everything in the surroundings with intense attention. This state is seen in contrast to relaxed wakefulness. It has been described as hypervigilant or as a state of heightened attentiveness.

Directed, focussed attention

Example

A father is driving a car at moderate speed on a highway. The car is being overtaken by many other cars. The driver notices that a blue car that has just overtaken him is a new car model that he does not be acquainted with. He says to his son, "Look, there's a car I've never seen before—I'll try to overtake it." He tracks the blue car among the cars in front of him and follows it with his eyes. ◀

In this example, although the driver is generally attentive while driving, his attention is particularly drawn to one car because it seems unfamiliar to him. He directs his attention to it. Here, as in the first example, attention is reactively triggered, but it involves focussing attention on something. Directed attention also involves action preparation, but more with the concrete control of actions. When a person wants to attentively perform a routine activity, perhaps because they previously made a mistake, it means that, in contrast to automatic execution in everyday life, they now pay attention to all details of the action: both the direction of the actions, the sensorimotor feedback, and the speed and skill of executing motor acts.

In a person with intoxication from sedatives or alcohol, a change in attention is noticeable. A police officer called to the scene speaks of disturbed attention, as any layperson would in describing people with such syndromes—even if they could not define what attention is. Everyone interprets the turning towards an object and looking to it of people as their "being attentive" to what they might perceive there. If these attention-accompanying movements are absent or incomprehensible, we assume a disturbance of attention.

Spatial attention—Modality

So far, examples of directed and undirected attention have been presented—another distinction concerns the modality of attention, e.g., focused on a sensory channel or on thought content. Focusing on a single sensory feature occurs, for example, when a person is looking for a specific book on the shelf, knowing that it has a red leather cover. Attention can be directed like a selective filter to a sensory feature. This is an example of spatial attention.

Humans can also direct attention to their own body. For example, it is possible to successively direct attention to different parts of the skin with closed eyes, feeling how clothing or a chair touches the body. The reader can, for example, let the somatosensory attention wander. Attention should wander around the side of the body: First, it is directed to the right side of the head, then further to the right side of the neck, the shoulder, the arm to the hand, then back to the armpit and along the side of the chest to the hip, down the leg to the foot and back along the inner side of the leg; similarly on the left side over the leg, the chest, and the arm back to the head. They roughly trace the homunculus representation in the sensorimotor cortex. In doing so, one feels, for example, the skin tension in the head area, glasses or an earring, etc., a collar, a necklace, etc., on the neck, or clothing on the shoulder. This exercise takes some time, as the turning of attention with feedback from the somatosensory areas, usually the clothing on the neck, arm, hip, legs, and feet, each takes a little time.

This example illustrates spatial attention in the somatosensory area. Another example of spatial attention is the cocktail party phenomenon, where you can selectively focus auditory attention on conversations between different people around you.

Directed attention—mental form
Finally, the mental form of directed attention should be illustrated.

Example

A man is sitting on the subway and is not thinking about anything in particular. His thoughts are directed to taxes, and he remembers a tax deadline. Now he is startled by the thought, that a larger sum of money will additionally be due for a roof repair, and now the family will be financially overwhelmed. He considers how to manage the situation, such as through a loan, asking for help from relatives, overdrawing the account, drastic savings, etc. The initially free-floating, undirected attention has been focused on a topic. Initially, a shock occurred with the mental realization of the temporal coincidence of two payment deadlines, then a focused search for solutions. There is also a mental search for cognitive features, for example, in puzzles that require a specific word or a class of properties of words. ◄

Priming
A form of involuntary activation with high specificity is priming. An example should illustrate what is meant by this. If a person is told a word and it is attentively understood, then within the brain the word is stimulated in its cortical representations and also in its associative connections. If shortly thereafter the same or an associated word is to be found or recognized, for example, with a very short presentation time, this is easier after the pre-activation. For example, a gap word t_i_p_p_ is probably difficult to complete. If a car repair was mentioned beforehand, it is easier to find the word seemingly "spontaneously" because the semantic field of car, car parts, and then tailpipe has been activated. Priming seems to work only if the first stimulus is attentively noticed (Naccache et al. 2002).

Some scientists regard attention to cognitive content as "awareness," in contrast to consciousness. Cognitive focussed attention and "being aware that…"—e.g., being aware that certain people at a large party are related- can direct associations and ways of thinking.

Awareness as maintaining a certain pre-activation on constraints of a topic, enables, for example, quick argumentation in negotiations through the priming effect. Awareness of a fact is not the same as the attention focus: because a person can be aware of many facts simultaneously, but can only focus on one topic.

4.2 Definitions

The taxonomy of attention phenomena has not yet found an universal agreement. Psychological research has invested a lot of energy in defining the term "attention" (Prinz and Hommel 2002). Although everyone has a layman's concept of attention, how is attention to be defined? Some researchers reserve the term "attention" solely for selective attention. However, since one can be attentive not only to something specific but also more or less attentive without a specific object (see examples above), it seems better to keep the term broad. Most researchers also acknowledge that undirected activation processes, such as the startle reaction, have a function in attention regulation.

Attention always becomes apparent only in processes, that occur with more or less attention. Attention is realized in different mental functions. There are no pure attention phenomena. This circumstance is particularly important in the diagnosis of attention disorders; because an attention disorder can be feigned if the disorder does not affect the attention functions themselves, as suspected, but the processes in which attention is supposed to be realized, e.g., the visual processes being examined, etc. Like other psychopathological features, attention is not directly observable—like thinking, which can only be assessed through speech, or drive, which cannot be captured independently of other features, such as overt behavior.

Attention refers to various completely different issues, which can also occur more or less coupled. For example, inattention in traffic can occur because a person becomes tired or because they are busy eating or talking on the phone. In one case, tonic attention is reduced and will only improve after a sleep or after drinking coffee. In the other case, spatial attention is diverted from the road and directed to something else and can immediately be redirected to traffic.

Another example is the focussing of attention on a sought-after male person in a blue shirt among pedestrians on a busy street. In this case, spatial attention is diverted from traffic, and a specific attention function is activated, which is directed at a color feature and male body shape.

A final example of a group of attention functions concerns executive attention, such as attention to complicated parking or in the stage of learning to drive. In this case, executive attention to parking can be disturbed due to agitation. It is not clear whether a separate entity of executive attention needs to be postulated (see also Wu 2011).

Common to all states and processes that occur attentively, as opposed to non-attentive states, is that they occur in an activated manner—further below, in the neuroscience section, an attempt is made to describe various neural mechanisms involved. The activated processes are then often, but not necessarily, conscious. There is also a close inverse relationship to the automation of processes. Automated processes can occur without attention, in contrast to controlled processes (e.g., Cohen 1993). Here, too, there is an association to executive processes (Chap. 6).

Psychopathologically, corresponding to what has been said, there are disorders of different attention functions—mostly in the direction of either reduced or increased function. For example, hyperattentive symptoms occur in paranoid syndromes, showing transitions to states of increased agitation, or pathological fatigue in narcolepsy.

For the description of attention functions, it is useful to separate categorical distinctions from dimensional features. Categorical distinctions describe incompatible states like sleep or wakefulness, while dimensional features describe a quantitative gradation. In the case of agitation, for example, the degree of agitation must be assessed psychopathologically.

4.2.1 Categorical Distinctions

First, two categorical boundaries can be described:

1. A categorical boundary lies between non-consciousness (coma, sleep) and wakefulness, a person is conscious. A person cannot be attentive if he is not awake. Attention is thus dependent on wakefulness as a necessary but not sufficient condition (Chap. 8 consciousness).
2. The status of "being focussed attentive on object x" is a different status than "not being focused attentive on object x." Information processing occurs differently in the first status than in the second.

This concerns the "all-or-nothing principle" of attention. In undirected, wandering attention, one can notice the entire visual field, all incoming auditory stimuli, somatosensory, and bodily perceptions.

However, if a stimulus is processed that requires more complex information processing, such as when the gaze falls on a letter containing a number indicating the amount of debt, etc., the situation changes abruptly: The world seems to shrink to the written words and numbers, a message that wants to be mentally explored in its consequences. The environment is no longer perceived.

There is generally a difference between being attentive to an object and not being focused attentively, i.e., general attentiveness. In this case, the person is attentive but not specifically to an object or activity (as in our first example of the doorbell ringing).

The two categorical distinctions of attention states contrast with the quantitative gradations:

1. wakefulness, as observed in slow waking up from sleep or slow getting tired and falling asleep, furthermore
2. the arousal level or attentiveness and
3. the intensity of focussing attention.

4.2.2 Dimensional Characteristics

Normal and Pathological Attention Variance
There are overlapping areas of normal attention variance and pathological variance, a circumstance that complicates psychopathological assessment in this area:

1. The physiological variance refers, for example, to fatigue. If we experience many of the audience members taking a short "nap" in a lecture at 1 PM, it is annoying for the speaker—it can be explained by our normal midday tendency to fall asleep. This follows circadian laws (see below). Fatigue and the tendency to fall asleep, however, can be a pathological phenomenon in narcolepsy.
2. A second example is the physiological variance in focused attention to an object. This can be slight or very intense. This variance becomes evident in reaction time measurements. A subject may notice the stimulus to which he is supposed to react, but only slightly and without effort. Their reaction times will be slower than those of another subject who pays full attention to the appearance of the stimulus with all effort.

In the variance of focused attention, there are pathological conditions. For example, in psychopathological states, there is a pathological reduction in maximally focused attention. Some patients with mental illnesses cannot make an effort to pay attention to a stimulus. Here, the circumstance becomes evident, which is often observed in psychopathology: The pathological variance and the normal, physiological everyday variance overlap. In other words, I cannot tell from the individual reactions whether they were low due to slightly strained focused normal attention or pathologically low focused attention. It also becomes immediately clear that the diagnostic assessment of focused attention is not possible without the cooperation of the person who must direct their attention to a task and strain themselves maximally. This aspect of effort has been emphasized more recently.

1. The first, variance thus concerns the "attentiveness", the tonic unfocused attention.
2. The second variance is often equated with the "effort," the effort a subject makes to work quickly and correctly (Fig. 4.1).

In attention, it is difficult to separate normal and pathological variance components. Additionally, there are difficulties in differentiating various psychopathological phenomena in the area of attention: The variation in fatigue is not easily distinguishable psychopathologically from the quantitative variation in the level of tonic attention.

Additionally, there is variance in the control, adaptation abilities or flexibility of attention processes.

4.2.3 Control of Attention

Attention is regulated voluntarily and involuntarily. Selective attention can occur passively or be actively directed, for example, when searching for something. It can occur without effort or with effort.

Concentration is usually understood as sustained focussed attention. This leads to further phenomena. Active concentration performance results in ignoring distractors.

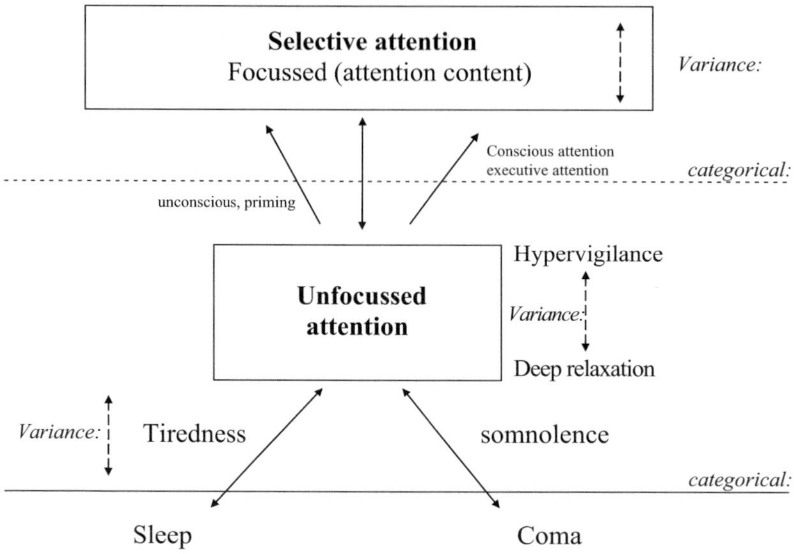

Fig. 4.1 Taxonomy of attention domains. On the one hand, two categorical distinctions arise: 1. between awake and not awake and 2. between focussing on an object or not focussing on it (or not focussing on any object). On the other hand, there are quantitative differences in the intensity of focussed attention, how much a person can be aware of at the same time, and also in the level of unfocused attention

Arousal refers to a phasic unfocused attention, usually with a startle reaction. Arousal is generally determined by external stimuli, but one can also self-induce arousal through thinking about a feared opponent, rival, or legal disputes.

The control of various attention functions is managed by different processes, which can be described as voluntary, active, and involuntary, passive. There is interindividual variation in control processes. Dysfunctional attention regulation can also be observed (see below).

Control of Agitation
Since antiquity, it has been considered an ideal for a person to be able to keep emotions in check, i.e., to plan and prepare actions without being excited and becoming hectic (today often colloquially referred to as "cool"). In the psychopathological field, one often encounters the opposite: A patient shows activation and agitation without focussed attention, without action plans. There is nothing but undirected agitation. This is seen in affective states, such as aggression or anxiety attacks (Chap. 11 Emotions/Affects).

Control of Fatigue
Usually, a person tries to counteract a decrease in vigilance due to fatigue. However, this is not always successful and especially not completely, leading to a particular state of attention with simultaneous fatigue and selective attention. This state is familiar to many people from driving at night when beginning to feel tired.

The compensation endeavor just described is also observed in the study of somnolence. When a somnolent patient is awakened, voluntary attention to certain environmental events is acitvated before the patient sinks back into the state of apparent sleep.

4.2.4 Course of Attention Processes

Awakening of Attention
Turning to an object, which arouses interest, is the passive beginning of focused attention. Attention is awakened by the perception of the object, "bottom-up." In contrast, when searching for an object, such as a salt shaker on a crowded table, an attention process is initiated "top-down" by cognitive processes.

Dimensions of Attention

Pathological distractibility—Failure of focussed attention

First of all, attention can be distracted if the person voluntarily or involuntarily develops another focus of interest. The initial focus of attention on the object may be insufficient. In the example of searching in the kitchen, the ringing of the phone can interrupt the search process.

Fatigue—Decline or Failure of Attention

Being awake and attentive has its price. The "costs" of attention are fatigue and declining effort ("effort consuming"). The word fatigue within this context does not distinguish between the need for sleep and reduced vigilance on the one hand and the failure of selective, focussed attention on the other. The effort to invest focussed attention decreases. Fatigue from strenuous activity is to be distinguished from tiredness at night and drowsiness.

Experimental psychology has examined the performance course in attention-demanding tasks and found a generally moderate decline in performance (Broadbent 1971). Long ago, the task of tracking a clock with error detection (sudden double advancement of the hand) was introduced as a vigilance task and is still used today, the Mackworth clock. Besides a slight variance within the normal range, there are outliers in terms of reaction time and error frequency. These are mainly found in sleep regulation disorders. Attempts are made to distinguish the decline in performance in terms of declining targeted attention from fatigue and falling asleep (see below).

Attention Dimensions

Table 4.1 shows attention dimensions: Directed/Undirected; the distinction between phasic/tonic for voluntary and involuntary attention phenomena in attention to sensory perception and thought or imagination contents.

4.3 Disorders of Attention, Clinical Syndromes

In psychiatry, disorders of attention are common. Attention is an Achilles' heel of information processing in the brain. It is necessary for orderly information processing and for the functioning of the organism in the environment.

Disturbances of Sustained Attention, Wakefulness

In narcolepsy and in acute medical conditions with somnolence, it is examined whether a patient, on the one hand, suffers from increased fatigue and shows a lack of sustained attention, which is also referred to as vigilance disorder. On the other hand, it must be clarified whether he is in the stage of somnolence, with the risk that he might "slip" into a coma. In the examples (see above), a disturbance of the level of sustained attention in paranoid disorder has already been addressed.

Disturbances of Phasic Attention

Patients report being easily scared, i.e., an increased phasic, not voluntarily controllable attention activation, such as severe fright at the slightest provocation; each time, it leads to a vivid arousal with vegetative and motor characteristics.

4.3.1 Examples of Impaired Attention Functions in Psychiatric Disorders

Schizophrenia

- distracted by internal experiences that are not always comprehensible to others.
- in paranoid experiences, a person can be hyper-attentive, undirectedly attentive, hypervigilant, suspicious. In this state, the person cannot complete any task, gets nothing done, disturbance of executive functions.

Table 4.1 Attention Dimensions

	Phasic		Sustained		Comment
	Decreased	Increased	Decreased	Increased	
1 Fatigue				Daytime drowsiness, tendency to fall asleep (imperative)	Quality of feeling tired
2 Undirected	arousal reduction, not reacting to new stimuli	easily startled, increased exitable arousal	arousal level reduction, persistent hypoattentiveness,	arousal level increased, persistent hyperattentiveness,	Attentiveness, nonspecific arousal, internally or externally triggered
3 Directed sensory	Decreased sensory focus	Increased sensory focus, e.g., suspicious, distractible	Decreased sensory focus Errors in monitoring	Increased sensory focus Fixated on an object, "tunnel vision"	Focussing on stimuli in one of the sensory channels
Directed Cognitive	Decreased focus on thought contents	Increased focus on thought contents	Decreased thought focus, Errors in cognitive processing	Increased thought focus Hyperfocussed, restricted thinking flexibility	Focussing on thought contents or on imaginations

- in negative symptoms, reduction of attention in the sense of hypoattentiveness.

Mania
- hyper-attentive, tireless. The focussing of attention can be reduced, for example, due to permanentely new ideas.

Depression
- Unable to focus on a task or a test in a prescribed way;
- unable to exert sustained attention (even when relatives urge the depressed person to "activate all effort"); usually, in a depressive episode, there is already a failure of the compensatory effort applied in the previous development of depression.

Delirium
- Reduced alertness, decreased directed and undirected phasic attention and fluctuating attentiveness. Although the person often appears awake and attentive in acute delirium, they cannot activate focussed attention or can do so only inadequately. Disturbed allocation and focussing of attention. At the same time, due to impaired consciousness, there is a lack of cognitive integration of perceived information.

Attention Deficit Syndrome (ADS)
- impaired direction of attention to tasks with too low reward expectancy low expectation of reward; during longer activities increased distractibility and interruptions—(usually with impulsivity, as well as reduced frustration tolerance)—relationship to the disorder of becoming motivated—for example, the expectation of reward for monotonous tasks for school/work is not sufficient.

Autism
- Attentive to specific things (hyper-focussed) or inattentive to the environment, withdrawn,
- no attention directed to the social environment, to other people.

Somatization Disorder
- attention fixed on the experience of disturbance in one's own body, disorder of the flexible, adapted regulation of focused attention.

In many of these examples of clinical attention disorders, it is assumed that they are caused by factors that do not belong to attention, such as hallucinations, delusions, affects, etc. These arguments should be set aside for now, as the other sections of the book will address the specific aspects, such as executive aspects of attention, motivational aspects, and content-related aspects, e.g., thought contents that affect attention. However, it should also be considered whether one can explain with sufficient certainty why another disorder is more important and the attention disorder is only secondary. The different components of the sustained attention state, attentiveness, are clinically indistinguishable in many cases.

4.3.2 Disturbance of the Components of Attention

Fatigue

Sleep test. In somnology, a multiple sleep test is used to objectify fatigue. For this, a patient is given the opportunity to fall asleep in the sleep laboratory, and the time to reach the various stages of sleep is measured.

Fatigue and Disturbance of vigilance: vigilance does not refer to the spectrum from wakefulness to coma—it is to be distinguished between the reduction of attentiveness due to fatigue on the way to Sleep and due to clouding of consciousness with the transition to coma. With progressive brain damage, the patient eventually falls into somnolence or a sopor, where a combination of massively reduced attentiveness and disturbance of focused attention is present. Here, the EEG can distinguish a pre-comatose event from drowsiness. In most cases, fatigue is also observed in delirium, e.g., due to disturbances of the day-night rhythm.

Disturbance of sustained undirected (unfocsused) attention, attentiveness (arousal level)
The level of undirected (unfocsused) attention, the attentiveness, fluctuates. It may be best to imagine it as the sum of the current activity of the various attention processes (quasi as the integral of the individual associative activations with their feedbacks).

Reduced sustained attention
A patient is in a state of reduced inner tension regarding external stimuli and thought content despite being awake. It is not certain to what extent this state can be distinguished from a relaxed state voluntarily achieved through meditation exercises—only that the relaxed attention in meditation was achieved voluntarily and the reduction of sustained attention in psychopathological states is involuntary and even beyond the person's control. The person cannot free themselves from this state, for example, after being asked to perform an attentive task.

Phasic attention reduced—Disturbance of Arousal
When you get a puff of air in your eye, not only does the eyelid twitch and the eye close quickly, but changes also occur in the body—the muscle tone increases, the head is pulled back, and the body posture changes. This is called the orientation reaction (it is also referred to as the "startle response").
On the one hand, disturbance of arousal affects the orientation reaction, but general arousal can also be reduced: Attention is not phasically activatable, the patient does not appear excitable, not even by previously effective stimuli. As is often the case in the field of attention disorders, a potential assessment error must be ruled out: Naturally, the state must not be explainable by active diversion of attention or, for example, meditation.

The reduction of the level of unfocused attention is not easy to examine. The EEG provides clues, with the degree of desynchronization of the basic rhythm being related to the extent of unfocussed and focussed attention.

Increased—Enhancement of attention
An enhancement of attention can be observed both in normal psychology, such as during exams and job interviews, and as a psychopathological feature, for example, in people who perceive themselves as threatened, such as individuals with paranoid disorders. They are hyper attentive, constantly looking around without being selectively attentive to anything. This is also referred to as "hypervigilance"— this state often also accompanies reduced fatigue, e.g., in mania.

Phasically increased—disturbed phasic undirected attention
Too many stimuli lead unpredictably to agitation, such as in mania. Clinically, it is observed that a second manic patient in a ward may lead to an uncontrollable escalation of dynamics between the patients. One manic patient increases the agitation of the other patient, and the fellow patients are involved.

The increase in phasic attention is clinically often associated with increased distractibility, as e.g. in mania. The increase in phasic attention is also observed in paranoid, borderline, and post-traumatic syndromes.

Categorical Selective Attention
If selective attention is impaired, on the one hand, only the extent of focussing may be reduced, but on the other hand, the physiological process of focussing itself may also be affected—attention may be untargeted, not be directed to an agreed-upon object at all. The latter is the case when there is neglect on one side (see below) and the person cannot direct attention to an object located on that side. The disorder potentially affects voluntary attention focussing, which also occurs passively, for example, when following a primarily interesting object.

Possible reasons for the lack of attention focussing:

a) spatial: neglect,
b) content-related: a disturbance in the activation of thoughts or sensory features that enable focused searching,

c) if attention focussing is expected, for example, during a test examination, focussing may fail due to various causes, with other psychopathological factors dominating:
   - motivation and willingness to cooperate are lacking,
   - distraction,
   - fixation on other contents— e.g. thought insertion in schizophrenic patients: sudden inspiration of new contents with a change in the attention focus.

How can it be diagnosed whether focussed attention is absent?

- The patient may indicate that they are not paying attention to something.
- When observing the patient, it may be noticeable:
  - looking around, which is not directed at the agreed-upon object,
  - not turning towards an object, not following an agreed-upon object with the eyes. Just as the teacher in school pays attention to the students' attention-based behavior, so it applies, for example, to behavioral observation during tests: the fact that the patient has directed his attention to the test object at all is essential for the validity of the results.

Reduction of Selective Attention

Maximum focussing is not achieved. This is investigated, for example, by means of reaction time measurements, for example, in tests of psychomotor speed: the patient is supposed to be quick in a simple task, for example, in the reaction time experiment: because the subjects master the task well, for example, recognizing a specific stimulus, they can try to fulfill this task with reaction to a button as quick as possible.

In the evaluation of selective attention, distraction must be considered, as the distraction of focussing itself also determines reaction time performance. A patient may be capable of quick reactions but is distracted, e.g., by psychopathological phenomena, such as hearing voices. This is one of the reasons why reaction time measurements usually have low diagnostic validity, especially in patients with mental disorders.

Another disruptive factor in the diagnosis of the quantity of selective attention, which is even more important, is the high variance in motivational states. If a person is slow in reaction time measurements or other speed-dependent tests, it must first be clarified whether they were sufficiently motivated. Behavioral observation in neuropsychological tests is indispensable for the interpretation of findings for this reason alone.

In addition to objective distraction, for example, by disturbing noises, distractibility as a disposition of the subject, as a psychopathological phenomenon, plays a role. Often, "concentration" is used as a poorly defined term precisely to denote resistance to distracting stimuli. A person who can solve difficult puzzles in a noisy café is considered highly concentrated.

The quick completion of mental tasks requires effort, and thus exhaustibility is another factor in considering the quantity of selective attention. Clinically, the speed of the decline in attention is noted. For example, in the d2 test, where specific marked letters are sought, it is evaluated how many correct stimuli are found in each time segment. Usually, the exhaustion of selective attention occurs over periods of hours rather than minutes.

4.3.3 Content-Related Attention Disorders

In addition to the formal aspects of attention, there are also content-related aspects, which have already been addressed in the discussion of focussed attention. A pathologically increased focus of attention on a goal occurs clinically. This is especially observed in delusional syndromes, in overvalued ideas, and in mania. The attention is indeed intensified but completely inflexibly directed at a specific object. An example from everyday experience is the rapt attention on a person one is currently mourning the loss of. Here, the subjective focus of attention does not align with the attention goals in the social environment: The patient, thus fixated in attention, will only briefly or not at all glance at someone entering the room, whom everyone around the mourner immediately looks at. This is important for a psychopathological examination. The patient pays attention to something, but not to what the examiner wants to direct the attention to.

This phenomenon is closely related to narrowed consciousness (Chap. 8). The involuntary nature of the symptom, which contrasts with the voluntary concentration efforts of healthy individuals, is important.

In the case of increased focussed attention, another feature of attention comes into play: the disengagement of attention from a focus. There may be a reduced ability to disengage attention from a topic.

These attention disorders affect several mental illnesses:

- somatoform disorder,
- somatization disorder,
- dissociative disorder,
- acute stress reaction.

4.3.4 Attention and Age

In old age, reaction times become longer, with not only the motor component being delayed but also the central component (Kliegl et al. 1994). Selective attention is reduced, as shown in speed tests.

Some very old and particularly demented people are found in a state where they "just sit around," with reduced attention to the environment, attentiveness is reduced without fatigue. When asked if they are engaged in remembering something or thinking about something, they deny it. This state, purely superficially, seems to come close to a Buddhist ideal because the individuals are in great calm without thinking about anything.

Dementia patients often have a lowered arousal level. The discrepancy between the memory impairment of Alzheimer's patients, the "non-recognition" when, for example, new, unknown people appear, and the attention disorder—the lack of arousal—has not been intensively investigated: A young person would look at a person entering the room, i.e., first become aware of them, whereas a demented person, for example, does not even look up.

In delirium, a form of increased arousal and one with hypoarousal—an inattentive type—is described (Reischies et al. 2003).

4.3.5 Neglect

Neglect refers to the inattention to objects on the left or right side of the patient. Neglect of the left side is often observed after a right-sided stroke. Neglect also applies to purely mental processes, for example, in the imagination of a spatial scene. In this case, memories of spatial relationships on one side do not succeed.

Meanwhile, many neuroscientific findings on this clinical phenomenon have been presented (Driver et al. 2004). The movement tendencies of the eyes, with the coordinates of the head, but also of the hand with the coordinates within the "grasping space", are represented in the parietal cortex. These movement tendencies to the opposite side are missing in parietal neglect (Chap. 5 Central Motor Skills; Fig. 4.2).

4.4 Diagnostics

It has become clear from the first sections: In the area of attention, we are dealing with closely related phenomena that cannot simply be considered in isolation.

People differ in the variables of attention, almost as personality traits: There are always highly attentive people and others who always appear almost meditatively relaxed. The conditions for tiredness and falling asleep, for fatigue, for arousal and the investment of selective attention are individual. For this reason the area of attention functions is often not adequately examinable in a clinical setting,

Neglect: large re-sided infarction

a

b

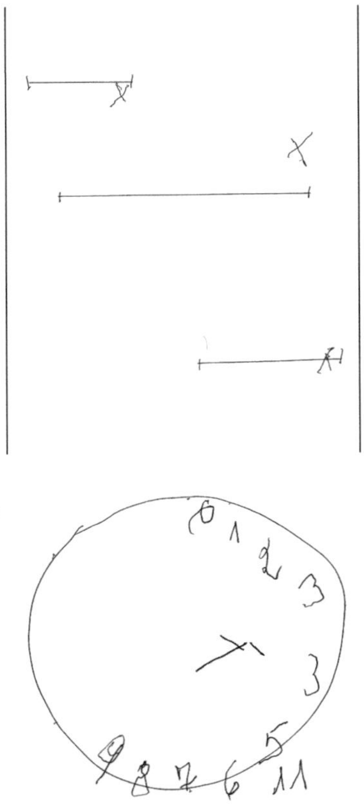

Fig. 4.2 a, b. Neglect—Example of a patient with a large right-sided brain infarction. a) Lines of different positions and lengths are perceived only in their right part. When the person is asked to mark the lines in the middle, the markings are thus placed too far to the right, b) when drawing a clock, only the right part is drawn

especially because in the clinic, patients are initially diagnosed only once in a cross-sectional manner. Through direct observation and testing, only a part of the attention variance can be covered. A history taken from other persons about the level of attention preceding the disease syndrome is difficult to get and often not reliably obtainable. Therefore, information from relatives must also be relied upon, who should be asked to describe in detail how the behaviors in everyday life were.

Additionally, test examinations must sometimes be conducted. Unfortunately, there are only insufficient methods to test attention functions. For example, e.g. only selective attention is tested, assuming that all other areas of attention are undisturbed—such as vigilance, the voluntary activation of attention on the test, arousal, etc. In other words, poor performance in attention tests often leaves the question open as to which of the attention functions is disturbed. Another problem that must be considered when a patient's attention seems disturbed and is to be examined: Is it a disturbance of attention in the sense of the inability to engage the attention function, or is it that the person is not investing attention in the task at that moment: Is this deliberately so or lack of motivation to cooperate or just a random distraction at the moment of the examination (Fig. 4.3).

- Sustained attention tests (Mackworth clock);
- Reaction time proceedures;
- Search tests, (e.g. d2 test);
- Pathfinder tests, non-verbal variant (Reischies and Berghöfer 1995);
- Cross-out tests;
- Stroop test (Chap. 6),
  - executive attention,
  - suppression of an information processing channel.

Performance factors in attention tests

- attentiveness: tiredness, arousal, agitation;
- interest, motivation;
- Selective attention: cooperation;
- Affects, e.g., aggression, anxiety (agitation);
- Rule out: neglect, Balint syndrome;
- Disturbed information processing of the basic task—rule out: other neuropsychological syndromes; peripheral: eye muscle disorder etc..

Schema for Diagnostics

1. Fatigue :
   - Falling asleep (nodding off at a rest)
   - e.g., slowness of blinking
2. arousal
   - increased arousal

   being easily scared, heart rate, galvanic skin response

   (are triggering conditions specific?)
   - decreased arousal

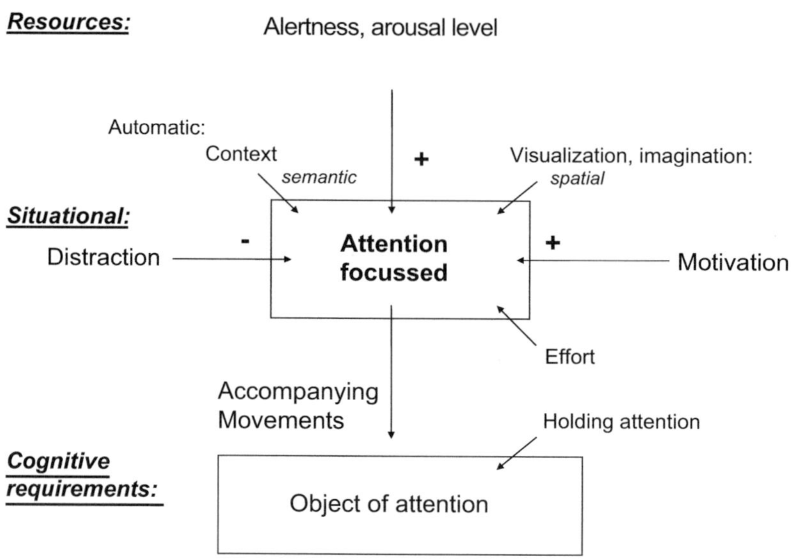

Fig. 4.3 Clinical factors for attention assessment: resources and situational factors. Resources are, on the one hand, attention processes, and on the other hand, the capacity for information processing, which should proceed attentively. Situationally, distracting factors may be present. These are only partially observable by an examiner: The distraction can be caused by mental processes or emotions. Also, the effort that the person exerts in focused attention is a variable that cannot be fully assessed by the observer.

3. unfocused attention, attentiveness e.g., amount and speed of eye movements
   - increased attentiveness
   - decreased attentiveness
4. attention not focused on an agreed content, the patient should pay attention to: Fixation of the eyes, attention-accompanying movements,
   - distracted, uncooperative (deliberately?)
5. disturbed quantity and quality of focussed attention
   - extent of distraction effect in tests, concentration
6. differential diagnosis:
   - reduced motivation
   - clouding of consciousness (Chap. 8)
   - drowsiness
   - somnolence

   (when waking a person with somnolence, basic cognitive functions are disturbed, e.g.
   working memory, fluency etc.)

4.5 Neuroscience

So far, attention has been referred to as activation, which initially means a psychological concept of activation. At the neurophysiological level of consideration, however, it is, for example, about the triggering of action potentials (see Posner and Petersen 1990; Posner and Rothbart 2023; Parasuraman 1998; Treue 2003). One principle of attention functions is approaching the membrane potential to the threshold for triggering an action potential. This is achieved within the neuron by excitatory postsynaptic potentials. Example: Sensory neurons are engaged in processing a stimulus in a reaction experiment. The membrane potential of the neurons is altered by the stimuli, i.e., the primary probability of the occurrence of an action potential. A baseline shift of the membrane potential takes place (Kastner et al. 1999; Hopfinger et al. 2000), it is under the control of excitatory and inhibitory postsynaptic potentials caused by the afferent neurons. The decrease in the "baseline" sensitizes (pre-sensitizes) the neurons processing the stimulus. Errors can occur due to preactivation: The neurons "report a stimulus" and initiate a reaction without the stimulus occurring—a false positive error, as investigated in reaction time psychology (see Aston Jones et al. 1999; Fig. 4.4, see also Parr and Friston 2019).

Usually, a neuron gets input by a wide variety of synapses on the dendritic tree. Some of these originate from activating systems that are considered to belong to the attention system. When these "inputs" arrive, the triggering of the action potential shortly thereafter becomes faster and more efficient due to the specific triggering input. We must therefore assume a twofold information processing:

1. one of attention, which ensures a nonspecific pre-activation, and
2. one of the current content processes—in the above example, the information processing for the reaction time task or the mental process (such as a thinking task or a cooking procedure).

Each of these information processing steps is accompanied by an activation and pre-activation of the specifically involved task-elements, for example, the activation of the semantic units for the objects being used, etc. Activation in the everyday psychological sense is neuroscientifically more of a pre-activation; which can be more or less specific.

Organization of attention in special neuronal systems and in the network functions of the cortex

As with other functions, the organization of attention occurs in several different mechanisms and regulations. These can partially complement each other, so that one of the mechanisms can fail without the entire system collapsing. For example, several transmitter systems exist in the reticular formation, the ascending reticular activating system, ARAS—with brainstem areas for the origin neurons of the respective transmitter system. Psychiatry and psychopharmacology deals in important parts with the functional disorders of various of these transmitter systems.

A fundamental distinction between special attention systems and attention effects of information processing itself must be made here. On the one hand, there are neuronal systems like the noradrenergic system, which is involved in activation tasks, predominantly of a phasic nature. There are special neurons with a special transmitter,

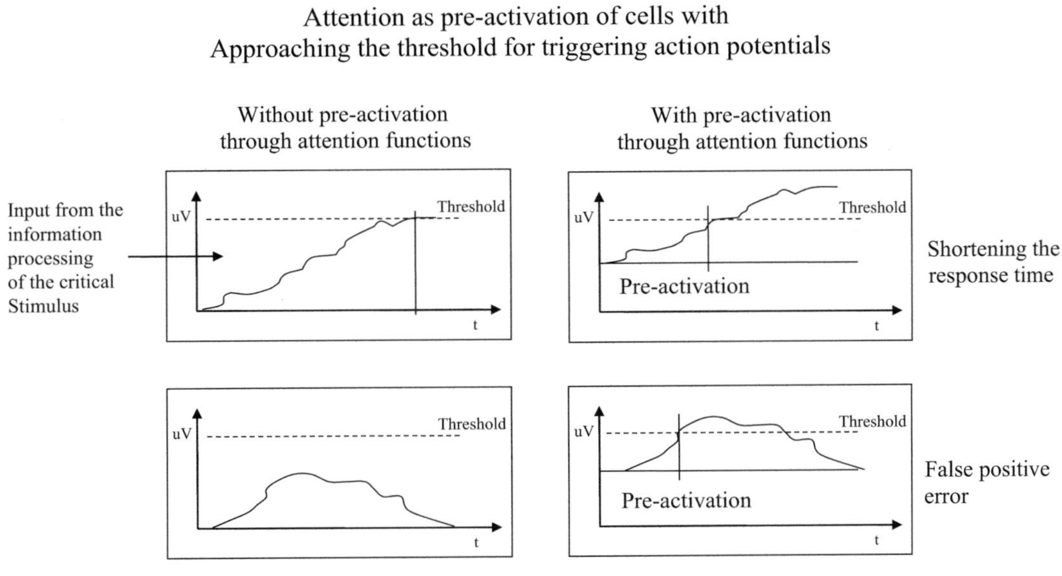

Fig. 4.4 Attention processes involve the preactivation of cells, which then respond with higher probability, or faster. However, this comes at the cost of a higher rate of false positive reactions

which is released at the synapses, noradrenaline. On the other hand, the brain also has selection processes that lead to pre-activation through the ongoing information processing. Illustratively, in the semantic system, the activation of a word will activate the semantically related "neighborhood," however distributed it may be represented in the brain. This leads to faster and more effective information processing of the related semantic units. These are priming effects that have been mentioned above. This example shows that the "focus of consciousness" always includes the process of specific pre-activation.

▶ This information processing does not occur solely through systems found in special brainstem nuclei and equipped evolutionarily with various transmitter systems. Rather, the information processing of a significant part of selective attention and the focus of consciousness emerges between the cortical neurons in terms of network functions.

Although attention is safeguarded against damage through various mechanisms in the basic functions, it remains the Achilles' heel of the human information processing system. For if the attention functions are critically disturbed, perception selection, thinking, and memory searching are disturbed, and as a result, the person can no longer behave intelligently in the environment.

The neuroscientific data and model concepts are presented under three headings:

1. vigilance (Sect. 4.5.1),
2. attentiveness and arousal state (Sect. 4.5.2),
3. selective or focussed attention (Sect. 4.5.3).

First, we assume that the mechanisms of the three areas can be separated in psychopathology. However, it is not yet ultimately certain whether there are not significant overlaps. One theoretical position is that, for example, arousal mechanisms could also be necessary for selective attention or waking mechanisms for attentiveness. We hold the position that we are dealing with physiological individual mechanisms that evolved separately and have been tried and tested in evolution. However, they cause patterns of changes that cannot be exactly separated from each other psychopathologically. In this case, the presentation at least follows certain main functions of the individual mechanisms.

4.5.1 Vigilance and Fatigue

The regulation of sleep, specifically falling asleep and waking up, is specifically controlled by brainstem systems. These systems are already quite well known and depicted in physiology books (see Saper et al. 2005). For psychiatry frequent psychopathological symptoms occur that relate both to attention and to sleep disorders.

First, the circadian tendency to fall asleep should be described. There is a first peak around noon, during which the tendency to take a short sleep is high. The most important, incomparably higher and broader peak of the circadian tendency to fall asleep is after midnight. This has the important function of ensuring that sleep is not interrupted too early. Because the sleep pressure that accumulates over the day is already reduced during the first hours of sleep. When sleep pressure decreases, the circadian tendency to sleep sets in after midnight and ensures continued sleep until the morning. Therefore, two mechanisms are essential for sleep:

1. the circadian tendency to fall asleep and
2. the sleep pressure that accumulates over the time of wakefulness.

In severe depression, we find a disturbance of continuous sleep, or the symptom of early awakening. This could be explained by a disturbance of the circadian brainstem mechanisms affecting vigilance regulation and thus the control of fatigue. Sleep is disturbed in the second half of the night because sleep pressure has already subsided after a few hours of sleep due to wakefulness during the day. This can also explain the symptom of lack of feeling rested and fresh in the morning and the disturbance of feeling awake during the day.

After sleep deprivation and in narcolepsy, a state can be examined that is referred to as fatigue, in which a reduction in attentional functions is observed. Fatigue is a subjective item. However, the tendency to fall asleep is objectively examinable. Electrophysiological examinations can help diagnose the state of fatigue, i.e., the EEG is diagnostically valuable in this situation. Subvigil stages can be characterized in the dynamic EEG status fluctuations (Ulrich 1994). The "multiple sleep latency test" in the EEG, which is conducted in the sleep laboratory, can objectify the tendency to fall asleep.

Conclusion
Decreased vigilance in fatigue is characterized as the state of increased tendency to fall asleep. It ranges in the EEG from subvigil stages with fleeting attainment of sleep phases to awake alpha-EEG with eyes closed. Pupillographic examinations can also capture wakefulness.

A specific regulation is known from the study of narcolepsy. Hypocretin or orexin (OX1, OX2) is pathologically reduced in narcolepsy (see Saper et al. 2005). It apparently acts on the one hand in the lateral hypothalamus and can be modified in its effect there (this is currently being discussed for the vigilance-promoting effect of medications, e.g., Modafinil).

The serotonergic neurons of the raphe nuclei of the brain stem are active in wakefulness. The decrease in their activity apparently also interferes with the processes of sleep-wake regulation. The model of the "seesaw" of sleep-promoting and wakefulness-mediating neuronal groups in the brainstem and hypothalamus applies here (Saper et al. 2005).

A differentiation of a disorder of wakefulness from clouding of consciousness seems possible. By examining cognitive functions after awakening a patient, a differentiation between fatigue and clouding of consciousness can apparently be achieved. Patients in delirium who appear more sleepy than other delirium patients tend to have fewer disturbances in cognitive performance than patients who are classified as having clouded consciousness (Gabriel 2007).

4.5.2 Arousal, Attentiveness

The neurobiological model of activation is (see above) the decrease of the membrane potential; this induces an approach to the threshold for elicitation of an action potential. This has been demonstrated for the noradrenergic system (Aston Joned et al. 1999). The noradrenergic system cause an arousal, e.g. after painful stimulation. Various inputs of neurons can effect the described decrease of the membrane potential. It represents a more or less unspecific pre-activation. This mechanism seems evolutionarily useful as a reaction to the occurrence of a dangerous situation.

Brainstem-cortex connections
Neurons of the activating part of the reticular formation, which are referred to as ARAS and belong to various transmitter systems, are involved in phasic arousal, an activation following either pain stimuli or new stimuli (see Saper et al. 2005; Fig. 4.5).

Cholinergic Neurons
Cholinergic synapses are involved in many different functions, such as in the circuitry of the Basal ganglia and they are also necessary for hippocampal function. Several cholinergic nuclei in the brainstem and basal forebrain have a specific role in arousal functions.

The nucleus basalis Meynert in the basal forebrain is the nucleus that selectively activates the cortex in a region-specific manner. Thus, to a certain extent selective activation is already possible through the cholinergic system. In the basal forebrain, the frontal cortex can influence these neurons. This allows the activation level of the cortex to be under its own control. This is important, for example, for the trainability of relaxation, mediation and psychotherapeutic procedures, etc.

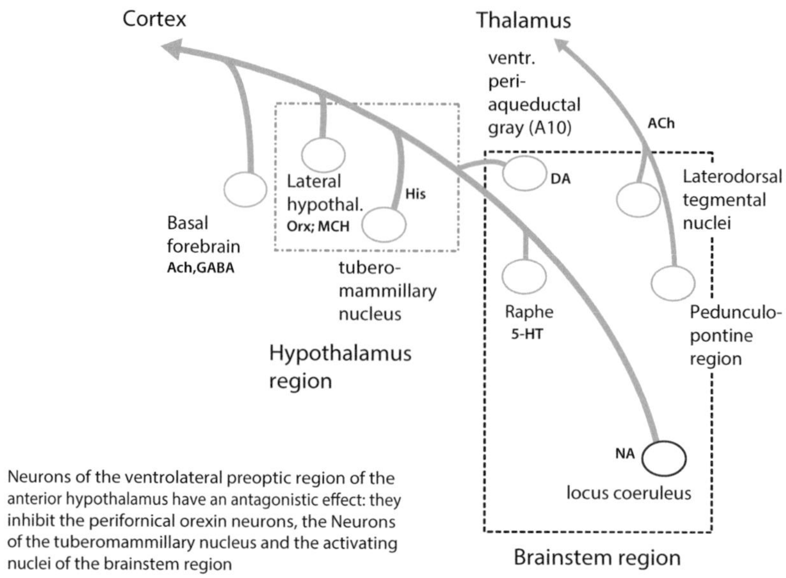

Fig. 4.5 Brain regions or nuclei that mediate wakefulness, arousal, and attention (predominantly unfocussed). In Sleep areas are reduced in their activity in the ventrolateral preoptic nucleus of the hypothalamus (Saper et al. 2005). BF Basal forebrain (Ncl. basalis Meynert etc.), LH Lateral hypothalamus, vPGA ventral periaqueductal gray (tegmental area, or A10), TMN tuberomammillary system, Raphe Raphe nuclei, LC Locus coeruleus, PPT pedunculopontine region

Cholinergic activation is necessary for the desynchronization of the EEG during arousal, as well as for other attentional functions. A reduction in cholinergic input leads to the occurrence of attention disorders and memory system disturbances.

Due to the regionally differentiated cholinergic innervation, a certain selectivity of activation is possible. Accordingly, this system could play a role in selective attention. However, is less about specific associative attention and more about the activation of "channels" such as acoustic information, somatosensory information, etc. The attention can be directed to the modality of the stimulus information through preactivation in these sensory areas.

The innervation by the Ncl. basalis Meynert does not extend to the occipital cortex, which has been used as an explanation for the occurrence of visual hallucinations in some syndromes (see there).

A group of neurons in the pedunculopontine region (and in the laterodorsal tegmental nuclei) is involved in the activation of the thalamus within the framework of the ascending activating system (ARAS). It is under the control of the ventrolateral preoptic hypothalamus, whose neurons are active in Sleep and suppress the neuron groups involved in attentional reactions (Saper et al. 2005).

An important mechanism is the reciprocal inhibition of the nuclei. The monoaminergic nuclei inhibit the neurons of the ventrolateral preoptic hypothalamus during the day. In turn, these neurons inhibit the monoaminergic nuclei of the ARAS at night (Saper et al. 2005), the transmitters GABA and Galanin seem to be involved.

Noradrenergic Neurons

Arousal functions are partly carried out by noradrenergic neurons. There are only about 20,000 cells, which are located in the locus coeruleus (LC). These diffusely innervate the cortex. However, they also activate the other brainstem nuclei, so that complex interactions between the arousal centers can be observed. The noradrenergic neurons have an excitatory effect; the membrane potentials of the cortical neurons are relatively decreased by EPSPs (see model Fig. 4.4).

The activity of the LC is related to the error rate in speed-dependent attention tests (Aston Jones et al. 1999). This is consistent with an decrease in the membrane potential of executive neurons, which are thereby brought closer to the threshold of the action potential. In response to a pain stimulus, the magnocellular part is stimulated (Aston Jones et al. 1999).

Serotonergic Neurons

To what extent serotonergic neurons, which are found in the raphe nuclei of the brainstem, are necessary for arousal is currently not certain. As mentioned above, they are largely tonically active, namely in wakefulness. However, a contribution of serotonergic functions to the desynchronization of the EEG during arousal is assumed.

Triggering of arousal

Arousal is triggered not only by pain stimuli but also by a new stimulus, i.e., after passing the familiarity check (Chap. 3 Episodic Memory). The triggering of arousal does not occur only spinally, for example, after pain stimuli. Rather, an intense arousal can also be triggered, for example, by neurons for visual recognition when they report a threatening stimulus. They may activate the brainstem via the amygdala. The locus coeruleus can also be activated by the amygdala.

In addition, there is a, albeit weak, incompletely effective, top-down control of activation. The well-known psychological example is the mother who is not awakened by various lous noises from sleep but by a low noise from the child sleeping in the next room. Therefore, there must be a programmable filter that can automatically trigger arousal when specific, trained information arrives. It is still unclear what exercises this filter function. For example, there is a frontal control of cholinergic cortex innervation (Sarter et al. 2005). Individual differences in the ability of top-down control of attention and arousal levels could be seen as a personality factor and thus mediate psychopathological reactions.

Models of Arousal

The neurophysiology of arousal in behavior has now been well studied in some models. The startle reaction is achieved, for example, by a targeted air puff to the eye, the cornea, and the involved neurons that cause the reactive eye closure have been characterized (Koch 1999).

Arousal from a state of low vigilance is studied in the orientation reaction, in which an animal stands up, looks around, and prepares to avert potential dangers. In many studies, the increase in heart rate has been measured as a sign of activation, etc.

In the EEG, the degree of desynchronization of the alpha baseline activity can be observed as a measure of arousal. Thalamic mechanisms are involved in this process.

Thalamic activation, ERTAS

Thalamic focal activation system, ERTAS, extended reticulothalamic activating system (Newman 1997). The cholinergic system can perform an initial selective function of attention through region-specific cortical activation, e.g., directing attention to sensory channels. The cholinergic attention function also influence the thalamic filter for the sensory systems that send information to the cortex. A patient with anticholinergic delirium can no longer direct attention or, in general, regulate attention. This can be explained in part by the disruption of selective regional cortical activation of brain areas.

Starting from pedunculopontine and laterodorsal tegmental nuclei, there is a cholinergic activation of the nonspecific thalamic nuclei, especially the intralaminar and reticular nuclei (see Mesulam 2000). The reticular thalamic nuclei are inhibitory in the cortex via GABA. They are excitatorily controlled cortically, but cholinergically controlled in an inhibitory manner. From this, it can be concluded that they reduce their control function during cholinergic activation and allow higher activation of the cortex by sensory stimuli (see Mesulam 2000).

The described activation could be demonstrated in studies: A change from relaxation to intense attentiveness was investigated. Both the reticular formation and the intralaminar nuclei of the thalamus were active during attentiveness, and a correlative relationship of the activity of the brain regions being shown (Kinomura et al. 1996).

Arousal level and attentiveness

While arousal represents a reaction to a significant event, the level of activation by the activating brainstem neurons is rather to be seen as a quantitative phenomenon that can vary from moment to moment. The arousal level is primarily intended to describe the extent of unfocussed attention, which is also referred to as "attentiveness".It is assumed that this arousal level is best understood as the sum or integral of the activations of various systems. Ultimately, a fluctuating level of unfocussed attention results.

The arousal level is predominantly regulated involuntarily: For example, the ascending reticular activating system (ARAS) with its various transmitter systems plays a role in waking up. This also applies to arousal by a stimulus that causes a surprising activation.

Arguments suggest that unfocussed attention is controlled by processes that operate in two domains. The partitioning of the psychological dimension of attentiveness into two domains is comparable to the sensation of temperature into hot and cold, which is physiologically partitioned into different receptors, for warm and cold sensation, although it physically belongs to a single temperature dimension. Comparable to the perception of hot and cold, there exists not only one dimension of the attention level, but a bidirectional deviation of a baseline level of unfocussed attention should be assumed—one direction towards the reduction of attentiveness to sleep, fatigue, and the other towards the highest arousal, an attentional excitation state.

This would also imply that wakefulness, characterized by a regular alpha EEG, is to be described as a baseline state maintained by many processes, from which there are deflections in one direction towards sleep and in the other towards increased, excited arousal. At least, this is supported by the fact that there is a phylogenetically old behavior pattern of sleep preparation in fatigue.

It is probable that arousal systems and attentiveness are regulated differently. Accordingly, more separate systems could be conceivable, interacting with each other: One would be the vigilance system, which regulates wakefulness and is most active in wakefulness, and another would be the arousal functions, which are stimulated by external stimuli and content with which the person is dealing.

4.5.3 Focussed Attention

Since the Middle Ages, the imagination has existed that an "inner eye" moves when a person is thinking and pays attention to something in thought. Jaspers mentions in his Psychopathology (4th ed. 1942) the image of the spotlight for attention on the stage of consciousness. In this mental image, focussed attention becomes vivid when one thinks of the brightness and focus of the stage spotlight and, in addition—as an image of attentiveness—considers the background lighting.

These mental images lead us to false physiological expectations. Besides the thalamic and cholinergic mechanisms of selective activation of brain regions and larger groups of neurons, there is no structure that could correspond to the beam of attention. Contrary to this popular analogy, the autopoiesis of the attention focus in networks is something very abstract (see below).

The simplest mechanisms of selective attention are turning away versus turning towards something, etc. Eye movements are the most important effectors of attention control. The psychopathological diagnostician observes them during the examination. The control of eye movements is closely linked to the control of focussed attention.

Focussed attention, stimulus-driven; Spatial focussed attention

Every visual neuron has a receptive field, this is already selective in a certain way. Visual activation by an object therefore already results in a focussing.

Spatially focused attention is a special case due to the mechanisms of eye movement; normally, we turn eyes, head, and body together (Astafiev et al. 2003). After discovering an interesting object at a certain location, neurons of the superior colliculi and frontal eye fields are pre-activated along with parietal brain areas. The shift of attention—initially without eye movement—functions to prepare the next movement, in this case, the movement of the eyes (see Kustov and Robinson 1996). Studies indicate that during the activation of saccades for a target area, the reactivity for stimuli there is simultaneously increased, meaning attention is focussed there (Moore and Armstrong 2003). The direction of spatial attention to a location is closely linked to the readiness to look there, i.e., directly with the mechanisms of eye movements. In focussed visual attention to the environment, particularly the posterior inferotemporal cortex and the visual area V4 are involved (DeWeerd et al. 1999).

The model of focussed attention has been established in the investigation of two competing visual stimuli and described as "biased competition" (Desimone and Duncan 1995).

1. The fundamental initial finding is that a visual receptive field is specialized for a kind of stimulus, for example, an oblique bar. The neuron fires particularly intensely when this stimulus enters the receptive field.
2. Now, the activation decreases when, in addition to the specific stimulus, a non-specific stimulus is also shown in the receptive field, i.e., two stimuli (besides the oblique bar, a vertical bar). The competition weakens the specified response of the neuron. Here, inhibitory neuronal connections apparently become effective.
3. Focussed attention on the oblique bar can now restore the old specialized response of the neuron, despite the competition from the vertical bar.

The examination situation of presenting two stimuli in the receptive field may initially seem somewhat artificial—but upon closer inspection, it is precisely the isolated presentation of a stimulus that is the artificial situation, which practically never occurs in the environment.

Model of the Emergence of Attention through External Stimuli

Particularly based on the works of Koch (2005), there is a perspective according to which attention and conscious sensory perception develop in the process of perception. Starting from a concept of attention resources, it is argued that the vast majority of stimuli presented to the cortex in the visual system are not perceived because they are not able to bind attention resources. Only stimuli that represent something, which in some way relates to meaning, interest, instincts, and innate releasing mechanisms, or of course the current conscious interest and the focus of the currently valid focus of attention, have a chance to be attentively perceived—i.e., not to disappear unnoticed in the perceptual processes. Naturally, stimuli that conflict with the aforementioned interests and instincts also attract attention.

The model can demonstrate in a particularly impressive way for psychopathology how, in the process of perception, what is important for the person is already filtered through an interplay of sensory analysis (bottom-up) and top-down processes, or what the structures inherent in information processing promote or filter out. This can explain how content fixations in psychiatric disorders affect sensory filtering. For example, employees in crowds at work involuntarily pay attention to their superiors. Strangers, however, who do not know this relationship among the people, pay attention to other people.

From the above, the selectivity of perception becomes clear, which always exists and normally practically filters out everything that does not seem necessary. When a person practices »mindfulness«, attentively dedicating themselves to all modalities and directions of the sensory systems, it becomes clear to them how much information is usually ignored. This primary selectivity occurs through sensory analysis (bottom-up) and interactions with inherent or trained systems, but without the need for the process of top-down focussing or strenuous concentration effort.

Conclusion
Internally generated and externally generated attention share a weighting structure. This determines which mental, internally considered objects attract the attention focus, but also which external stimuli are preprocessed and can thereby bind attention resources to maintain the attention focus. Proto-objects have been mentioned (Resnik 2000). These preprocessed objects can quickly attract attention but can also fall back into inattention.

This is related to the everyday experience that even very important things escape our perception with a magician, who skillfully manages to distract us by directing attention to other events (Mack and Rock 1998). This model can also explain interindividual differences in what is perceived, which, for example, become apparent for a couple walking through a city unknown to both of them. Furthermore, regarding the psychopathology of schizophrenic patients, the relation to gestalt psychological results on the distortion of their perception can be seen. Content-distorted perceptions are also observed in anxiety and personality disorders.

Dynamic Changes in the Activation Maximum
The maximum of activation in a neural network constantly changes when other contents, sensorily stimulated or in the course of thought, come to the forefront. This is apparently achieved by pre-innervation, which changeses the membrane potentials of the target neurons without action potentials having to be triggered—however, the triggering of action potentials in these neurons is subsequently facilitated. At the behavioral level, this is shown in priming experiments, where pre-stimuli cause a certain anticipation of the following stimulus. In schizophrenia, changes in specific semantic activation have been shown (Spitzer 1993).

Recently, pre-activation in a »global workspace« (Baars 1998) has been discussed. The selective pre-activation of ensembles in the neural network can be seen as a correlate of selective attention.

The associative connections for automatic associative focussed attention are, like for spatial attention, plastically adaptable to environmental conditions through feedback to the neural network. In this context, disturbances in the semantic processing of schizophrenic patients without neuroleptic treatment are found - in the effort to rationalize the delusion:

- Incoherence of thinking in schizophrenia,
- Patient appears distracted by voices,
- in the patient's thinking, associations that cannot be predicted by the person are seen as new information coming from outside.

How is attention directed?
In everyday life, it is about controlling attention when relevant sensory stimuli occur; think of a combat situation. A stimulus activates an attention focus; for example, the fighter initially pays attention to the opponent's fist, which is pulled back and could be accelerated for a punch—but is also prepared to fend off a kick.

In martial arts, action sequences are trained. Attention adjusts to the expectation of subsequent stimuli. The process is involuntary, and the action decisions are unconscious. The involuntary, sensory-controlled attention just described is to be distinguished from other forms, especially conscious, voluntary, non-sensory-controlled focused attention. This will be discussed further below (sections about motoric and executive functions).

An example is a person who sits down with friends in a crowded bar. After locating the seat and sitting down, there is a switch in spatial attention. It shifts from center-focused (when sitting down) to digit-focused (when grabbing a cup and a sugar cube from a bowl) to allocentric (when explaining who is sitting next to the person opposite) etc. Different cortical regions are activated, and specific groups of neurons are pre-activated for this.

1. A sensory stimulus initially activates a neuron ensemble, which is to be understood as a representation of its semantic unit.
2. According to Mesulam's ideas (2000), this input information activates an attention network that causes the attention focus optimally adapted to the content in the context. This causes the activation of neurons responsible for locations spatially corresponding to the stimulus. Consequently, the eyes, head, torso, and extremities are directed according to the input information. Additionally, the activation of situation-appropriate action readiness occurs, etc. Mesulam proposed a neural network that can process input information to output information like a parallel-distributed-processing network through layers of interneurons and which can learn. Success (or failure) reports are used as modifiers of the connectivity of neurons in the different layers (input, computational layer of interneurons, and output layer) (see below; McClelland et al. 1995). Thus, we are initially dealing with involuntary attention direction through situational cues: They cause the adapted direction of attention. The change of adapted attention targets occurs automatically in the transition of situations. Information from episodic memory can also be involved in these situations, but this is not primarily a function of the attention system and often leads to interruptions of automatic attention orientation.

Associative, cognitive attention

In the associative domain, for example, with thought content, there is no dominant influence of eye movements as with spatially focused attention. In associative focussed attention, the activation of semantically close units occurs. However, this is already a rough illustration, as each semantic unit is already to be imagined as a distributed neuron ensemble: Firstly, elements of a neuron ensemble representing a semantic unit also belong to ensembles that encode closely associatively related semantic units. Secondly, elements of an ensemble activate elements of other—semantically more distant—neuron ensembles.

▶ An important issue becomes clear from the descriptions: In every neural network, there will always be a maximum of activation. This is distributed but more or less specifically directed at the representation of a single content.

In brain imaging studies, specialized regions for object classes are demonstrated. A certain centering of a focus on a brain area, which is demonstrated in imaging studies, results from the functional specialization of brain regions for certain stimulus qualities and also certain classes of objects.

In associative directed attention, another psychopathological interaction arises: If the attention focus is, for example, directed at a fact, it is referred to that a person is aware of a fact—"being aware of a certain fact" (see above).

Arbitrary focussed attention—not stimulus-driven

The preactivation of semantically related units happens automatically, as experimental psychological studies show. In contrast, there is also an deliberate control of the attention focus. This can function without a stimulus. The arbitrary intention of the person can be programmed to focus on abstract stimulus features, memory contents, etc. It can also be directed towards something - according to instructions in a test. An example is paying attention to specific stimulus features during a quick reaction task, where the sought stimulus appears only rarely. The optimal attention setting results in a faster reaction.

On the one hand, we can physically turn towards an object or a location in space where an object is expected—for example, by "following the gaze," looking where others are looking. We can also do this in the somatosensory area, for instance. Voluntarily, we can pay attention to the touch of socks/stockings/shoes.

In this process, thalamic mechanisms of the activation of cortical areas are likely involved. They cause a change in the information processing of sensorimotor representations. Thalamocortical connections of the finger representation are altered when attention is directed to the fingers.

Attention and mental effort

The examples of attention tasks immediately make it clear that they involve more or less strenuous mental activities ("effort"). These are impaired in certain syndromes, such as in severe depressive episodes. It is not yet clear how this phenomenon occurs. For example, the frontal organization of focussed attention tires, meaning it apparently consumes resources. The exhaustion of limited capacities, which might be found in the activation of brainstem neurons, is a model. It is thus possible. that a person can activate brainstem nuclei in arbitrary attention situations ("top down"), and these additional attention effects wane after a certain, variable time.

Attention and executive functions

Since we are dealing with the preparation of motor actions in everyday behavior, a relationship to executive functions must also be considered (see also Wu 2023). An example can illustrate this. A task that requires a strong focus of attention is the Stroop test; it is exceptionally exhausting. The interference task requires naming the color of a word, which, however, denotes another color: The color of the letters of the word "yellow" is, for example, "red," and "red" must be said. It must not be read; instead, the name of the respective different color in which the color word is written must be said. The crucial circumstance is that highly automated reading solves the task faster compared to the less common, and therefore slower, color naming. For this reason, the interfering reading information must be inhibited so that the naming information can be implemented motorically undisturbed and quickly. This leads to a conflict in action control. In this arduous test, the anterior cingulate is activated (Barch et al. 2001). Reacting quickly also requires effort, as shown in the physiology of reaction times (Winterer et al. 2002).

For the aforementioned reasons, the Stroop task is classified as an executive attention task. In this process, attention is directed to a category of sensory processing, and other channels of sensory information are suppressed. Anyone who has ever performed the test feels the effort that quick processing requires. This also explains why the validity for psychopathological examinations can only be given in highly motivated individuals (see Salthouse 2005).

In addition to the features of voluntary control and effort, the active maintenance of an attention focus without a stimulus should be highlighted. This results in a close relationship to the functions of sustained-activity neurons, which are particularly found in the frontal brain (Fuster 1990). In other words, there is an overlap of voluntary, focused attention without a stimulus and working memory functions (Chap. 6 Executive Functions and Working Memory).

A sensory filter has also been mentioned before. A programmable filter allows only the stimulus features that the program has previously defined to pass through. To some extent, experimental psychological tasks of selective attention can best be described in this way. An example from everyday life is the—already mentioned—search for a person who is blonde and wearing a red shirt in a busy shopping street. Filters are implemented in information technology, and the question is whether the concept of the filter from this analogy leads to false expectations of physiological mechanisms.

How is the programming of a selection filter achieved physiologically? First, we have seen in associative attention that the activation of specific contents via the neuronal network causes a pre-activation of relevant neurons. This already addresses one mechanism. But there is another mechanism.

The functions of the projections from the cortex to the basal ganglia and back to the cortex via the thalamus, the "frontal loops" (see Fig. 7.3, Lichter and Cummings 2000), are diverse, but one function seems to be the selection and maintenance of the activity of neurons in the frontal brain (Gao et al. 2001; Gao and Goldman-Rakic 2003). This can build up frontal cortex activity, which is needed for the control of motor processes, but also for the top-down control of sensory processes and thus for selective attention. The function of the sustained-activity neurons mentioned here can be compared to the function of programmable sensory filters in holding addresses needed for searching in memory. When the correct address appears, either sensory or during memory search, the filter reports the occurrence of the event. In delayed-response tasks, among other things, holding specific sensory information is essential for completing the task after the delay (Fuster 1990).

Dopaminergic Neurons
The dopaminergic neurons of the brainstem have significant psychiatric importance:

1. they mediate neuroendocrine effects,
2. they act in the circuits of the basal ganglia (see below), and
3. they innervate the cortex, especially the frontal cortex.

In the cortex, cortical innervation primarily concerns the subtype of D1 receptors. The sustained-activity neurons of the frontal cortex are reduced in their activity by this innervation (Gao et al. 2001; Gao and Goldman-Rakic 2003). A role in maintaining attention on an object is suspected. Apparently, dopaminergic cortical innervation is less responsible for undirected activation in arousal than for the establishment of finely tuned cognitive filtering, working memory, and motor control.

Apparently, the sustained-activity neurons are essential not only for the temporal aspect in motor processes but also for the control aspect of attention, i.e., maintaining attention in situations where no stimulus directs attention. An evolutionary example is in animals the attentive waiting during prey catching. Attention is maintained on a location over a period of possible distraction—due to the chance of discovering prey there.

Attention disorders occur not only after brainstem and thalamus lesions, which also affect vigilance and arousal, but the role of attention disorders after frontal brain lesions was also noticed early on. Especially the frontal brain areas are involved in the effort to organize the top-down control of attention. A disturbance of programmable, voluntarily focussed attention is often clinically tested and is particularly noticeable in schizophrenia.

For the top-down control of visual attention, the thalamus, particularly the relatively large nucleus of the pulvinar, seems to play arole (LaBerge and Buchsbaum 1990). In the neuropsychological literature, neglect, the neglect of perception objects on one side, has been well studied (see Fig 4.2, Karnath 2001). For psychopathology, it is important that the disturbance of attention direction also relates to the representation of memory images of visual imagination.

This became clear through the famous Bisiach experiment: Patients with neglect also neglect their imagination of the affected side, for example, when Italian patients were asked to imagine standing in front of the Milan Cathedral. They described only the non-neglected side, not the neglected one. This changed abruptly when they were asked to imagine turning around, so now the representations of the previously neglected side were reported alone.

Since in psychopathology, less often lateralized lesions than constitutional disorders and degenerative changes of the critical regions are responsible for the pathological phenomena, something more general can be inferred: From the disruptibility of attention direction to internal representations, it can be deduced that the processes of recall of mental representations can generally be disturbed, while the representations themselves remain undisturbed; in other words, in most psychiatric conditions, a disturbance of access to mental representations is to be expected.

Concluding Remarks
In hardly any psychiatric field are the discrepancies between the diverse clinical phenomena, the neuroscientific findings of subsystems, and the uncertainty of what can be used neuropsychologically or experimentally for diagnosis as large as in the field of attention functions.

Attention disorders underlie psychopathological phenomena in other areas such as consciousness disorders, thought disorders, and affective symptoms. The connections will need to be examined more closely in the coming years.

4.6 Psychopathological Symptoms of Attention

Fatigue Intensified
Definition. The person feels tired over a longer period and has an increased tendency to fall asleep. Thereby, the intensity and control of attention are disturbed.

This is shown by the fact that tasks requiring attention can no longer be performed as before. Cognitive function is undisturbed after waking. Subjective quality of fatigue as opposed to the feature "hypoattentiveness".

Example

- A patient has not been able to sleep sufficiently for 3 days. In the interview, he is inattentive and fidgety. When left alone, he tends to sit quietly and limp and doze off.
- A patient has excessive daytime sleepiness. Although he tried to sleep sufficiently, he feels tired all day and ready to fall asleep at any time (he dozes off during breaks without any demands on him).
- A patient feels tired after reading just one page, he puts the book away, although the content might interest him. He can no longer muster the attention and needs to rest. ◀

Position in Psychopathology. AMDP 105.

Related Terms: Daytime sleepiness.

Psychopathological Interactions
- sensory restriction over a long period,
- overload, e.g., due to work,
- sleep disorder.

Differential Diagnostic Distinctions
- consciousness disorder (lowered vigilance according to AMDP)—differentiation from clouding of consciousness as a disturbed awareness of the matters currently concerning the person,
- concentration disorder and distractibility during long-lasting tasks,
- apathy, stupor, motor retardation.

Further Characterization
- reduction of pure wakefulness,
- characteristic reduction of undirected attention—in addition to the subjective characteristic of tiredness, the objective impairment within the framework of tiredness (e.g., reduction of undirected attention) is also included here—e.g., important for patients who want to deny tiredness, which can be investigated, for example, by the tendency to fall asleep.

Self-/Other Person's Judgment. More self- than other person's judgment.

Interview for Rating. Interview about introspection and especially the experience of falling asleep, dozing off.

Neuropsychology/Objectification
- behavioral observation,
- reaction to wake-up stimuli—a single wake-up stimulus only leads to a temporary increase in attention, then the previous state returns,
- preferably external observation of sleep times and sleep quality,
- work samples.

In the past, clocks were used that had to be followed and whose irregular jumps had to be noticed (see above).

Severity
1. From occasional and slightly increased readiness to sleep to imperative need for sleep (as in narcolepsy),
2. From slightly reduced workload without tiredness occurring to complete incapacity to perform due to fatigue with the slightest exertion.

Pathognomonic for: Overtiredness, narcolepsy.

Specifications
1. Increased daytime sleepiness,
   - after sleep restriction vs. without,
   - acutely newly occurred vs. habitual,
2. Fatigue after shorter exertion (increased fatigability),
   after even slight activities, there is fatigue in the mental domain with a decrease in attention—and potentially additionally in the somatic domain with the feeling of fatigue,
   - as pure reduction of attention, decreased vigilance,
   - with somatic fatigue.

Conceptual problems of the feature. We have the belief that we can correctly identify fatigue in everyday psychology through introspection. However, we use the tendency to fall asleep as a criterion, which is a behavioral variable.

Neuroscientific/cognitive neuroscientific models
1. Not yet known reduction of tonic attention functions in preparation for sleep behavior,
   - one factor can be the monotony of the environment or motivational disorder,
2. Neuropsychological studies have been able to show the disturbance of attention and the disturbance of (executive) frontal lobe functions in fatigue,
3. arousal can only temporarily improve attention,
4. undesirable drug effect, e.g., with neuroleptics,
5. possibly specific pathophysiology of increased fatigue and fatigability in depression syndromes,
6. Orexins can promote the function of brainstem nuclei, including the locus coeruleus—the orexin system is disrupted in narcolepsy.

Hypoattentiveness
Definition. Lowering of the level of undirected attention or arousal level, despite sufficient stimulation from the environment.

Example.

A patient is passive but not asleep; he cannot be sufficiently activated by calling him by his name or touching him, although he is not opposed to the examination. ◀

Related terms. Hypoarousal—does not include other types of attention control .

Psychopathological interactions. Motivation, fatigue, clouding of consciousness.

Differential diagnostic distinctions. Refusal, mutism.

Self-/other persons's judgment. other persons's judgment.

Interview for rating. Observation of the perception of environmental stimuli: inquiries.

Neuropsychology/objectification. Attention-related movements such as looking, turning towards something, pointing, etc., are reduced.

Severity
- mild: a reduction in the undirected attention is noticed, is not impairing,
- severe: a non-activatable state in which the patient, who is motivated, cannot engage in communication.

Conceptual Problems of the Feature. The delineability of decreased vigilance in terms of fatigue or tiredness is yet to be verified.

Neuroscientific/Cognitive Neuroscientific Models

The bottom-up activation by stimuli is disturbed. One possible mechanism is that the ARAS nuclei of the reticular formation are disturbed, or their afferent or efferent connections. Alternatively, the transmitter or receptor metabolism of the brainstem nuclei of the arousal system may be disturbed.

Furthermore, the top-down activation of attention may also be disturbed because new stimuli are not recognized as important stimuli for the person. "Novelty" is not reported further as a reason for arousal.

Hyper Attent—Hyperarousal

Definition. Increased level of undirected attention.

Example. A patient is excited, looking around restlessly, listening intently, in anticipation of something indefinite. The patient waits eagerly but cannot say exactly what for.

Related Terms. Sometimes misleadingly referred to as hypervigilance, the term hyperarousal also limits the state to temporary arousal states.

Psychopathological Interactions. Suspicion, delusional mood, state of excitement, state of anxiety.

Differential Diagnostic Distinctions. Anxiety, aggression.

Self-/Other Person's Judgment. Other person's judgment.

Interview for Rating. Questions about motivation, emotional quality of the increased arousal level.

Neuroscientific/Cognitive Neuroscientific Models

State of increased undirected attention, elevated levels of arousal. From this state, attention can at any time intensely focus on something indefinitely expected, in the sense of directing selective attention to something. In such a state, everything in the environment is repeatedly briefly checked. Relationship to anxious and aggressive agitation.

Reduced Focussed Attention

Definition. Maximum focussed attention is reduced. The ability to activate oneself for a task, despite interest, to mentally turn towards an object is impaired.

Activation of focussed attention also includes the turning of attention. This, in turn, involves turning away from the last focus of attention if one existed . Flexibility includes turning away from one stimulus to turn towards a new object of interest.

Example.

- A patient pays not attention to the respective mental task while working on simple tests in the psychopathological examination, which can be seen from eye movements, gestures, and also distracting verbal expressions. However, the patient says that she wants to solve the tasks.
- A patient cannot actively turn his attention to the examiner's questions, although he understands them and makes some effort. He cannot perform tasks that involve a sequence of laborious information processing. ◀

Position in Psychopathology. Attention and concentration disorders were usually undifferentiated summarized, see AMDP 10.

Psychopathological Interactions. Motivation, tiredness, clouding of consciousness, incoherence.

Differential Diagnostic Distinctions: Attention tests are only to be evaluated after excluding elementary neuropsychological deficits that could also explain the performance disorder.

- Incompliance (diagnostic), motivational problems,
- Concentration disorder as a special problem with long-lasting tasks; can be caused by disruption of thought, impaired control in the domain of drive and drive increase or depressive thoughts about meaninglessness or anhedonia,
- Fatigue, see above,
- Clouding of consciousness—the person cannot fully grasp the entire situation with all its aspects and requirements and act accordingly,
- normal variance of attention.

Neuropsychology/objectification.
- Patients cannot activate themselves to complete a simple series of mental routine processes, such as repeating numbers, saying months backward,
- Tests like cancellation lists, where a feature must be searched for, which are evaluated by time and errors, and "continuous performance tests" are used—with and without a working memory component,
- Tests of psychomotor speed like trail making tests (Trail Making Test) are often used, but can only be evaluated after excluding purely motor slowing and motivational disorder,
- The test of executive attention like the Stroop test (see above), where reading information from words must be suppressed to effectively say the different color naming,
- Short tasks of attention and concentration like counting months backward or serial subtraction (100 minus 7, subtracting 7 again from the result, etc.) are routinely performed. However, they are only to be evaluated after excluding elementary neuropsychological deficits that could also explain the performance disorder (e.g. calculation disorder),
- Routine tests like serial subtraction and saying months backward, etc., have different difficulty, which can be used in cases of suspected simulation.

Specifications. *Disturbed areas are:*

- spatially focused attention,
- associatively focused attention,
- voluntarily focused attention.

Distractedness
Disturbance of focussing and maintaining attention to a sufficient extent, i.e., keeping focused on an interesting goal (sensory goal or thought content) without getting distracted.

Sensory or thought focussing is reduced.

Example.

A patient immediately loses track while reading and cannot engage in even a slightly demanding task like a game, as he is easily distracted by minor interruptions, such as a person entering the room, leading him to mentally engage with other things and become absorbed by this. ◀

Related Terms. AMDP (10): Concentration disorders, reduced ability to sufficiently direct attention to an activity or mental topic.

Concentration disorder, inability to maintain the attentional span.

Psychopathological Interactions. Motivation, fatigue, clouding of consciousness, disruption of thought, thought pressure.

Differential diagnostic distinctions. Lability of interest and motivation as well as the number of objects of interest, e.g., in mania, is high. In contrast to the intensity of focussed attention when working on a task, it is more about the effectlessness of distraction.

Self-/other persons's judgment. Report from relatives.

Interview for rating. Question about reading and playing, observation during daily activities, in the ward routine.

Neuropsychology/objectification. Course of attention-related movements such as looking, turning towards, pointing, etc.

- Work probe in case of suspected sustained attention disorder, e.g., calculation sheets, etc. (for shorter stress: d2 test).

Severity. Mild disorder (possibly only in case of divided attention) at the border of normal attention variance and stress in sustained attention, especially against strong distraction.

Neuroscientific/cognitive neuroscientific models
Several mechanisms may be impaired. A disorder of frontal lobe functions is assumed. The function of the frontal sustained-activity neurons is impaired, making it impossible to willfully maintain attention on objects against distraction (Fuster 1990).

Content-related attention disorders
Narrowing of attention. It is usually assumed that attention is related to content at any given moment, whether it is a stimulus from outside or a mental content. However, attention is seen as a function available for all content. Nevertheless, some psychiatric symptoms can be characterized as content-related attention disorders - because attention is pathologically fixed on certain content. This is the case with delusion. But in content-related attention disorders, delusion is usually not present (Chap. 13 Delusion).

Examples are:

- reduced ability to detach attention from a certain topic,
- somatoform disorder,
- somatization disorder,
- dissociative disorder,
- acute stress reaction.
- Regarding the content-related disorders that manifest in attention, one can assume a group of attention-narrowing syndromes.
- usually dealt with in anxiety or neurotic disorders or in consciousness disorders.

Justification:

1. Narrowing of attention leads to secondary psychopathological phenomena,
    - somatization, hypochondria—associated with anxiety,
    - stupor and dissociation disorder of the integration of experiences—experienced as unpleasant, but not necessarily with anxiety,
    - acute stress reaction.
2. The narrowing of attention can be conceptualized neuroscientifically as a disorder in the ability to detach from one special feature and focus on another topic.
3. Narrowing to one topic as a defense mechanism—against the painful confrontation with another topic that is to be avoided.

References

Astafiev SV, Shulman GL, Stanley CM et al (2003) Functional organization of human intraparietal an frontal cortex for attending. J Neurosci 23:4689–4699

Aston Jones GS, Desimone R, Driver J et al (1999) Attention. In: Zigmond MJ, Bloom FE, Landis SC et al (Eds) Fundamental neuroscience. Academic, San Diego, pp 1385–1409

Barch DM, Braver TS, Akbudak E et al (2001) Anterior cingulate cortex and response conflict: effects of response modality and processing domain. Cereb Cortex 11:837–848

Broadbendt DE (1971) Decision and stress. Academic, London

Cohen RA (1993) Neuropsychology of attention. Plenum Press, New York

Cummings JL (1993) Frontal-subcortical circuits and human behaviour. Arch Neurol 50:873–880

Desimone R, Duncan J (1995) Neuroan mechanisms of selective visual attention. Ann Rev Neurosci 18:193–222

DeWeerd P, Peralta MR III, Desimone R, Ungerleider LG (1999) Loss of attentional stimulus selection after extrastriate cortical lesions in macaques. Nat Neurosci 2:753–758

Driver J, Vuilleumier P, Husain M (2004) Spatial neglect and extinction. In: Gazzaniga MS (Ed) The cognitive neurosciences III. MIT Press, Cambridge, MA, pp 589–606

Fuster J (1990) Inferotemporal units in selective visual attention and short-term memory. J Neurophysiol 64:681–697

Gabriel A (2007) Neuropsychologische Defizite im Delir unterschiedlicher ätiologischer Gruppen. Dissertation, Charité

Gao WJ, Krimer LS, Goldman-Rakic PS (2001) Presynaptic regulation of recurrent excitation by D1 receptors in prefrontal circuits. Proc Natl Acad Sci U S A 98:295–300

Gao WJ, Goldman-Rakic PS (2003) Selective modulation of excitatory and inhibitory microcircuits by dopamine. Proc Natl Acad Sci U S A 100:2836–2841

Hopfinger JB, Buonocore MH, Mangun GR (2000) The neural mechanisms of top-down attentional control. Nat Neurosci 3:284–291

Jaspers K (1942) Allgemeine Psychopathologie, 4. edn. Springer, Berlin

Karnath H-O (2001) Spatial awareness is a function of the superior temporal, not the posterior parietal cortex. Nature 411:950–954

Kastner S, Pinsk MA, De Weerd P et al (1999) Increased activity in human visual cortex during directed attention in the absence of visual stimulation. Neuron 22:751–761

Kinomura S, Larsson J, Gulyás B, Roland PE (1996) Activation by attention of the human reticular formation and thalamic intralaminar nuclei. Science 271:512–515

Kliegl R, Mayr U, Krampe RT (1994) Time-accuracy funcions for determining process and person differences: an application to cognitive aging. Cogn Psychol 26:134–164

Koch C (2005) Bewusstsein—ein neurobiologisches Rätsel. Spektrum—Elsevier, München

Koch M (1999) The neurobiology of startle. Prog Neurobiol 59:107–128

Kustov AA, Robinson DL (1996) Shared neural control of attentional shifts and eye movements. Nature 384:74–77

LaBerge D, Buchsbaum MS (1990) Positoron emission tomographic measurement of pulvinar activity during an attention task. J Neurosci 10:613–619

Lichter DG, Cummings JL (2000) Frontal-subcortical circuits in psychiatric and neurological disorders. Guilford Press, New York

Mack A, Rock I (1998) Inattentional blindness. MIT Press, Cambridge

McClelland JL, McNaughton BL, O'Reilly RC (1995) Why there are complementary learning systems in the hippocampus and neocortex: insight from the successes and failures of connectionist models of learning and memory. Psychol Rev 102:419–457

Mesulam MM (2000) Attentional networks, confusional states and neglect syndromes. In: Mesulam MM (Ed) Principles of behavioral and cognitive neurology, 2. edn. Oxford Univ Press, Oxford, pp 174–256

Moore T, Armstrong KM (2003) Selective gating of visual signals by microstimulation of frontal cortex. Nature 421:370–373

Naccache L, Blandin E, Dehaene S (2002) Unconscious masked priming depends on temporal attention. Psychol Sci 13:416–424

Newman J (1997) Putting the puzzle together: Toward a general theory of the neural correlates of consciousness I-II. Consciousness Studies 4(47–66):100–121

Parr T, Friston KJ (2019) Attention or salience? Curr Opin Psychol 29:1–5

Parasuraman R (1998) The attentive brain. MIT Press, Cambridge

Posner MI, Petersen SE (1990) The attention system of the human brain. Annu Rev Neurosci 13:25–42

Posner MI, Rothbart M (2023) Fifty years integrating neurobiology and psychology to study attention. Biol Psychiatr 180:108574

Prinz W, Hommel B (2002) Common mechanisms in perception and action: Attention and performance XIX. Oxford Univ Press, Oxford

Reischies FM, Berghöfer A (1995) Saccadic tracking test—normal data and reliability. J Clin Psychol 51:262–267

Reischies FM, Diefenbacher A, Reichwaldt W (2003) Delir. In: Arolt V, Diefenbacher A (Eds) Psychiatrie in der klinischen Medizin. Springer, Berlin Heidelberg New York Tokio, pp 259–284

Resnik RA (2000) Seeing, sensing, and scrutinizing. Vision Res 40:1469–1487

Salthouse TA (2000) Aging and measures of processing speed. Biol Psychol 54:35–54

Saper CB, Scammell TE, Lu J (2005) Hypothalamic regulation of sleep and circadian rhythms. Nature 437:1257–1263

Sarter M, Nelson CL, Bruno JP (2005) Cortical cholinergic transmission and cortical information processing in schizophrenia. Schizophr Bull 31:117–138

Spitzer M (1993) The psychopathology, neuropsychology and neurobiology of associative and working memory in schizophrenia. Eur Arch Psychiatr Clin Neurosci 243:57–70

Ulrich G (1994) Psychiatrische Elektroenzephalographie. Urban & Fischer, München

Treue S (2003) Neuronale Grundlagen von Aufmerksamkeit. In: Karnath H-O, Thier P (Eds) Neuropsychologie. Springer, Berlin Heidelberg New York Tokio, pp 259–267

Winterer G, Adams CM, Jones DW, Knutson B (2002) Volition to action an event-related fMRI study. Neuroimage 17:851–858

Wu, W (2011) Attention as selection for action. In: Mode C, Smithies D, Wu W, (Eds) Attention: Philosophical and psychological essays. Oxford UP, 97–116

Wu, W (2023) Movements of the mind: A theory of attention, intention and action, Oxford UP

Further Reading

Alexander GE, Crutcher MD (1990) Functional architecture of basal ganglia circuits: Neuronal substrates for parallel processing. Trends Neurosci 13:266–271

Baars BJ (1998) Das Schauspiel des Denkens. Klett Cotta, Stuttgart

Baars BJ (2002) The conscious access hypothesis: origins and recent evidence. Trends Cogn Sci 6:47–52

Dehaene S, Jonides J, Smith EE, Spitzer M (1999) Thinking and problem solving. In: Zigmond MJ, Bloom FE, Landis SC et al (Eds) Fundamental neuroscience. Academic, San Diego, pp 1543–1564

Knudsen EI (2007) Fundamental components of attention. Ann Rev Neuroscience 30:57–78

Mega MS, Cummings JL (1994) Frontal-subcortical circuits and neuropsychiatric disorders. J Neuropsychiatry Clin Neurosci 6:358–370

Noesselt T, Hillyard SA, Woldorff MG et al (2002) Delayed stiate cortical activation during spatial attention. Neuron 35:575–587

Rafal RD, Posner M (1987) Deficits in human visual spatial attention following thalamic lesions. Proc Natl Acad Sci USA 84:7349–7353

Salthouse TA (2005) Relations between cognitive abilities and measures of executive functioning. Neuropsychology 19:532–545

Central Motor Function

5

Contents

5.1 Demarcation and Overview

This section discusses the central control of movements. How can a living being search for food or defend itself in its environment? The first chapters dealt with the process of perception, memory, and how an important stimulus binds attentional resources to itself. Now, for example, a fly is to be shooed away or a berry eaten. In the movement repertoire, a thesaurus of available action schemes, the appropriate motor patterns are found.

The neurology of motor disorders includes not only muscle weaknesses or central pareses but also e.g., dyskinesias or disturbances in action control. Therefore, in the field of psychomotorics, the demarcation between neurology and psychopathology of motor skills is blurred, and there are overlaps. This section focuses on disturbances in the control of motor actions that occur in psychiatric conditions, e.g., alcohol intoxication with slurred articulation, or apraxic disorders in primary degenerative dementias. For example, a person tries to wash their hair with a facecloth or comb their hair with a toothbrush. In demented patients, disturbances in tool use and limitations in practical skills in everyday life are observed. Another example of an apraxic wrong action:

F. M. Reischies, *Psychopathology*, https://doi.org/10.1007/978-3-662-70293-2_5

Example

In a conference, an older specialist raises his hand to speak. Finally, he is asked to pose his question. The microphone is handed to him. He takes the microphone in his right hand and brings it to his head. He grasps the shaft of the microphone and holds it like a conventional telephone receiver between his ear and mouth. The routine of handling a telephone receiver is mistakenly applied to a microphone. ◀

Psychopathologically, impulse control disorders and compulsive acts, i.e., disturbances in action control, continue to be significant.

This chapter deals with learned motor actions, usually routine actions. Non-routine actions, which are performed consciously under the control of focused attention, should will be considered in executive disorders (Chap. 6). A taxonomy of different classes of motor actions has not yet been established.

5.1.1 Reactive Movements

First, however, an overview of the different classes of actions to which the psychopathological categories refer should be given. Rolls (1999) distinguishes between a) implicit actions, especially reactive movements, and b) explicit actions, which proceed through linguistic-smeantic and reward evaluation. The execution of a learned movement on command from outside is a first distinguishable category.

Reaction Time Model

In reaction time measurements, the movement for the reaction is first determined or trained. When the agreed triggering stimulus comes, the movement should be executed as quickly as possible; for this, a stimulus-response channel must be set up or activated: Stimulus 1 to Movement 2. For motor neurons, the model of the critical membrane threshold can provide an explanation. Pre-activation reduces the reaction time, as shown in Chap. 4 »attention«, but also increases the proportion of false positive errors (activity in the locus coeruleus, Aston-Jones et al. 1999; Wu 2011).

5.1.2 Spontaneous Movement

Besides the externally induced reactions, there are learned actions that are internally initiated and controlled. Even in spontaneous motor acts, CNS activity prepares the movement. Surprisingly, findings showed that frontal brain activity is already measurable when the person has not yet consciously decided to perform the movement, i.e., before the conscious decision (Libet et al. 1983). These results have sparked the discussion about the unconscious components of human spontaneous actions.

5.1.3 Action Motivated by Expectation of Reward

In clinical everyday life, neuropsychological examination procedures are conducted—e.g., memory tests, attention tasks, etc. Usually, the person agrees to perform this task. This is not a given. In clinical practice, such a test is occasionally refused or not performed with serious motivation. If a person exerts themselves during the execution, they meet the expectations placed on them, or they behave according to the requirements of the situation, and they receive confirmation. This is, for example, the relative reward for "participating" in a clinical test (due to this issue, those clinical neuropsychological examination procedures are selected which are less influenced by motivation effects).

If a strenuous or complex action is planned, the expectation of reward comes to the forefront for the question of whether and how the action will be carried out. The dependence of spontaneous actions on the relative expectation of reward becomes evident through psychopharmacological experiments. For example, numerous studies have been conducted in which a person is given a blocker of dopamine action (e.g., the neuroleptic Haloperidol). After taking the medication, the person can no longer perform self-planned actions as before. Generally speaking, they "can't do anything" with themselves. However, actions performed on instruction can be carried out. These aspects of the reasons for actions are discussed in Chap. 7 Drive (self- and externally motivated drive).

5.1.4 Errors in Routine Motor Skills—Apraxia

Concept of central action schemes or motor act scripts

The concept of motor act scripts is widely accepted today: patients with apraxias, especially in dementia, confuse entire movement units, as in the example of confusing the handling of a microphone with that of a telephone handset (Sect. 5.1). Gesture confusion also occurs. In graphemic apraxia, elements of writing letters are confused. Apraxia involves errors in automated actions that are highly overlearned. They are no longer performed under the control of selective attention. For example, in an apraxia list, the patient is asked for a series of learned movements or generally known gestures. This can lead to the execution of incorrect gestures.

It applies to apraxia that even under attentive execution, errors in the selection of central motor act scripts occur—focussed attention is no longer involved in the details of movement planning, as this was the case when it was learned.

So far, errors belonging to ideomotor apraxia have been discussed. In addition to errors in object use or learned gestures, there are errors that belong to other forms of apraxia; notably, isolated disturbances of grasping or touching, where actions are disturbed in terms of seeing or touching, should be mentioned.

5.2 Hierarchical Levels of Spontaneous Movements

The emergence of spontaneous movements occurs at several hierarchical levels: different classes of actions require different demands on the individual levels. An overview will be provided here.

5.2.1 Emergence of an Intention to Act

For a spontaneous movement, that is, a movement initiated by the person, the intention to act is developed in the person's CNS. Usually, various intentions compete at any given time, such as reactions to perceived stimuli, routines, affect-induced actions, or, in thinking, plans arising from factual considerations. Relative reward expectations are considered—this level also involves motivation. Intention selection is discussed in Chap. 7 Drive. At this first level, the intention formation level, one intention prevails. What happens with the intention until the execution of the action is considered in the following section.

5.2.2 Concept of Action and Sequence of Motor Acts

The planning of actions is addressed before the presentation of action execution. A) Action planning is initially a cognitive process (see e.g., Chap. 10 thinking). An action is conceptualized with the recall of context-appropriate action schemes. Many mental processes are involved in this: visual-spatial intelligence aspects, experience—thus a specific memory—as well as verbal thinking operations. B) After evaluating the action options, the selection of the appropriate motor acts follows. The prerequisites are that intention and action goal are determined and held in working memory. The control is carried out with the help of executive functions and working memory (Chap. 6). C) Under conscious focussed attention, sequence control with feedback control takes place. This applies at least to non-routine actions.

This attentive non-routine action includes the syndrome of dysexecutive disorder. Patients with this syndrome are reported to "get nothing done" (Chap. 6 Executive Functions and Working Memory). The dysexecutive syndrome is not identical with ideational apraxia, as this refers to a disorder specifically in explicit action—in contrast to ideational apraxia, which refers to disorders in sequences of routine actions (see below).

Retrieval of Action Schemes

The selection of learned action schemes for the action plan takes place on the one hand experimentally in the planning during the "playing through of an action". This planning of conscious actions takes place under focussed attention (see above). On the other hand, the selection of movements and movement-parts also occurs in routine actions. If faulty elements are selected in the process, it is referred to as apraxia. Incorrect selection of movements on objects or incorrect movements in gestures are observed.

This type of error is comparable to incorrect phoneme sequences in aphasia. Here, too, cortical brain damage is responsible for the fact that highly overlearned words are spoken with an incorrect sequence of phonemes, inserted or omitted phonemes. Rothi and Heilman see a close relationship between ideomotor apraxia and aphasia (1997), at least with regard to the selection error from an action "lexicon".

▶ The concept of an action lexicon is helpful because it clarifies that apraxia is a disorder of the selection of movements from a repertoire of learned actions.

The level of selection of action schemes is thus involved both in the executive control of actions and in selection disorders that occur in apraxia.

In apraxia, there is a disorder in the selection of trained central motor act scripts. A disorder of executive functions is difficult to assess in the presence of apraxia because it is not clear whether an error occurred due to a disorder of the executive control function or due to the selection of learned movements.

5.2.3 Elementary Movements and Complex Movement Sequences

Actions can be very elementary like "hitting the table with a fist" or very complex like a repositioning maneuver by a doctor when a joint is dislocated. The question has been raised as to what the neurophysiological unit of movement is for the central motor act scripts, essentially the "element" of motor skills? It is certain that it is not the level of motor neurons, nor the level of individual muscle fiber movement, not even the individual muscle group of a joint. Presumably, the elementary units of motor skills are short sequences of patterns of muscle activations and inhibitions that control an elementary movement, such as an action on a limb. This motor element is an automated action. Through practice, series of elementary movements become a learned sequence, like the elementary movement of striking a piano key and the sequence of a melody that the pianist masters.

Errors in routine movements also occur in elements of a gesture. An example is the military salute. The arm movement is performed correctly, but the hand is mistakenly placed with the back of the hand to the side of the forehead. Again, in comparison with aphasia (see there), the alteration of an element in a word, a paraphasia, can contribute to clarification.

The syndrome of ideomotor apraxia describes the occurrence of selection errors of learned elementary actions: the prerequisite for the diagnosis is the proof that the sensory system and muscle function are intact. Examples are confusion of object use (see above) or incorrect gestures. Clinically, lists of routine actions are examined.

5.2.4 Control of Motor Processes

The general use of an object, such as a hammer, is usually trained. In the specific situation, adaptation to the subject's situation and the environment takes place. What is the person's body position and what strength of hammer blow does the task require? This adaptation affects the skillfulness of the execution.

Before the movement begins, it must be checked how the action scheme can be executed in the current body posture and position relative to a possible object. A gesture like waving can be performed independently of the current body posture—but a targeted hammer blow cannot, e.g., on a board at knee height; for this, information about the exact position of the torso, the extremities, etc., must be evaluated: the relation of the arm to the nail, the bending of the torso, and the balance must be calculated beforehand.

Current Implementation of the Action Scheme
A adaptation of motor innervation for the position of body parts and the specific location of the object must take place. This requires the cooperation of many brain regions with their specific processes (Rizzolatti and Wolpert 1994).

Sensory information is needed for the adaptation of the action scheme to the specific situation. This is particularly evident when grasping. Accordingly, there are forms of apraxia that involve a disturbance in the inflow of visual information to movement control. Grasping is disrupted (Binkofski and Fink 2005).

The cerebellum is also involved in the implementation of the action scheme. Information about joint mobility and the trajectory of movements to a target as well as the speed distribution over time (acceleration, deceleration) must be calculated. When the person, after the preplanning that occurs implicitly, initiates the hammer blow, a ballistic movement is triggered that either hits the target or not—i.e., it can no longer be changed in the course of the movement.

Process Control with Integration of Sensorimotor Feedback
If a movement is adapted to the current situation and executed, feedback through the skin or via sight or hearing can usually be integrated into the adjustment of the movement even during the movement. Tactile apraxias refer to a disorder in the feedback of information from the somatosensory receptors for the control of fine motor skills. This particularly leads to a disturbance of groping.

Imprecise, Slow Movements
In addition to disturbances in the inflow of necessary information for the adaptation of the action scheme, there is also a disturbance that consists of the defective precision of the innervation of the extremity muscles. This leads to clumsiness. Movements of the fingers become worm-like, slow, and seemingly aimless. They miss the targets, and in many cases, it is not clear in the clinical examination whether the necessary sensory target information was missing or whether the activation of the motor neurons was executed too imprecisely.

5.3 Clinic of Disturbance of Central Motor Act Scripts or Action Schemas

The disturbance of motor skills can be caused in various areas:

1. Drive disorders with drive poverty and drive increase—level of intention formation (Chap. 7 Drive),
2. Disorders of executive functions with errors in the conscious and attentive organization of complex action sequences (Chap. 6)
3. as well as the disturbances of central motor act scripts or action schemas presented in this chapter.

Here, the disturbance of activation and adaptation of action schemas is first addressed. Examples from the clinic have already been given in the justification of a hierarchical division of action or motor levels. This chapter deals with the types of disturbances in the selection of action schemas and the specific visual-spatial adaptation of motor skills, which, for example, plays a role in dexterity.

Disturbance of Selection of Action Schemas
An example is errors in the task of (1) flipping a coin with the thumb so that it (2) randomly (heads or tails) lands on the palm, as a referee does before a soccer game. In the first part of the task, for example, all fingers are extended instead of just the thumb (Haaland et al. 2000; Fig. 5.2), or the extension of the hand to catch the coin is omitted.

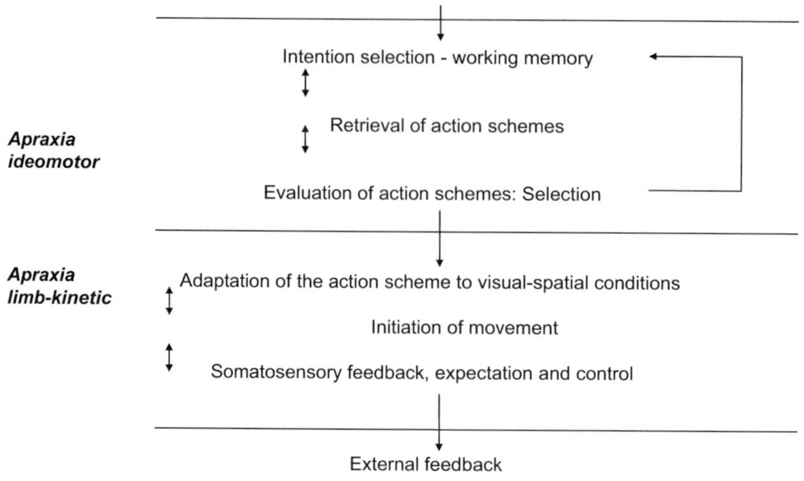

Fig. 5.1 Schema of central motor skills: A selection of movement elements of an action scheme is followed at the next level by the adaptation of the movement scheme to the current joint positions and body posture in relation to the target object

Apraxic errors are regularly observed in moderate dementia. Apraxias following focal brain lesions are depicted in the textbooks of neurological neuropsychology (Schnider et al. 1997, Goldenberg 2003).

Disturbance of Visual-Spatial Adaptation of Motor Skills, Limb-Kinetic apraxia
In the meantime, specific disturbances of execution control of action schemas have been better studied (Binkofski et al. 2005; Goldenberg 2003; Fig. 5.1). Clumsiness in everyday activities is noticeable, for example, in the use of cutlery or in trimming fingernails. In the examination of finger opposition, worm-like movements occur more frequently, for example. The syndrome of melokinetic or limb-kinetic apraxia also exists in automated actions.

Examinations

- Finger opposition, the fingers of the hand must be touched in sequence with the thumb.

5.4 Diagnostics

5.4.1 Examination of Apraxia

The diagnostics of apraxia are depicted in textbooks of neuropsychology. They are not discussed in detail here.

Errors in Tool Use
It is about recognizing object-use confusion errors (or errors in sequences). In the history taken from other persons, such errors must be inquired about, as their occurrence is characteristic of apraxia, but these errors overall occur rarely. They may be missed during the examination of a short apraxia task list. However, relatives can report spectacular wrong actions from everyday life. Lists for history taken from other persons: "Do errors occur in the following movements …?".

Automated Movements of Object Use and Gestures

- Lists (Poeck-Apraxia list, Poeck 2002) "Please show how to use a hammer; show how a soldier salutes; or: please show how to flip a coin with your thumb, like a referee before a soccer game", etc. (Fig. 5.2) Instructions are given a) or b) imitations are required.

Sequential Hand Movements
Fist-edge-flat hand sequences: It is examined whether the person can imitate sequences of 2, 3, or more hand positions. As with finger opposition, both clumsiness (see below) and sequence errors or completely wrong movements can be observed. An example is the instruction to first hit the table with the fist,

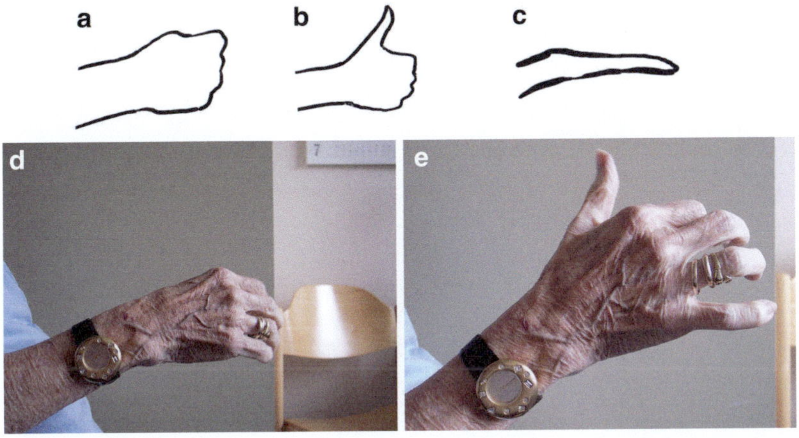

Fig. 5.2 a–d. Examples of ideomotor apraxia. **a, b** The person is supposed to perform the movement as it occurs when flipping a coin with the thumb, with the coin then being caught on the palm. Incorrect spreading movements are visible (Haaland et al. 2000) **c, d** in the patient with dementia and apraxia symptoms, the subsequent catching movement is missing

then with the edge of the hand, and finally with the flat hand, with the movements first being demonstrated for imitation. In gerontopsychiatry, errors frequently occur (Barry and Riley 1987; Reischies 2005). Follow instructions: Three steps of an instruction are given: to take a sheet with the right hand, fold it in the middle, and place it on the floor (Mini Mental State Examination—MMSE).

These tasks test complex functions. Often, language comprehension disorders, paralysis, or severe working memory disorders cannot be excluded as alternative reasons for errors, so errors should not be readily attributed to apraxia disorders.

Drawing: copying of figures
The copy of the 2 pentagons of the MMSE, which must at least overlap with a square, allows a rough estimation of the patient's visuospatial constructive abilities.

Copies are also required in the neuropsychological battery of CERAD, where a wire model of a cube must be drawn. Visuospatial dysfunctions become particularly evident here (Fig. 5.3). Rey Complex Figure (see Lezak et al. 2004): A complex line drawing must be copied. A simpler version is the Read variant (element by element is copied, Reischies and Lindenberger 1996).

Clock drawing test
In the clock drawing test, in most variants, the circle is provided by the examiner. The following should be drawn:

- 12 digits of the clock face and the 2 hands showing the time "10 past 11 o'clock".

First, visual-spatial criteria for the drawing are checked. Furthermore, whether the indicated time is recognizable, etc. The assessment can be done according to the rating by Shulman et al. (1986).

The clock test examines a variety of functions

a) in the domain of visual imagination,
b) the thesaurus of visual object concepts, and
c) visual-spatial practical skills in drawing, arranging on the clock face, and the angle of the hands.

> ▶ If an old person has not drawn for decades, they may possibly draw the clock incorrectly without a serious praxis disorder being present. However, by observing the drawing process and the finished clock, one can often find features of disturbed central action scripts.

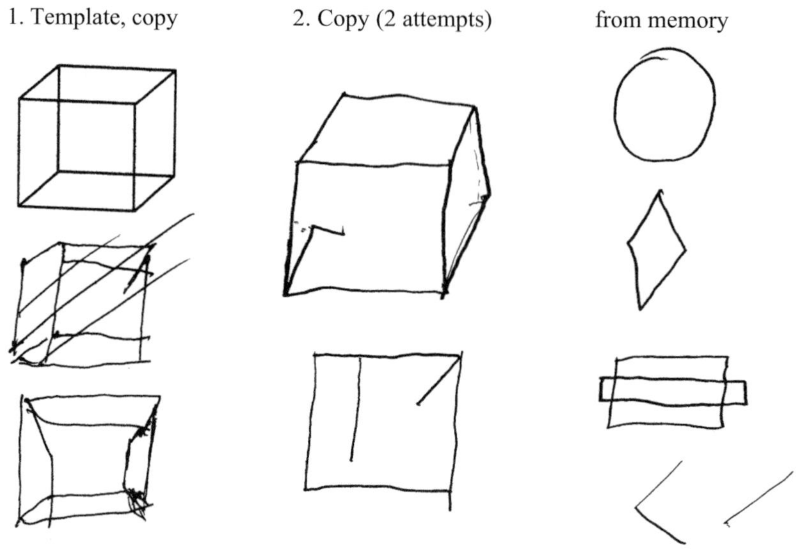

Fig. 5.3 Examples of constructive apraxia: The spatial aspects of the wire model of the cube cannot be drawn by the patient. Various attempts are made, but each fails to capture the spatial relationships. After distraction, he remembers the other simple figures he was able to copy, but not the details of the wire cube

Some investigators have given the task of the laying of a star with matches or the drawing of a five-pointed star.

5.4.2 Specific Forms of Apraxia

Ideational apraxia. It is more frequently observed in dementia syndromes. Complex, previously mastered sequences of movements can no longer be performed. To test this, complex activities are requested, such as putting a paper in an envelope and sticking a stamp on it or preparing filter coffee with a pot of cold water and an immersion heater.

Callosal apraxia. In this form of apraxia, verbal commands to perform actions can be executed with the right hand but not with the left hand, as the motor script activated in the left hemisphere does not reach the right hemisphere via the corpus callosum (for left-side language-dominant individuals). The occurrence of unilateral apraxias after disconnection, for example in callosal apraxia, indicates the disruptibility of the transmission of selected action schemes to the specific motor cortex and parietal areas, which are supposed to adapt and execute the schemes (Fig. 5.4).

5.5 Neuroscience

In the context of this presentation, a detailed description of the neuroscience of overall motor function and its disorders cannot be provided. Only fundamental findings will be described here, which can help to understand how a person performs targeted motor actions, which in turn can be disturbed in the various forms of apraxic symptoms.

First of all, the physiology of motor function appears to be clearly divided into the levels of cortical and spinal motor neurons. At the level of cortical motor function, the planning and initiation of actions, as well as the accompanying changes in posture, in collaboration with the cerebellum, are controlled. The level of spinal motor function concerns the control of muscle contraction and the details of joint positions.

Motor actions always occur in a coordinated manner, i.e., the activation of motor ensembles for a joint movement simultaneously involves a

Apraxia - Taxonomy

Action concept system

Polymodal apraxia
extremities, buccofacial

Ideomotoric
Learned gestures (with/without meaning)
Learned tool use

Ideational
Complex learned sequences

Action production system

"frontal", production - apraxia

Limb kinetic apraxia
Speech apraxia

Sensorimotor interface

"posterior", input - apraxia
Unimodal apraxia
Tactile (buttons)
Optical (touch-sensitive)

Fig. 5.4 Taxonomy of apraxia: Forms of apraxia are (1) on the one hand caused by disturbances of the action concept system. These are disturbances of learned or even routine actions, where the selection or sequence of movements is incorrect (limb apraxia). These can also affect mouth and tongue movements (buccofacial). (2) Psychopathologically, disturbances in the action production system are common, especially in the goal-directedness of movements and articulation. (3) A third group of apraxias is closely related to perceptual disturbances, such as a disturbance of grasping, which is under optical and tactile control.

retardation an inhibition of ensembles that encode the alternative direction of movement or possibly interfering posture motor function.

5.5.1 Motor Cortex

For a long time, the central unresolved question was what the motor neurons in the cortex encode. Are they specialized to trigger the contraction of individual muscle fibers, the contraction of entire muscles, or the movement of antagonistic muscle groups at individual joints? It was found that although a homunculus map for motor functions exists, on the other hand, individual neurons activate very different muscles. The solution that was achieved was surprising: The control of a movement apparently occurs through a population vector in the motor cortex. If the hand is to reach a target, not just a small group of cortical neurons fires to directly control the movement to the target. In a population of motor neurons, each motor neuron has a preferential direction of movement. Many neurons are activated when a specific movement is to be executed; the other neurons either fire less for this direction or are even inhibited for this direction—because they are specialized for the opposite direction (Georgopoulos et al. 1986; Ghez 1991). Thus, each neuron is responsible for a direction of movement in space. This can be illustrated by the image of a hedgehog. The spines of the hedgehog point in every direction and are meant to represent the possible movements of the hand in space. In a specific movement, the neurons responsible for that direction are the most active. In the image of the hedgehog, the spines are longer in one direction. The neurons are most strongly activated in a specific direction of movement when the intended movement targets their specific direction in space. The neurons that encode the opposite direction of movement are inhibited. The direction of movement to be executed is represented by the neurons that encode this direction, as these neurons show the highest activity in the population.

▶ Only through the interaction of all neurons in the population does a precise movement signal emerge. In a population of motor neurons that transmit information to the spinal level, the activation of a direction of movement, the population vector, predominates at any given time. This specific direction of movement is executed by the spinal motor neurons.

The spinal level is to be understood as a local network that outputs a coordinated joint movement to the muscles according to the activity of the motor cortex population.

Disturbance of the Motor Cortex
If the cortical motor neurons are damaged, either a paresis of the limb results in the case of complete damage to the motor neurons for a limb, or only a slowing and coarsening of movements. Incomplete damage to the motor cortex still allows movement to be executed, but not as precisely as before the damage.

A dedifferentiation of motor functions occurs. For example, in intoxications and degenerative dementia diseases, coarsening of movements occurs, which can be referred to as limb-kinetic apraxia (or melokinetic apraxia).

Prefrontal Motor Regions
In the prefrontal hand area, neurons are found that represent action schemes of grasping. The neurons are active in specific types of grasping, seizing, etc. (Rizzolatti et al. 2004; Gottlieb 2002).

In collaboration with the "where" units of the parietal lobe, the location of the object and the type of grasping are specified (Pause et al. 1989). After that, the prefrontal hand area is activated, which accomplishes the action scheme for the motor cortex.

According to this model, a repertoire of motor action schemes is stored in the prefrontal cortex, which has been trained over the course of life. The action schemes can be retrieved for routine tasks, as has already been investigated in single-neuron recordings in the example of grasping. The action schemes exist for the use of tools that a person needs in everyday life and in their profession.

Damage to the Representation of Action Schemes. If the action schemes are damaged, errors occur in retrieving specialized movements such as grasping.

Errors in the Sensory Control of Action Schemes. A specific disturbance of grasping or touching is found in high parietal lesions, which must provide the sensory control for the action schemes (Binkofski et al. 2005).

Handlungssequenzen
How is a trained action chain organized? Reseach findings on the coding of the sequence of movements are instructive for this (see Halsband et al. 1994). When a simple square is to be traced, a sequence of simple movements is executed. The individual movement with its direction is represented in the primary motor cortex, as shown above. It is apparently irrelevant whether the line is drawn by the movement of the arm, wrist, or just the fingers. Four movements are needed for a square, two movements in the forward and two in the backward direction. It is not a routine action, but also not a movement that must be under complex executive control. In studies on monkeys performing these drawings, neurons in prefrontal motor areas could be characterized (Averbeck et al. 2002). In an ensemble of these neurons, the coding of the sequence is found. The individual neurons show activity that is closely related to a stage of the sequence of actions. These neurons can apparently also realize the imagined trial run of a movement sequence without movement success, like a skier mentally training the various turns of the slope.

During the attentive first execution of an action sequence, the individual movement is selected in the areas of the frontal cortex. In contrast, however, in learned complex movements, the selection is taken over by automated network functions that no longer fall under executive attention. In apraxia, this network activates errors in the sequence of action schemas when it is grossly damaged. This leads to an increased error rate, which is proportional to the extent of the damage to the neural network.

5.6 Psychopathological Symptoms of Central Motor Function

Apraxic Disorders
Definition. Disorder of central action organization, which manifests in wrong automated actions without paralysis of the extremities.

Example

- An old woman shows incorrect use of an object: washes her hair with a facecloth, even though she understood the task.
- A man draws a letter, a clock face, a house, a star, or a stick figure incorrectly, even though he could draw these objects correctly before.
- A man cannot imitate a simple sequence of hand movements, even though he could do it before. ◀

Position in Psychopathology. Not in AMDP, but as a dementia feature in AGP.

Psychopathological Interactions. Clumsiness, aphasia: problems with understanding the task.

Differential Diagnostic Distinctions
- Paralysis and especially motor clumsiness must be excluded as the sole cause of the wrong actions (also sensory deficits that can lead to errors in object use),
- Clouding of consciousness—the person cannot clearly understand and imagine the task,
- Simulation, conversion symptoms
- explainable solely by the interactions of the mentioned factors,
- Refusal or demoralization with a devitalized condition and action attitude: the motivation for the action must be clarified for the diagnosis of disturbed motor control,
- in new tasks (not errors in routine object use or gestures), a deficit may become apparent due to executive dysfunction.

Further Characterization. Individual action scripts are executed incorrectly or in the wrong order because the central action script was incorrectly activated.

Self-/other persons's judgment. other persons's judgment—since these features occur rarely, partner statements are very helpful.

Neuropsychology/objectification
Behavioral observation and inquiry in daily activities:

- Apraxia lists: Various verbal action prompts or prompts to imitate actions and gestures,
- Drawing or copying objects or copying complex nonsense figures.

Severity. Rare errors up to frequent, everyday-relevant disturbances.

Specifications
- isolated disturbance of: grasping or touching,
- gestures,
- object use,
- dressing dyspraxia,
- grapheme: apraxic agraphia,
- drawing,
- especially spatial relationships (constructive apraxia).

Conceptual problems of the feature
Belongs to the so-called brain tool disorders, i.e., disturbance of information processing that affects one of the "modules" of the mind (Fodor 1983), i.e., with automated—implicit information processing.

Neuroscientific/cognitive neuroscientific model concepts
Disturbance in the area:

1. central action plan,
2. central action script that includes the routine execution of the action plan,
3. visuo-tactile control,
4. adaptation to the current environment and own body posture—relationship to limb-kinetic apraxia,

5. implementation and activation of execution—relationship to central paralysis and limb-kinetic apraxia.

Motor clumsiness—melokinetic apraxia
Definition: Simple movements, previously performed skillfully by the person, can now only be carried out slowly and uncertainly, with the target accuracy of individual movements significantly reduced.

Example

A man with alcohol intoxication can no longer perform the—previously skillful—control of finger motor skills, the movements are performed slowly and imprecisely, they are incertain and aimless. From the life history it is known that he previously had undisturbed fine motor skills, so it is an acquired disorder. ◀

Differential diagnostic distinctions. Incorrect movements, disturbance of the influx of sensory information in the adaptation of the action scheme .

It is not the reduction of strength of the muscles that leads to the slowing down and uncertain execution. It is not an incorrect selection of elementary movements, as in ideomotor apraxia.

The mechanisms of action selection in motivated action selection—that is, for non-routine actions—are discussed in drive functions.

Excessive non-targeted movements, as in ataxia, are not the cause of clumsiness.

References

Aston Jones GS, Desimone R, Driver J et al (1999) Attention. In: Zigmond MJ, Bloom FE, Landis SC et al (Eds) Fundamental neuroscience. Academic, San Diego, pp 1385–1409

Averbeck BB, Chafee MV, Crowe DA, Georgopoulos AP (2002) Parallel processing of serial movements in prefrontal cortex. Proc Natl Acad Sci U S A 99:13172–13177

Barry P, Riley JM (1987) Adult norms for the Kaufman Hand Movements Test and a single-subject design for acute brain injury rehabilitation. J Clin Exp Neuropsychol 9:449–455

Binkofski F, Fink G (2005) Apraxien. Nervenarzt 76:493–511

Fodor JA (1983) The modularity of mind. MIT Press, Cambridge

Georgopoulos AP, Schwarz AB, Kettner RE (1986) Neuronal population coding of movement direction. Science 233:1416–1419

Ghez C (1991) Voluntary movement. In: Kandel E, Schwartz JH, Jessell TM (Eds) Principles of neural science, 3. edn. Elsevier, New York, pp 609–625

Goldenberg G (2003) Apraxie. In: Karnath H-O, Thier P (Eds) Neuropsychologie. Springer, Berlin Heidelberg New York Tokio, pp 337–347

Gottlieb J (2002) Parietal mechanisms of target representation. Curr Opin Neurobiol 12:134–140

Haaland KY, Harrington DL, Knight RT (2000) Neural representations of skilled movement. Brain 123:2306–2313

Halsband U, Matsuzaka Y, Tanji J (1994) Neuronal activity in the primate supplementary, pre-supplementary and premotor cortex during externally and internally instructed sequential movements. Neurosci Res 20:149–155

Lezak MD, Howieson DB, Loring DW (2004) Neurospychological assessment, 4. edn. Oxford Univ Press, Oxford

Libet B, Gleason CA, Wright EW, Pearl DK (1983) Time of conscious intention to act in relation to onset of cerebral activity (readinesspotential). The unconscious initiation of a freely voluntary act. Brain 106:623–642

Reischies FM (2005) Die Stellung von Screeninguntersuchungen und neuropsychologischen Markertests in der Demenzdiagnostik—allgemeine Aspekte. Z Gerontopsychologie & -psychiatrie 18:105–114

Reischies FM, Lindenberger U (1996) Grenzen und Potentiale kognitiver Leistungen im hohen Alter. In: Mayer KU, Baltes PB (Eds) Die Berliner Altersstudie. Akademie Verlag, Berlin, pp 351–377

Pause M, Kunesch E, Binkofski F, Freund HJ (1989) Sensorimotor disturbances in patients with lesions of the parietal cortex. Brain 112:1599–1625

Poeck K (2002) Apraxie. In: Hartje W, Poeck K (Eds) Klinische Neuropsychologie. Thieme, Stuttgart

Rizzolatti G, Wolpert DM (1994) Motor systems. Curr Opin Neurobiol 15:623–625

Rolls ET (1999) The brain and emotion. Oxford Univ Press, Oxford

Rothi LJG, Heilman KM (1997) Apraxia: The neuropsychology of action. Psychol Press, Hove

Schnider A, Hanlon RE, Alexander DN, Benson DF (1997) Ideomotor apraxia: behavioral dimensions and neuroanatomical basis. Brain Lang 58:125–136
Shulman KL, Shedeletsky R, Silver IL (1986) The challenge of time: Clock-drawing and cognitive function in the elderly. Int J Geriatr Psychiatry 1:135–140

Further Reading

Wu W (2011) Attention as selection for action. In: Mode C, Smithies D, Wu W, (Eds) Attention: Philosophical and psychological essays. Oxford UP, 97–116

Executive Functions and Working Memory

6

Contents

6.1 Introduction

In the last chapter, highly automated actions such as routine object use and routine action sequences were described. How does a person organize a conscious action that is not routine? How does he plan actions? A person does not live only in the past and the present but also in the future—he plans actions. This chapter is about non-routine action (Shallice 2002); we proceed to the self-initiated and consciously supervised action of humans (Fuster 1990).

Executive functions help to organize actions. An example should illustrate this: A person wants to draw a square. First, he copies it, draws a square. In doing so, under focussed attention, a side line is first drawn, which corresponds in length to the model, then at a right angle to it, the second line, which should be of equal length. Then, again at a right angle, the first movement is performed in the opposite direction, and finally, the two free ends are connected. The simplicity of the task lies in the repetition of the visual model, which provides the template or makes it clear what is still missing. If such a sequence of movements is to be made without the template, a system must take control. The instruction must be stored in working memory: "(1) A straight line, (2) at a right angle an equally long line, and (3) then at a right angle the first movement back in the opposite direction and (4) finally connect the ends." The intermediate results are compared with the project goal. For many people, visual imagination will provide the model—it is, so to speak, copied from the imagination. This no longer works for non-visual action sequences. Then the executive organization of action sequences is indispensable.

Beyond the organization of new actions and simple action sequences, executive control according to the view of many researchers encompasses more. It is generally about the regulation of a person's activities. The classification

F. M. Reischies, *Psychopathology*, https://doi.org/10.1007/978-3-662-70293-2_6

by Das et al. (1997), which comes from the discussion about artificial intelligence, Shallice (2002), is illustrative:

- »zero order«: a stimulus is analyzed by a one-dimensional processing with a response determined by it, example: thermostat regulates the target temperature on one dimension;
- »first order«: »zero order« plus a model of the environment, which allows a more flexible adaptation of the response schemes;
- »second order«: There is the possibility to compare several alternative models. This allows evaluating different response schemes (and outcomes) between which one can choose;
- »third order«: Maintenance of a model of one's own ways of acting (meta-model). This allows a hierarchical organization of response schemes—e.g., (a) in relation to the higher level of individual beliefs, (b) their justifications, and (c) predictions of the consequences of one's own actions.

In addition to the elementary organization of action sequences, executive functions thus also concern the entirety of a person's ways of acting. One must distinguish between elementary executive functions and their disorders on the one hand and complex executive regulation on the other.

Executive functions include:

- Planning of partial goals,
- Maintaining the plan, updating the plan in case of modifications, and
- Monitoring which partial goals have been achieved,
- Inhibition of (still) inappropriate activities,
- Error detection,
- Organization of the reaction to errors.

Examples of executive tasks:

- »Tower of London« test, in which discs must be rearranged on rods,
- Puzzle, 2 complex spatial objects to be assembled,
- Series of tasks that require time management. Errors arise because a person devotes too much time to one of the tasks and overlooks that they can no longer adequately handle the others.

Salthouse has criticized the concept of executive disorders as they are usually assessed in neuropsychology. He argued that tests of executive functions are closely related to perceptual speed and judgment ability (Salthouse 2005).

Working Memory

Working memory represents a function clearly distinguishable from episodic memory. On the one hand, it refers to involuntarily operating buffer storage in various modalities (e.g., acoustically: counting the chimes of the church clock from buffer storage). On a second level, the organization of the buffer storage and the retrieval from it is included.

Example: A cook puts down a knife during his cooking procedures, then needs it again, and confidently reaches for the—from buffer storage—remembered place where the knife is located.

The importance of working memory is familiar to most people from intermediate results in mental arithmetic: e.g., 56 + 17 (6 + 7 "13 in mind", 50 + 10 plus the result in the buffer store).

6.2 Disruption of Executive Functions and Working Memory

Executive functions and working memory are necessary for the organization of complex everyday actions. For example, the work plan must be kept in memory. After the first stages, an update occurs during monitoring, indicating which subtasks have been completed. Subsequently, it is determined which new sub-goal must be tackled to efficiently pursue the overall goal.

Far-reaching consequences arise from the disruption of basic executive functions.

An important aspect is the overlap between the fields of executive dysfunctions and formal thought disorders. A disruption of working memory is also reflected in thought disorders, Chap. 10 Thinking. For instance, the forgetting of the thought goal, which is relevant in a communication situation, can be observed in circumstantiality or the disruption of thought, where the person suddenly loses the thread. In the tradition of psychopathology, formal thought disorders are presented as a separate chapter. Here, only a reference is made to it, and the main focus is placed on the practical symptoms of executive dysfunctions.

A person attentively plans an activity or considers which arguments are appropriate at which point in a negotiation. The overlap of dysfunctions of executive motor functions, attention, and thought disorders arises from the commonality that they involve non-routine actions or attentively performed actions.

A disruption of the executive levels can be diagnosed through detailed observation of the behavior of patients with the possibility of inquiry and additionally through neuropsychological examination procedures. The psychopathological analysis of behavior also considers how differentiated the person controls their actions.

The disruption of complex executive regulation can be described as a reduction in effective organizational levels according to Das (Das et al. 1997). For example, a person may be described as "simple-minded." A relative notices that the partner is only guided by sensory impressions. Thus, actions in some brain damage syndromes are predominantly guided in the sense of stimulus-response automatisms.

In the context of executive dysfunctions, the concept of **prospective** *memory* also plays a role. In a test session, a task must be completed at a specific point. It may come to "forgetting to remember", for example, that there was a particularity at the specific point. Symbolically, the knot in the handkerchief is a signal that the person should still remember something—a call or a purchase. Prospective memory is tested, for example, with an assignment:

- at the end of the session, please still …
- when x is announced, then …

6.3 Neuroscience

The neuronal control of complex actions is still insufficiently investigated. However, research has now at least explained elements of planning, control, and execution of individual movements.

6.3.1 Control of Spontaneous Movements

Spontaneously generated movements seem to have a different control region within the brain than reactive movements. Spontaneously generated movements have correlates in the cingulate cortex (Schieber 1999). Actor-related neurons were also found there (Shima and Tanji 1998). When a primate selects the other of two possible motor actions due to changed reward assignments, these neurons are active. They are not active when only reactively the alternative movement must be performed, e.g., after a signal prompts a change of movement. These neurons thus seem to become active only when the actor decides to perform a different movement because the old one is no longer rewarded. The orbitofrontal cortex is closely connected with the cingulate cortex, so that the concrete expectation of reward and the relative value of the reward can be conveyed. In an experiment with a primate choosing between two types of movements the value of the reward (which consists of food, e.g., sugar water) can decrease due to satiation. By changing the reward scheme on the part of the investigators, the expectation of reward can decrease.

In executive functions, prefrontal brain areas and those of the anterior cingulate have been found to be activated in fMRI studies. The neuroscientific investigation using electrophysiological single-neuron recording is still in its early stages.

6.3.2 Working Memory

If there is an action plan, as described e.g. in drawing a square, on the one hand, the goal of the action must be stored, and on the other hand, monitoring must take place to determine which subtask has already been completed.

Let us again consider the example of drawing. The monitoring of what has been completed is very simple when drawing, as it is given by the already drawn line. However, if no such documentation takes place, for example, if a square is to be drawn in the air, then other functions must step in. This section on working memory deals with the attentive organization of actions without direct sensory control.

Working memory is associated with the sustained-activity neurons of the prefrontal cortex (Fuster 1990; Goldman Rakic and Selemon 1997). How can sustained-activity neurons organize actions? Fuster's conception was initially that these neurons realize the temporal dimension of information processing in the brain. Classic examples were delayed-response tasks. A monkey sat in front of a curtain and had the task of searching for food under one of two pots. For example, food was shown under the right red pot. Then the curtain was lowered. After several seconds, the curtain was lifted, and the monkey had to retrieve the food, which had meanwhile been swapped, from under the left blue pot. The alternation (»delayed alternation task«) was introduced to make the task as specific as possible for the memory of the side and independent of the memory of sensory impressions.

Fuster described neurons in the prefrontal cortex that maintained the direction of movement for the interval time, which must be taken after the curtain is opened to reach the food. If the monkey is distracted for even a short time for another action, i.e., it performs another task attentively in the meantime, the task can no longer be executed without errors. It is assumed that the information actively maintained by such sustained-activity neurons is crucial for working memory.

In the dorsolateral prefrontal cortex, the described sustained-activity neurons for working memory are primarily found. They maintain a tendency to act even against intermittent interruption of sensory control, i.e., when the animal can no longer see the moving object. Visual and verbal working memory in the human brain can be differentiated in functional imaging studies (Gruber and Cramon 2003).

The manipulation of the contents of working memory

Updating working memory plays a central role in the organization of executive functions. An example is the monitoring of information about the project status, which sub-goals have been achieved, what is the next sub-goal, etc.

The feedback of movements is integrated into a monitor to update the information about the main action. In the example of the complex action, ensembles of sustained-activity neurons must be assigned to a unit, for example, a sub-goal. If something changes in the unit, the latest current information is maintained.

Tests examine for example the monitoring of intermediate sums in an arithmetic task at two locations—, two stacks of cards. The unit is called: left or right stack, the task is performed (addition or subtraction of a certain number), and then the new result is stored until it is called again.

In tasks that require manipulation of working memory, a different brain region of the dorsolateral prefrontal cortex was found compared with simple storage tasks.

Example

A task that requires the organization of material in working memory and in which patients with schizophrenic psychosis perform poorly is the number-letter-span the number-letter range. A sequence of numbers and letters is given, and the person is asked not to reproduce them in the given order but to sort them by numbers and letters in numerical and alphabetical order. For example, 4 J 3 B 9 K is given, and the person should then say 3 4 9 B J K. This requires a variable manipulation of items in working memory for each sequence. ◀

6.4 Neuroscience of Complex Executive Regulation

Little is known about this field of neuroscience. Above all, it is still unclear how the regions of the prefrontal cortex work together for this regulation.

On the one hand, analyzing the consequences of actions and the flexible assignment of reward and punishment (negative consequences) is a task of the orbitofrontal cortex. Apparently, a probability of the occurrence of reward is calculated. The incoming reward is controlled in collaboration with the ventral tegmentum and ventral striatum (Schultz 2004, Brooks 2001). If the expected reward falls short of the expected value, the behavior is changed. It is precisely this behavioral flexibility that is impaired after lesions of the orbitofrontal cortex.

In addition, there is the control of attention on newly performed actions. On the one hand, it must be recognized that a task needs to be worked on with attention. There exists a "bottleneck" of information processing because only one object or process can be in the focus of attention. The Supervisory-Attentional-System has been proposed as an organizational unit for this (Shallice 2002).

Furthermore, the initiation of actions must take place, which is associated with the function of the dorsal and medial region of the prefrontal cortex. The neurons associated with the actor role have already been mentioned above. If there is a disturbance in this region, disturbances in action initiation result, which are also described in Chap. 7 about drive. Behavior with a lack of drive is observed.

The various functions of the prefrontal cortex are involved in the control of the person's actions. Further research into these functions will only make it possible to explain complex executive regulation (Reischies 2005).

6.5 Psychopathological Symptoms of Executive Control

Disorder of Executive Control
Definition. Disorder in the sequential organization of multi-part actions, for example, tasks in everyday life.

Example. The patient cannot complete a more complex task, he fails in the organization of the task, although he has the motivation to complete the matter and is not clumsy in the individual actions. He starts multiple times. However, the activity fades at various stages of completion. The caregivers report, "he can't get anything done."

Position in Psychopathology
The feature has now been included in the AMDP system (AMDP 11th edition, 2023).

- Concept from new neuropsychological studies,
- especially common in the clinic of schizophrenic negative symptoms and in the acute symptoms of disorganized schizophrenic patients,
- remotely related to ideational apraxia.

Related Terms. Disorganised, ideational apraxia.

Psychopathological Interactions. Drive disorder, thought disorder, concentration disorder, control disorder in the drive domain.

Differential Diagnostic Distinctions
- explainable solely by the above mentioned interactions,
- refusal or demoralization with a reduced vital state and reduced action disposition: the motivation for the action must be clarified

for the diagnosis of the disturbed executive control.

Further Characterization. Disorder of action organization, especially because the activation of sub-tasks, which is due at certain points, e.g., after feedback, is not worked out.

Self-/Other Person's Judgment. Other person's judgment.

Interview for Rating. Question about efficiency in everyday life, history taken from other persons.

Neuropsychology/objectification

- elementary: tasks such as folding a sheet, putting it in an envelope, and sticking a stamp on it,
- complex: behavioral observation and inquiry regarding activities such as withdrawing money at the bank or transferring money, preparing an application at an department,
- tasks like the "Tower of London" test, where discs must be rearranged on rods.

Severity. From mild disorder, which manifests in more complex everyday or professional tasks, up to severe inability to manage one's affairs.

Neuroscientific/cognitive neuroscientific models
Disorder in the area of

1. working memory—subtasks and their sequence, disorder in "procedural memory",
2. "feedback processing"—the implementation of the next subtask does not occur because the completion of the preceding task is not processed,
3. disorder of inhibition of alternative action intentions, disinhibition,
4. the reporting of the completion of a subgoal cannot be processed—inefficient "collateral discharge", faulty deletion in case of negative feedback, etc.

Disorder of working memory
Definition: Disorder in the automatic intermediate storage of information during complex action sequences.

Most probably underlying dysfunction in psychopathological features such as the disruption of thought, circumstantiality of thinking, and also in forms of comprehension disorder—on the other hand, disorder in the organization of solving extensive everyday problems.
Tests:

1. Elementary:
   - Digit span (a sequence of single-digit numbers is to be repeated; procedure: test each sequence length a maximum of 2 times, stop after 2 errors),
   - Corsi block-tapping (a sequence of blocks distributed on a field is to be repeated).
2. Attention-related:
   - "continuous performance test" with memory component—e.g., react to X when A was given before or two consecutive odd numbers (e.g., Attention-Levine test),
   - N-back tasks: A sequence of numbers are given: do not repeat the current number each time, but say the last (−1) or the second last (-2) number.
3. Memory Updating:
   - on 2 or more fields (cards), arithmetic operations appear, e.g., (+3) (−1), and the results for the fields must be given at the end,
   - number-letter-span (see above),
   - incremental addition: serial calculation 10 + 1, +2, +3, +4, etc. In the sequence, the result must be given each time (11, 13, 16, etc.).

References

AMDP-System (2023) Manual zur Dokumentation des psychischen Befundes in Psychiatrie Psychotherapie und Psychosomatik, 11. edn. Hogrefe, Göttingen. Engl. translation: W Guy, TA Ban 2012, Springer Berlin

Brooks DJ (2001) Functional imaging studies on dopamine and motor control. J Neural Transm 108:1283–1298

Das SK, Fox J, Hammond P, Elsdon D (1997) A flexible architecture for autonomous agents. J Exp Theoret Artif Intell 9:407–440

Fuster J (1990) Inferotemporal units in selective visual attention and short-term memory. J Neurophysiol 64:681–697

Goldman-Rakic PS, Selemon LD (1997) Functionsal and anatomical aspects of prefrontal pathology in schizophrenia. Schizophr Bull 23:437–458

Gruber O, von Cramon DY (2003) The functional neuroanatomy of human working memory revisited. Evidence from 3-T fMRI studies using classical domain-specific interference tasks. Neuroimage 19:797–809

Reischies FM (2005) Psychopathologie. In: Förstl H (Ed) Frontalhirn. Funktionen und Erkrankungen, 2. edn. Springer, Berlin Heidelberg New York Tokio, pp 83–101

Salthouse TA (2005) Relations between cognitive abilities and measures of executive functioning. Neuropsychology 19:532–545

Schieber MH (1999) Voluntary descending control. In: Zigmond MJ, Bloom FE, Landis SC et al (Eds) Fundamental neuroscience. Academic, San Diego, pp 931–1049

Schultz W (2004) Neural coding of basic reward terms of animal learning theory, game theory, microeconomics and behavioural ecology. Curr Opin Neurobiol 14:139–147

Shallice R (2002) Fractionation of the supervisory attentional system. In: Stuss DT, Knight RT (Eds) Principles of frontal lobe function. Oxford Univ Press, New York, pp 261–277

Shima K, Tanji J (1998) Role of cingulated motor area cells in voluntary movement selection based on reward. Science 282:1335–1338

Further Reading

Georgopoulos AP, Caminiti R, Kalaska JF, Massey JT (1983) Spatial coding of movement: a hypothesis concerning the coding of movement direction by motor cortical populations. Exp Brain Res 7(Suppl):327–336

Pasupathy A, Miller EK (2005) Different time courses of learning related activity in the prefrontal cortex and striatum. Nature 433:873–876

Drive, Intention Formation—Action and Movement Disorders

7

Contents

7.1 The Construct of Drive (Antrieb)

In the last sections, it was about the advance planning of an action, the selection of motor schemas, and their implementation.

Even before the planning and execution of an action, the motives for actions are important; in a way, the degree of interest can be disturbed. For what reason, with what desire and interest is one acting?

Whereby not motivation for a single action is in focus, but a drive level that is, for example, reduced in a depression.

It is about the general level of Intentions, which are further developed into action plans with the selection of motor schemas. We do not yet know what an action intention is. We can assume

F. M. Reischies, *Psychopathology*, https://doi.org/10.1007/978-3-662-70293-2_7

that it is something that a person, who is confronted with an action option, more or less has.

Here, for example, the feeling of energy, the feeling of interest, or in contrary a resistance, not being ready to act, come into play.

These complex processes of drive, drive regulation are important in psychiatric everyday life; many psychopathological symptoms refer to the drive concept.

However, the drive concept itself is vague; it is not used in all psychopathological schools.

We try to define it: The concept of drive state is that of the amount of promoting influences on action initiation and targeted activity in everyday life—predominantly spontaneous activity, whereby the drive state does not have to be conscious. In certain situations, the influences can have a negative, inhibiting effect. It is a psychopathological Construct of not directly observable mental Action Dynamics.

Example

A 40-year-old depressed man had stayed mostly in bed or on the couch for weeks. He had neglected his apartment because he couldn't manage anything anymore and recoiled from even the smallest everyday tasks. This happened not only because the tasks became a burden to him, but because he felt anxious, insecure, and inhibited in all actions. He had not opened his letters and therefore had not paid his bills. Today, he suddenly appears transformed. The reason is that a "switch" from depression to mania has occurred, i.e., in a bipolar affective psychosis, a shift in drive state and mood from one day to the next.

He jumps out of bed, skips breakfast, but after washing, shaving, and choosing his best suit, he rushes out of the apartment and goes to the bank to withdraw money because he has an idea to buy a new, particularly powerful computer. In the bank, he feels superior to the bank employee and is condescending. He is aware that with the computer he plans to buy, he will make a lot of money—because he has a business idea and quickly calls two old acquaintances to arrange a lunch meeting with them. It is known from his family that several members suffer from bipolar affective psychosis. ◀

In addition to the mood "switch," several other areas are suddenly changed in the example, including the various dimensions summarized under the concept of drive.

If we are looking for the level of disturbance, one finds the level of intention formation and the level of action readiness, which is discussed here—the drive level.

Since there is not only psychopathological variance in the direction of an increase in drive but also in the direction of a decrease, we must assume these two directions of change for the concept of drive—which also appear in bipolar affective disorder as mania and depression—a positive pole and a negative pole. This contrasts with attention, where there is only one direction, that of activation. In drive, it is about a threshold of action initiation with facilitation of action initiation and also with a decrementing function, with inhibition.

Example

A patient acted with strong manic drive disinhibition after being admitted to the hospital—he showed highly dynamic, and aggressive behaviors—uttered insults with elements of devaluation and indiscrimination, mixed with sexual uninhibitedness in insinuations and concrete accusations.

We consider the drive area for spontaneous mental activity and everyday actions. In addition, there are many other motor activities that, unlike the person's everyday actions, can be initiated and controlled differently and only partially appear correlated with the drive level: we think of eye movements, clearing one's throat, scratching, instinctive reactions to alarm, nutrition and sexual behavior, etc.

The drive level is complex and it is not certain to what extent it must be divided based on future neuroscientific analyses. It encompasses such diverse domains as intention formation and selection, motor action readiness, interest, expectation of reward, and anxiety-related retardation as well as motor and mental effort.

Explanations that prefer motivation in the sense of reward incentives to explain the phenomena fall short—or the reduction of anxiety-inducing expectations.

For everyone knows the variance of drive through caffeine, alcohol, or perhaps also drugs like amphetamines, cocaine. The aforementioned genetically influenced psychiatric illnesses like mania and bipolar depression affect the drive. The best example is bipolar affective disorder, which can be accompanied by a maximum increase and elimination of one's own drive.

7.1.1 One's Own Drive Versus Externally Motivated Drive

Sensory impressions stimulate thoughts and reactions, but even such reactive mental activity ceases if there is no own drive. Patients in stupor can no longer be stimulated to internal activity by external impressions, that would be externally recognizable. Not even based on eye movement can it be seen that these persons "take part." The separation of one's own drive from externally motivated drive is clinically meaningful, e.g., in a depressive episode, it is primarily one's own drive that fails. This distinction is described in detail by Klages (1967)—(see below).

7.1.2 Unconscious Drive Variables

Decisions for spontaneous acts are mostly not made consciously. Many of the activities of everyday life, following a need, catching up on a postponed action, etc., happen without conscious evaluation of whether and if so, when they should be carried out (it is said that the walk to the refrigerator is almost always not consciously decided). The person experiences themselves as acting out of routine or for understandable reasons, only in some cases is retardation inhibition or driven behavior experienced. The drive state and its disturbances are mostly not conscious.

7.1.3 Amount of Targeted Motor Actions as a Parameter of the Drive State

How appears what we call drive? The amount of spontaneous actions of a person shows us the current drive strength in everyday life. It can fluctuate within the physiological range or be pathologically reduced or increased. This can form a pragmatic basis for clinical drive assessment. In the psychopathological examination, we can observe the amount and dynamics of spontaneous, i.e., obviously person-initiated movements, which are observable in dealing with the person—this includes eye movements and verbal expressions—spontaneous contributions in the interview.

First, the number of spontaneous movements. It is about the amount of actions or movements and with what energy and speed they are carried out—repetitive movements are not counted.

A possible objection is: If one only pays attention to the pragmatic variable of the amount of spontaneous actions, actions that, for example, occurred due to disinhibition (see below) or increased impulsivity etc. also come into play. In these actions, intention formation and decision processes are disturbed.

Principle uncertainty about the influencing factors of observed actions

We do not know in clinical everyday life in most cases whether a consciously matured consideration of reasons led to a planned action or a less controlled impulse, a thoughtless routine. There is a principally uncertainty about the influencing factors of observed actions, which determined a person in his decision. In everyday life, every person pays attention to and assesses the reasoning levels of the actions of others—they try to figure out the intentions and are often wrong.

Another possible objection is that there are rarer situations in which mania does not show itself as described above in restless activity, but in tense dynamics, i.e., not an increased number of spontaneous movements, but a tense expectation, the preparation of a "strike" that the person is determined to carry out, is noticeable.

It should be noted that, as a rule, the amount of spontaneous actions of a person in everyday life gives a good indication of the drive state.

7.1.4 Action Dynamics and Effort

Drive is further assessed based on the dynamics with which a person acts. An example is the dynamics in asserting interests. It describes the concentration and effort in actions and the repeated initiatives, even when setbacks are experienced. This dynamics requires effort. Patients who are in a manic phase invest this effort and pursue their goals with high energy. Information about the dynamics of the action can already be obtained from the force and speed of individual movements of the extremities and the trunk.

Sustained and Phasic Aspects: High dynamics can be observable in a highly motivated single action. This circumstance leads to diagnostic problems. The clinical concept of drive refers to the amount of activities over a certain period, to the characteristic of action readiness of a person that lasts over a certain period—the concept refers to the drive state, the drive level. The drive state cannot be assessed from a single action; because in a single action, it may be a matter of exceptionally high action dynamics due to high specific motivaton for this one single action—with otherwise rather reduced drive state. In the special case of a persistently high motivation—e.g., in an application situation—a persistently high action dynamics must be diagnostically distinguished from a high drive state that cannot be situationally explained.

Motivation is seen as only one factor in the process of premotor integration, as a factor of drive. Motivation is assumed to be psychologically explainable—briefly represented as an effect of goal-related reward expectations. Besides the situational character of high motivation mentioned above, there are apparently biological differences. If only motivation is considered, the phenomena of modification of the amount of spontaneous actions by psychopharmacological effects or drugs respectively cannot be explained—or it would lead to an inappropriate expansion of the concept of motivation. Drive variation occurs in psychiatry in many cases independently of changes in motivation.

The premenstrual syndrome as a hormonally caused disorder usually involves not only emotional changes but also a disturbance in action organization and control. In mania, it even seems that the increased drive incessantly finds new occasions for action, which in turn act as further—temporary—motivators. Many depressive patients feel motivated to act but cannot bring themselves to do so, have no energy left ("battery is empty"), or are immediately maximally exhausted. This is dramatic in highly motivated individuals with depression who suffer from experiencing themselves as tormentingly inhibited, inactive.

The drive is not conceptualized in this way in the Anglo-American language. Rarely is there talk of "urge" or "drive" (Sims 2003).

In cognitive neuroscience, a distinction is made between effortful mental operations and automatic ones. The focus is less on the effort of motor execution, the muscle level, and more on the effort of mental control. Effortful processes are, for example, conscious, while automatic ones usually run unconsciously; effortful actions are controlled by focussed attention. This distinction is important for psychopathology because in depression, effortful mental processes are disturbed, but automatic actions are less so. Fatigue effects also impact automatic processes less than effortful ones.

For applying neuropsychological examination procedures, the question always arises as to how much a patient engages with the task, makes an effort by trying to perform well. This particularly affects performance in effortful tasks. The question is fundamentally important for the interpretaton of test results—but difficult to answer in clinical everyday life.

Conclusion
The level of drive can be clinically assessed best by the amount of spontaneous actions and the dynamics, the energy with which the actions are performed.

7.1.5 Various Factors of the Level of Drive

It is not yet clear which factors determine the extent of the level of drive or, what components the construct "drive" consists of. Therefore, we first consider influencing factors on the everyday variance of drive. Besides the extremes of drive increase or drive decrease, there is also a smaller range of drive variance in actions in everyday life.

What causes a strong level of drive and high action dynamics in everyday life?

a) The group of physiological needs or instincts and their subjectively perceivable side.
b) The group of motivators for reward-related behavior regulation; this group is also related to interest (see below), an entity attributable to affects.
   - Emotional: interest,
   - Intention
   - Reasons that appear to the person as a necessity for action
   - expectation of reward
c) In addition, action readiness should be high, i.e., the availability of action schemes and the willingness to exert oneself.
   - Executive: planning and effectiveness of execution control,
   - action readiness and joy in the execution, willingness to exert effort, discipline
   - effort, concentration (exertion)—physical—mental.

In the listing, the term willpower is replaced by, on the one hand, the willingness to exert effort and, on the other hand, discipline, i.e., the expectation of being able to rely on oneself regarding the performance to be delivered.

It must be assumed that all these influences are integrated into the initiation and dynamics of action, the above-mentioned premotor integration. The forces promoting action in premotor integration are referred to as drive. Mental processes responsible for the amount and dynamics of targeted motor actions thus represent a complex of many dimensions: In the following, we start from stimuli that the person processes, thereby arriving at more or less spontaneous intentions up to actions.

At which points in action preparation is the dynamics of an action modifiable?

A perception
- inspires,
- triggered emotion, ideas/impulses, knowledge about the stimulus, one's own abilities regarding possible actions, general attitude. emotion: interest, curiosity.

The person evaluates
- primary internally generated interest, reasons
- curiosity for exploratory actions.

Current drive strength
- Expectation and hope to achieve values that seem attainable at the moment,
- in the various roles a person plays in everyday life,
- in relation to primary vegetative motivators.

Vegetative needs, instincts etc. (unconscious or conscious)

a) Increase of positive events: motivators in general—in relation to needs and the personal value profile see below, immediate reward, symbolic positive feedback (e.g., receiving praise).

b) Reduction of negative events: defense of anxiety, frustration defense, self-defense, fear of shame.

Energetic Functions

- agitation in the sense of arousal, dynamics, in relation to the primary vegetative motivators drive/instinct, e.g., aggressiveness (Lorenz 1963), hunger, etc.
- Number of ideas, action ideas
- Availability of action associations and action schemes with the readiness to put in an effort for them.

Complex Information Processing for Action Decision

If the amount of spontaneous targeted everyday actions can clinically be considered as a parameter of the drive level, the factors that promote action readiness and initiation must act in the sense of an increase in drive.

Positive

Values and extent of the concrete expectation of reward for the action,

Reward attainability seems high (in relation to resources)—comparison of expectation with the last success (reward prediction error),

Negative

Ambivalences—inner conflict tension, intervening negative intentions, ambivalence in "urge tension" vs. conscience; certain forms of drive disorder can prevent the preparation of the action from being fully completed, so that initiation, the activation of motor units, does not occur,

- motor thresholds are increased,
- action scripts are not available
- Personality factors: Overcontrolled (e.g., overcompensated impulsivity, aggressiveness)
- increased inhibition, anxiety.

Conclusion

The action readiness of a person can thus be both promoted and inhibited at many points of premotor integration.

7.1.6 Ambivalence and Uncertainty of Information about the Process of Intention Formation

In some cases, we come to the assessment that a person has experienced "ambivalence," i.e., the person was torn between two intentions to act. This is referred to as ambitendence. Ambitendence refers to the difficulty in deciding between two action options, while ambivalence refers to the simultaneous presence of two interests or emotional tendencies, e.g., being torn between two feelings or emotional evaluations.

Ambivalence is suspected when observing the person's actions and secondly supported by consistent statements from the person. However, a complete clarification of the factors that led to an intention cannot be expected. We often suspect ambitendence and ambivalence but cannot obtain clarifying information. A person might also be acting out an intention.

7.1.7 Will Versus Drive

The concept of will as an instance in action preparation has practically been abandoned (see above). People feel the sensation of wanting to do something during conscious action decisions.

Here, attention should be drawn to the difficulty or impossibility of sufficiently analyzing action organization into subcomponents. The feeling of wanting to do something is probably a—albeit weakly effective—subcomponent.

7.1.8 Attention and Drive

How does the nonspecific drive state relate to unfocussed and focussed attention (Chap. 4). In states of increased drive, one typically finds clinically hyperattentive states and increased arousal. It is characteristic that people with a depressive syndrome cannot activate themselves and quickly tire when trying to maintain their normal daily activities. Thus, a certain influence on drive by unfocused attention is likely.

For the planning of complex, non-automatic actions, focussed attention is needed, here in the role of executive attention. The planning, control, and motor execution of an action is precisely what characterizes it as an effortful action—and is responsible for the rapid fatigue experienced by the person.

7.2 Clinic

7.2.1 Disorders of the level of drive

Quantitative Change

Undoubtedly, we must distinguish on the one hand a normal variation in the daily amount of targeted motor actions as well as the dynamics with which they are carried out, and on the other hand a pathological variation—pathological reduction or increase in drive level.

Disorder of one's own drive

In brain damage syndromes of the basal ganglia and the prefrontal cortex, clinicians observe a reduction in spontaneous actions, while reactive actions—as execution of instructions—are still carried out.

In abulia, no spontaneous movement is observed (Berrios et al. 1995—akinetic mutism see Förstl and Sahakian 1991). It is considered the most severe disorder of drive. Usually, only simple commands are followed, such as the command to open the eyes, etc. The one's own drive is completely extinguished—in contrast to better-preserved ability to act with externally motivated drive, movement on command. For abulia, also referred to as "state witout will," the problems associated with the concept of will apply: For many of the psychopathological symptoms, the concept of will is dispensable.

Ambitendence

In addition, there are drive disorders that relate to ambivalence. In ambitendence and ambivalence, at least two alternative intentions to act become active. This can be reported by the person, for example, or it becomes clear from observable action approaches. For instance, a patient lingered on the threshold of the ward for a day because he could not decide whether to be admitted or to leave the clinic.

Disorder of intention formation and impulsivity

When a child is distractible in school, it follows, e.g., both the stimuli of the environment and spontaneous ideas. On the one hand, there is a disorder of focussed attention in everyday life. In testing, patients with "attention deficit disorder" usually do not show neuropsychological attention disorders, although the picture of disturbed behavior in school would suggest this. Accordingly, the students are persistently attentive in their preferred hobbies. They can also attentively devote themselves to a matter in a critical situation; however, they fail in everyday routine—for example, school—when it is experienced as boring and laborious. The allocation, in a sense the investment, of focussed attention on the currently relatively low expectation of reward of school activities, does not succeed. This seems to be particularly true for young male students.

A second area of disorder in Attention Deficit Syndrome is impulsivity and disinhibition. This also applies to manic syndromes. In mania, for example, disinhibition of control by reward incentives may occurs, which come to the person's mind and are then pursued for a short time until new goals determine the actions.

The disorder of behavioral control can involve the lack of suppression of actions that a person would reluctantly perform but feels involuntarily drawn to, and that would be

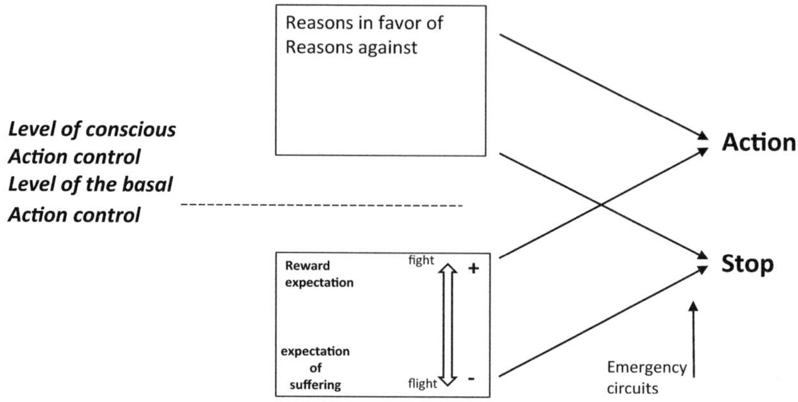

Fig. 7.1 Influences on the one hand on the initiation or on the other hand the stopping of an action—on the one hand at the level of conscious action decision—on the other hand at a basal level of action tendecies: At the first level, the person consciously weighs the reasons for or against the action. At the second level, the—mostly unconscious—control of actions is dominated by several axes of antagonistic influences: e.g., fight—flight, expectation of reward—anxiety, high rank—low rank (high self-esteem—low self-esteem), approach—withdrawal (interest—disinterest), sense of competence—incompetence, readiness to act—not ready to act

automatically performed without conscious control. Impulse control is often disturbed in psychiatry, but the term seemingly describes homogeneous psychopathological phenomena.

Conclusion

Disorder of the drive level is a pragmatic term for a heterogeneously caused change in the amount and dynamics of spontaneous actions, which often cannot be further specified. (Fig. 7.1).

When assessing a person's action, it is possible to diagnostically narrow down which of the possible influencing factors were effective. However, ultimately, one will not be able to reliably identify the decisive influencing factors in detail in that case; this is a problem for the forensic assessment of crimes—especially those committed by mentally ill individuals.

7.3 Diagnostics

The components of generating spontaneous actions mentioned above correspond to those of the psychopathological examination. Thus, it makes sense to address the dimensions of drive in interviews and to observe them in behavior. This results in questions that are included in the interview for psychiatric exploration. For example, in a patient voluntary actions may be absent for one of various reasons or a bundle of different deficits.

When securing a characteristic, a number of situational marginal factors must be excluded differential- diagnostically to arrive at a reliable psychopathological evaluation. Situational marginal factors of the drive level are motivation or demoralization, fatigue, and somatic illness behavior as in heart failure, or diagnostically disturbing marginal factors such as restriction of cooperation (especially in neuropsychological examination procedures), possibility of simulation, etc. Many people do not like to talk about their reasons for action; in addition, they often do not consciously or falsely experience these reasons for action.

Action tendencies and actions that do not occur purely reactively (such as chasing away a fly) are assessed. The assessment of action dynamics is based on observations of how decisively, attentively, determinedly, and effortfully the person acts. In doing so, the premorbid level of everyday activity and action dynamics must be determined through third-party anamnesis.

Dimensions

- Reduction or increase in interest in actions, appreciation, and motivators that lead to absent or increased amount of actions,
- specific disorders in the initiation of actions (impulsivity, manipulative behavior, etc.).

Differential diagnostic attention is paid to 2 domains:

1. Specific other disorders of the activation of action executions, executive disorder, lack of planning, etc. Disorder of the control of the organization of actions,
2. Disorder of central motor skills or executive function— motor characteristics of an absent action (Chap. 5).

Understandable reasons for actions

In every psychiatric exploration, an attempt is made to work out to what extent the decisions or actions of a person are understandable from their life circumstances. In doing so, demoralization and fear, etc., or hopes and understandable prospects of success are sought as reasons for active actions or the omission of activities.

Content factors of drive

Attempts are often made to understand the reasons for changes in drive from the biographical background information known about the patient. In psychoanalytic literature, groups of factors are assumed into which drive factors can be categorized. For example, there is acquisition (or wanting to have), search for familiarity, desire for physical affection, cleanliness, social respect or recognition, and sexual needs. In behavior therapy, such factors are considered in behavior analysis. The clinical examination of these motivators or drive factors lies beyond what can be described in this clinical psychopathology.

Observation at actions for assessing the level of drive

Emotion

- interest, eye movements (in part during the interview),
- joy in activities.

action readiness

- motor: action latency, motor dynamics
- cognitive: movement, action ideas (in part during the interview).

Motivation

- extern: expectation of reward (in part during the interview),
- intern: convictions etc. (in part during the interview).

effort

- motor: strength, acceleration, dynamics, dealing with environmental resistances
- cognitive: effort, concentration (in part during the interview, tests).

Planning (in part during the interview)

Planning

A person with a high level of drive who has planned an action can sit quietly and wait for a certain moment. They must wait to act further and are aware of this. Other people in such a situation walk around restlessly. This motor restlessness is not referred to as increased drive.

It is noticeable that in the psychopathology of actions, dimensions occur that are oriented against each other, such as impulsivity, which indicates action readiness, and planning, which can signal efficient organization with strong action readiness. Planning of actions can collapse in an impulsive person or in mania due to strong, intervening impulses by following the impulses.

According to the various dimensions of the drive level, several general domains of disturbance must be assessed:

1. In the emotional domain, the interest: disinterest, disengagement,
2. in the domain of motivators:
   - loss of reinforcers; or in motivation by anxiety of loss: decrease of anxiety,
   - internal motivators: loss of appetite, abandonment of dominance efforts, etc.,

3. effort: vital fatigue as in sickness behavior, exhaustibility,
4. action readiness and activation: hypoarousal, reduced focussed attention; disturbed action control
5. action planning: apraxia, dysexecutive states.

7.4 Neuroscience

In neuroscience, the drive and motivation area is attributed to frontal lobe functions (Rolls 1999). Only future neuroscientific research can differentiate the underlying frontal lobe functions. Despite the diversity of frontal lobe functions (Danek 2005; Reischies 2005), it becomes clear how difficult it is to explain a large number of phenomena with the few basic mechanisms known so far.

These arguments lead to the conclusion: Before the action, the representations of external motivators, internal reasons for action, and "drives" must be integrated into an information processing system to trigger the action of the person; we refer to this phase as premotor integration.

7.4.1 Neurophysiology of Self-Generated Actions

Considerable progress has already been made in the field of distinguishing reactive actions from self-generated actions. This was possible by examining the same actions in two different constellations:

1. the action occurs as a learned reaction to an external stimulus and
2. the action occurs without an external stimulus, thus internally generated.

It became convincingly clear that different brain regions are involved. Here, the self-generated action is of particular interest. It almost always occurred after the »Supplementary Motor Area« (SMA) was activated (Mushiake et al. 1991), which could be confirmed in imaging studies (Jenkins et al. 1994). This led to the concept that self-generated actions are planned in prefrontal brain areas and processed in the SMA. Apparently, motor discharges can be directly triggered from the SMA. The »Supplementary Motor Area« is connected in a frontal cortico-subcortical projection loop (frontal lobe) with the Basal ganglia.

The variables that manifest in the variation of drive must therefore affect the information processing before the release of motor acts in the SMA. The prefrontal brain areas and the Basal ganglia have already been mentioned as involved brain structures.

7.4.2 Neurophysiology of Drive Elements

The following will present the influencing factors of interest, value representation, concrete reward expectation, and action pressure due to needs. Intentions are also formed in the effort to avoid anxiety (Chap. 11 emotion and affect).

Interest in new events and action readiness
One approach to explain the variance in action readiness is based on emotions. According to neuropsychological conception (Frijda 1986), the various emotions are closely coupled with specific action readiness. In the case of interest and joy, this is in the direction of increased action readiness. Interest as a fundamental emotion (Chap. 11 emotion and affect) and curiosity behavior are still scarcely researched neuroscientifically.

Ccuriosity appears to be innate and shows itself early; it is crucial for the child's development. When a child is presented with something new, it seems to be delighted and approaches the new thing. This can likely be explained by a coupling between novelty and reward, which has been confirmed in neurophysiological studies. Dopaminergic neurons in the ventral striatum respond not only to reward but also to new things (Schultz 2004).

When a new stimulus is processed, initially a

1. »familiarity signal« will be absent, as the stimulus is not recognized. Therefore, in the second step, it must be identified whether the new thing can pose a danger. According to neuroscientific data, it is assumed that the stimulus information is processed by the
2. Amygdala. If it detects an object of fear or a context that suggests negative events, the so-called inhibition system is activated, which is also responsible for flight behavior (Chap. 11 emotion and affect; Fight-Flight Axis). If this is not the case, we can assume that the
3. dopaminergic neurons of the ventral tegmental area (VTA) activate the "reward" system. It activates, among other things, an approach behavior.

Action due to vegetative needs

A second approach is based on internal motivators. Instincts and drives have been discussed. Vegetative needs such as hunger or the urge to urinate prompt a person to make action decisions. An insightful example is that hunger changes the perception—the hungry person perceives food sources, approaches them, or becomes aware of them; however, when satiated, the food source is no longer perceived.

Action to reduce anxiety

Furthermore, a pressure to act is observed, into which a person enters in order to avoid negative emotions. Many actions are carried out to escape the negative consequences of inaction, such as sanctions, anger with parents, partners, or superiors. They are, like the reactions to expectation of reward, in a mediated sense, reactive actions, i.e., with knowledge of the person and the environmental events, the actions and also the energy in their execution are understandable.

Action based on values, motivation

Imagine, for example, a buffet where a person is standing in line and already surveying which dishes match their personal taste; they choose accordingly. On the second trip to the buffet, something may have changed: The person is already somewhat satiated and, above all, a concrete negative or positive experience with the dishes modifies the selection criteria. What has happened: The satiation changes the interest and the intention formation and the experience of the concrete quality of the dishes changes the selection criteria. There is a flexibility in the appreciation of dishes, the favorite dishes from the general value catalog are updated for the specific buffet.

Cortical neurons have been studied regarding their preference for objects. Neurons were found in the orbitofrontal cortex that showed a preference order for food.

Neurophysiological studies of prefrontal neuronal activity can explain why patients with damage to these brain areas have problems with spontaneous action initiation.

Orbitofrontal neurons encode reward after actions (Thorpe et al. 1983; Rolls 1999) and thus represent the values that can be achieved through actions. Reward is not represented solely in the orbitofrontal cortex but also, for example, in the amygdala. The neuronal activity of orbitofrontal neurons is more specific when the expected reward fails to appear, - in terms of the relation of rewards of different choice objects (Thorpe et al. 1983; Tremblay and Schultz 1999). The flexible change in behavior after a change in the reward assignment to actions is especially disordered after lesions of the orbitofrontal cortex (Wisconsin Card Sorting Test, clinically see Rolls 2000). It has been concluded that in the orbitofrontal cortex, the construction and adjustment of the expectation of reward can be achieved with the control of incoming or absent feedback after actions, and thus a significant part of the information processing for motivation.

Reward signals are information about the absolute values of an object or even just symbolic values (O'Doherty et al. 2001). In the case of symbolic values, the reward is not directly given by a reinforcer.

Expectation of reward in the specific situation

In addition to the value of an action category, etc., the expectation of reward of the current action execution is crucial at every moment for whether the action is carried out. The example of the buffet illustrated (see above) how the expectation of reward is adjusted at every moment.

> A systematic overestimation of the probability of reward is observed in mania and conversely, the underestimation with a pessimistic expectation of success in depression.

It seems that people with very severe depression no longer read and also do not think because the lost expectation of reward is also crucially necessary for cognitive activities. Without expectation of reward, nothing happens—the person also stops thinking—the expectation of reward is virtually the currency with which transactions are made in the CNS.

The role of the described dopaminergic influence on the expectation of reward is evidenced by the physiology of addiction, in which people are driven to repeatedly seek and consume addictive substances (This apparently also applies to non-substance-related addictions). Physiologically, this has been analyzed in self-stimulation studies (Rolls 1999). Dopamine might be necessary in the brain's information processing to highlight a stimulus among others due to its significance for a future reward—"incentive salience" (Berridge and Robinson 1998).

Reward prediction error

The orbitofrontal cortex is closely connected with the ventral striatum and the ventral tegmental area. Neurons of the ventral tegmentum have a function in the processing of expectation of reward related to an event (Schulz et al. 2004; Fig. 7.2). The level of neuronal activity of the dopaminergic neurons can be explained by the prediction error, the difference between the expected reward and the reward received after an action (reward-prediction error). When a living being desires a reward, an object, because this object promises, for example, to satisfy hunger, it will change its behavior. This behavioral

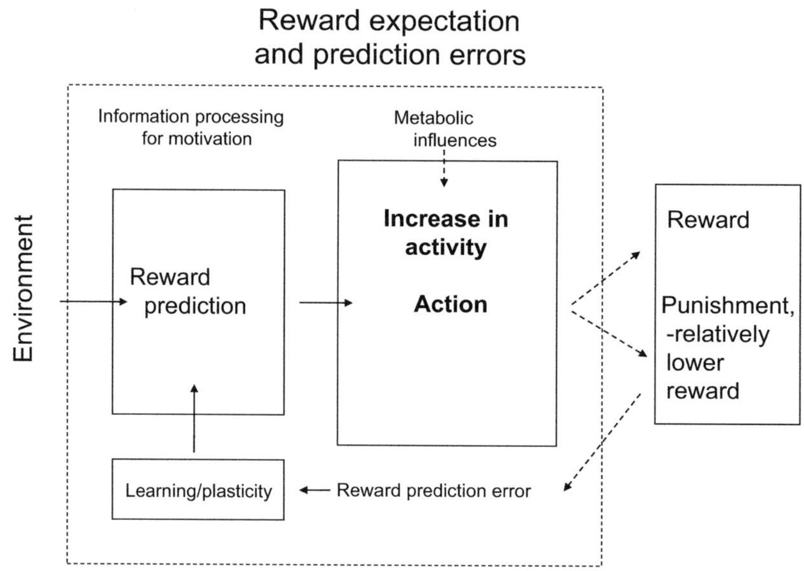

Fig. 7.2 A portion of the variance of drive is explained by variables of the reward system, especially with the expectation of reward. It is a behavioral learning model. In this process, the organism learns, after an expectation of reward has been determined, depending on the current feedback, whether the action needs to be changed or can remain the same. Here, the expectation of reward is particularly important, influencing whether and with what dynamics the action is performed. The neuronal systems, nerve cells, transmitters, and receptors that mediate the expectation of reward are disrupted in mental illnesses and can be pharmacologically/toxically modified

change will persist until it has reached the object or the expectation is reduced, for example, because the object is not attainable or not able to satisfy the hunger. The prediction error is the crucial variable for explaining the learning of behavior (Montague et al. 2004).

In recent years, the prediction error has been supplemented with the expected future reward in the description of the function of dopaminergic neurons. The special kind of future reward, the "reward saliency," is important in this context. Thus, not only the difference between expected and actual reward but also a weighted expectation of the next reward describes the behavior of neurons in the ventral tegmental area (Montague et al. 2004; Marschner et al. 2005).

Sequences of Frontal Loops in Premotor Integration

A series of frontal cortical-subcortical projection loops has been described, which are of particular importance for psychiatry (Cummings 1993). As a first frontal lobe loop, we consider the loop that involves the orbitofrontal cortex (see Middleton and Strick 2000). This loop runs through the ventral striatum (nucleus accumbens), the ventral pallidum, and the mediodorsal thalamus back to the orbitofrontal cortex. The connection of the mentioned brain areas has been investigated in more detail. The orbitofrontal cortex projects to the nucleus accumbens of the ventral striatum and to the ventral tegmental area. The nucleus accumbens, in turn, receives the psychiatrically important dopaminergic innervation from the ventral tegmentum. From the nucleus accumbens, the information is also projected back to the cortex via the ventral pallidum and the mediodorsal thalamus (Houk et al. 1995). It has been unclear so far why the connection from the ventral pallidum to the mediodorsal thalamus is only very sparsely developed. In any case, this loop seems less suitable for processing very large amounts of information simultaneously, and the data on the functions of the nucleus accumbens suggest that the structure is involved in the more general release of motor functions, etc., and not so much in the concrete detailed information processing of complex motor preparation.

Other loops involve the dorsolateral prefrontal cortex, which seems to be engaged in working memory and its updating, and the anterior cingulum (Tanji et al. 2002; Fig. 7.3).

The motor implementation apparently occurs in collaboration with the anterior cingulum. Its neurons have their function in preparing a specific alternative action—especially after the absence of reward for the first action (Shima and Tanji 1998). The reward information from the orbitofrontal cortex is conveyed to the anterior cingulum. It has been shown that neurons can be found there that are active when switching to the alternative action chosen after the absence of reward for the first action. These neurons do not encode an action switch that occurs "passively" on request. These data have been interpreted as an indication of a role for these neurons in voluntary action initiation.

The neurophysiological data presented here can explain the internally generated action triggering more closely: After the information that the expectation of reward for an action is high, this action is initiated. In doing so, the information is first passed on from the orbitofrontal cortex, ventral tegmentum, and nucleus accumbens via the orbitofrontal-ventral striatal projection loops to neighboring cortex areas. In the manner of screw threads, as a figurative illustration, the information is thus passed on to the next cortical-subcortical projection loops. In the process of premotor integration, the dorsolateral prefrontal loops are involved. This happens until the preparation of the motor action in the anterior cingulum. The inclusion of information from working memory and knowledge occurs in this way.

The neurophysiological data and concepts can help explain a deficit in patients with prefrontal brain damage in feedback-sensitive test procedures (Wisconsin Card Sorting Test, Object Reversal Test, Cantab-Shift-Test—see probability Object Reversal Test, Reischies 1999a, b). In many cases, the failure of actions directed at satisfying one's own needs is observed. A deficit in patients in the initiation of spontaneous actions can be explained with the data.

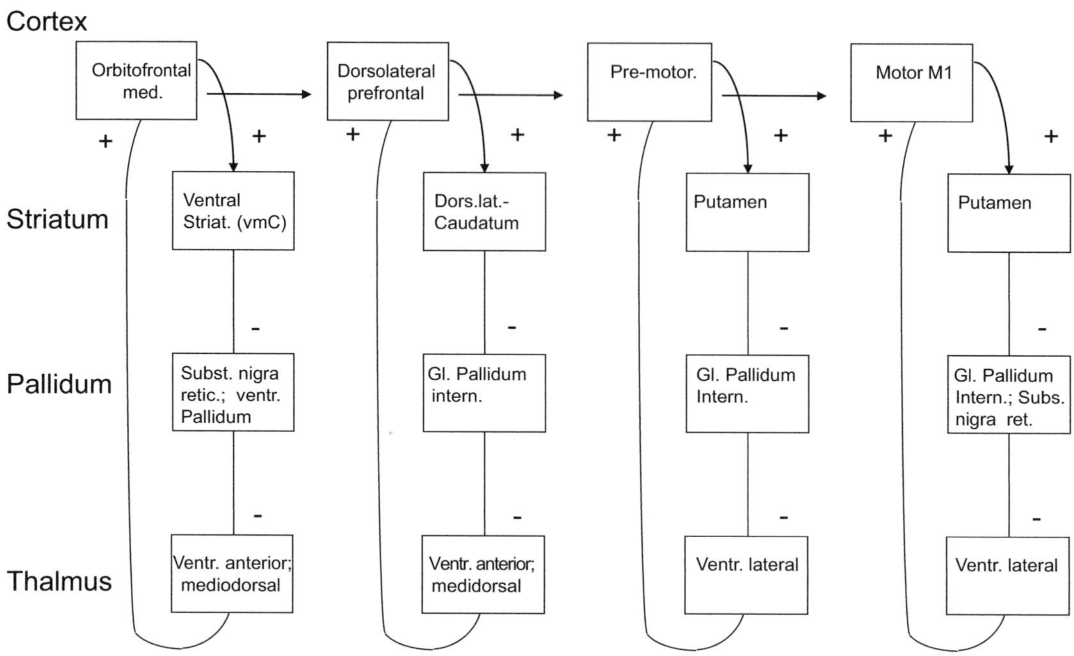

Fig. 7.3 Cortical-subcortical projection loops (frontal loops). Each cortex area is connected in a loop via specific areas of the striatum, pallidum, and thalamus with itself and the immediate surroundings. One of the functions of this system is to regulate the thalamocortical afferent to the cortex. For action initiation and drive, the orbitofrontal loops are apparently important. The model of a sequence of activation in the orbitofrontal cortex, in the next step an activation of the dorsolateral prefrontal loops, and then the premotor and motor loops is depicted. The dopaminergic system has a central activating effect here, acting in the striatum and pallidum (as well as in the frontal cortex).

Once an action is learned and can be performed implicitly, the absence of positive feedback (or negative feedback) in healthy individuals can lead to the development of a behavioral alternative. This does not occur after damage to the orbitofrontal network and can also explain why there is a disturbance in behavioral flexibility, especially why actions of these patients are still performed even when they are no longer rewarded.

7.4.3 Model of Neurons in Premotor Integration

Each neuron in the brain receives many excitatory and inhibitory influences at the synapses of the neurons connected to it. The neuron integrates this information for discharge at its axon, which transmits the information further. We can assume that the integrating function of activating and inhibitory influences is already inherent in the basic neuronal constellation (see textbooks of neurophysiology).

How can we conceptualize that in the preparation of an action, the signal of a neuron group in the motor cortex is ultimately processed to trigger the motor action (at least the initiation of the spinal motor action)?

Accumulators in Action Preparation

The study of the physiology of rapid movements has led to the model of accumulators: Motor neurons or other neurons directly influencing motor function accumulate the afference—both activating and inhibiting—over the preparation time of a planned action. Precursors were models of reaction time, which described the change of the membrane potential through the integration of excitatory postsynaptic potentials (EPSPs) until the threshold for triggering the action potential is reached. They modeled the temporal arrival of the EPSPs as a "random walk" of the membrane potential and attempted to describe these conditions mathematically. These models could explain the temporal relations and errors in rapid reactions (Smith and Ratcliff et al. 2004; Usher and McClelland 2001).

During the preparation time of an action, it is decided whether movement A or another movement (B) will be executed. The decision for action A thus results from the relative activation and thereby the speed of activating the neurons belonging to the action scheme A until the threshold of the action potential is reached. If a neuron is activated to trigger action potentials, it recruits the next neurons whose action scheme it represents, and the action is motorically realized. In the decision of whether reaction A or B takes place, errors occur, as observed in reaction time experiments.

According to the accumulator models, a separate instance does not decide which action is performed; rather, the decision is made by the neuronal motor unit. When the threshold is reached in the premotor integration phase, it then inhibits the alternative accumulating neurons ("the winner takes it all" principle). The accumulator model elegantly bypasses an otherwise demanding decision algorithm. This would have to perform the selection of action schemes. However, evidence for an independent decision apparatus has not been found.

According to an accumulator model, the psychopathology of drive with drive reduction and drive increase could play out in this process. A change in threshold or an inhibitory tone in the premotor integration process can lead to a reduction in the number of successfully initiated actions and vice versa. It must be assumed that a reset of the accumulators occurs after a preparation and action cycle.

In summary: Neurons involved in action initiation exhibit

1. a "random walk," i.e., the membrane potential shows a random variation of the membrane potential at rest at the many thousands of synapses of afferent neurons—but in action preparation, a systematic activation occurs only through the incoming information for the generation of a specific action. Therefore, the movement of the membrane potential shows a systematic drift due to the specific information for action preparation.
2. The system can force a decision: At the moment of decision, a general change of the membrane potential of many accumulators leads to an action. In a way, this forces the determination of the highest probability of the correct action. However, this leads to an increase in error probability, as depicted by the increase in arousal through noradrenergic neurons (Chap. 4 attention). These error probabilities have been described in the study of elementary reactions and reaction times.

7.4.4 Illusion of Self-Attribution of Action Initiation

In stimulation experiments, evidence was found for central action-organizing brain regions; it was examined how the subjective experience of passive movement is, which was triggered by CNS stimulation. (1) In subcortical/spinal stimulation with movement initiation, there was a denial by the person—they did not experience that they had initiated the movement. (2) When stimulation of the central action-planning cortex areas was performed, the person believed they had wanted the action; specifically: When the movement was triggered in the motor cortex, the person experienced it as imposed. However, if the stimulation that led to the movement was set in the supplementary motor area, the person said, "I was just about to perform the movement." The supplementary motor area is thus an area that lies at least near the region where spontaneous movements are triggered.

From such experiments, it has also been concluded that the introspection of drive, intention, and action organization is unreliable (example: advertising and purchase decision). This already points to the distinction between conscious and unconscious action initiation (Chap. 8 consciousness).

In spontaneously initiated actions, there seems to be a binding phenomenon that binds a correlated cortex event for the person to the moment of the subjectively beginning intention, although temporally disparate events have occurred (Libet et al. 1983; Haggard et al. 2002). The information processing from the first-person perspective is accompanied by mediofrontal brain activity (Vogeley et al. 2004).

7.4.5 Metabolic Effects on Action Preparation and the Amount of Spontaneous Actions

The data described above suggest that for the subjective side of the acting person, there is a connection to the experienced intentionality of a movement, whether self-initiated or induced as a fixed reaction by stimulation. However, it also follows that a lack of action due to a disturbance in this region is not experienced as a failure of one's own action, but not at all, i.e., the person does not notice that they are acting less. Apparently, there is no "meta" level that monitors the absence of spontaneous actions. This leads to the assumption that the felt intention must be identical to or strongly overlapped with the above-described preparation process of actions. A tormenting slowdown is reported by only a few Parkinson's patients, and the depressive retardation must be seen as a special problem of laborious information processing. These considerations are consistent with what is also suggested by the Libet experiments (Libet et al. 1983; Yazawa et al. 2000), which showed that the perceived intention occurs only after the beginning of the buildup of the prefrontal readiness potential in medial prefrontal brain areas (SMA).

Dopaminergic influences

The innervation of the basal ganglia has a decisive impact on the initiation of movements; in its disturbance, a bradyphrenia has been reported (Shipley et al. 2002). For a long time, the increase in drive in mania was treated solely with neuroleptics, i.e., through antidopaminergic effects. Additionally, the general sedative effect of neuroleptics was utilized. As a side effect, a pseudo-parkinsonian rigidity of the extremities is unpleasantly experienced.

Valproate as a medication that apparently generally reduces the initiation of action potentials, has a known effect on the increase in activity (Bell et al. 2005; in combination with lithium, Reischies et al. 2002). It is unclear at which point in the brain the decisive reduction in actions occurs. It is conceivable that there is a pharmacological effect on the distributed network functions required in the process of action preparation; whereby the cell membranes that cause the action initiation become less frequently suprathreshold.

7.4.6 Neurobiology of Psychomotor Disorders

What is the relationship of these neuroscientific findings to psychomotor disorders or disorders of voluntary motor function? We have seen how action initiation must influence the individual, quasi "elementary" processes of movement initiation.

For the reasons mentioned, it seems justifiable to present psychomotor disorders at this point. They can be explained by misregulations in the process of voluntary or involuntary movement initiation.

7.5 Psychopathological Symptoms of Drive and Psychomotor Function

Characteristics of Drive Reduction

The first symptom, the loss of interest, is usually represented in emotions. The interest represents one of the psychopathologically fundamental variables of drive, as described above. For this reason, this characteristic is classified in the drive section.

loss of interest
Definition. A person experiences himselve as less oriented towards the environment, feels less intentionality and action readiness regarding the things, people, tasks, or opportunities in his lifeworld. It is a subjective aspect, specifically the affective part of drive reduction.

Reduction in the triggering of attention; reduction in emotional expression (e.g., facial expressions and gestures)—on the cognitively conscious and communicative level and the action readiness.

Example

A patient who previously took an active interest in everything and paid attention to everything new, viewing it with interest—also in order to seek his opportunities, reports that he experiences less and less interest; he does not take part, sees no opportunities, sits motionless on a chair, and eventually hardly looks around the room. ◀

Position in Psychopathology. Subsumed under drive reduction in AMDP.

Psychopathological Interactions. Disappointment over loss, grief, loss of vitality, loss of energy.

Differential Diagnostic Distinctions. lack of drive, anxious inhibition, shameful inhibition.

Self-/other persons's judgment. Introspection data and observation, assessed by the examiner.

Interview for Rating. Question about the feeling of interest in everyday life, history taken from other persons.

Neuropsychology/objectification. Behavioral observation (interview, practice, clinic), also history taken from other persons; characteristic: attention-associated movements (eye, trunk movements, gestures, etc.); assessment of the reaction when trying to elicit interest.

Severity. Slight relative reduction from the old level—only to be assessed by close acquaintances—to complete loss of any interest.

Conceptual Problems of the Characteristic. To be isolated from depressive syndrome, as also in dementia and negative symptoms of schizophrenia.

Neuroscientific/Cognitive Neuroscientific Models
interest is one of the fundamental emotions (Chap. 11 emotion and affect).

Lack of drive
Definition. A person shows reduced targeted activity; the amount of spontaneous actions and action tendencies is reduced for actions that do not occur purely reactively (such as swatting a fly) or are based on external motivation.

Example

A premorbidly active, lively patient just sits around, responds curtly to address, and initiates neither motor activities nor verbal communication. In conversation, he neither follows up nor contradicts (except when very personally important conflicts are discussed).

The reduction is not attributable to another factor, such as deliberate, intentional omission of actions, refusal, motor impairment, consciousness disorders, etc. ◀

Position in Psychopathology. AMDP 80.

Related Terms. abulia

Psychopathological Interactions. Loss of interest, poverty of thought, retardation, anxiety.

Differential Diagnostic Distinctions. Apathy includes a deficit on the recipient side with fewer sensations, so the person also reacts less—often difficult to differentiate from lack of drive.

- depressive stupor, catatonic stupor (see below),
- akinetic mutism,

To be distinguished: language comprehension and perception disorders,
- Consciousness disorders,
- Motor slowing,
- Severe muscular weakness or, for example, inactivity due to severe heart failure,
- Active protective posture in, for example, psychotic experiences that would be experienced during activity (or, for example, commanded by phonemes),
- Active resisted, refusal (in externally motivated drive),
- Autism.

Further characterization. Differentiation of the lack of actions in various areas is often informative: spontaneous activity of the person, actions for oneself, activity in externally motivated drive, psychomotor reactions, reactive activity.

Self-/other persons' judgment. Other persons' judgment

Interview for rating. Question about self-assessment of the current "drive," discuss one's own drive and externally motivated drive, history taken from other persons necessary.

Neuropsychology/objectification. Behavioral observation in the interview or, for example, on the ward with the feature: interruptions and interjections of the patient (in relation to expected activity), behavior in everyday life.

Severity. Fewer activities than usual up to complete failure of drive in stupor.

Specifications: Attempting a pathogenetic specification
- Loss of reinforcement, lack of motivation,
- Lack of arousal,
- Executive deficit,
- Increased threshold of activities, lack of self-confidence, anxiously controlling inhibition,
- Emotional factors: reduced curiosity, aggression.

Social domain:
- Social withdrawal,
- Objective reduction of social contacts,
- Reduced eye contact,

Subjective:
a) Active—isolating oneself—(e.g. as a protection),
b) Passive—lack of maintenance of social contacts.

Professional domain (related to plans)

Conceptual problems of the symptom. Heterogeneity is considerable, see subjective drive domain often different from objective.

Neuroscientific/cognitive neuroscientific models
1. Motivation, values or rewards and/or their attainability low,
   - Reinforcer loss situation objectively or as a disturbance of the CNS mechanisms of motivation (organic reinforcer loss situation; Reischies 1999a, b),
2. Arousal level and dynamics low,
   - Arousal deficiency situation,
3. executive processing of action schemes cannot or cannot fully take place, so that the final activation of the motor units does not occur,
   - Executive deficit,
4. Motor threshold is too high, therefore weak impulses remain inefficient,
5. lack of self-confidence as part of the depressive syndrome,
6. endocrinological influences.

Stupor
Definition. State of massively reduced or abolished drive.

Example

Severe manifestation of drive reduction. A patient is admitted to a clinic lying down. He says nothing and does not comply with any requests, but seems to be awake as he has his eyes some times open. He can be made to sit up. Even then, he does not perform any spontaneous or induced movements. It later turns out that a bipolar affective disorder is known. ◀

Position in psychopathology. Not in AMDP.

Related terms. Lack of drive

Differential diagnostic distinctions: important distinction from sopor and transition to coma:
- When excluding sopor, pay attention to neurological symptoms: paresis or tone (weight of the arm when dropped onto the bed), peripheral reflexes;
- Brainstem symptoms: corneal reflex, pupillary reflexes, eye movement and doll's head phenomenon, breathing;
- especially signs of herniation; for details see neurological examination of unconscious patients
- Emotional stupor in severe emotions, or after trauma,
- Dissociative stupor:
  a) related to emotional stupor,
  b) caution: used manipulatively (see histrionic), consider history taken from other persons.

Further characterization. The patients blink very rarely.

Self-/other persons's judgment. Only other persons's judgment.

Interview for rating. Attempt simple, obvious requests, e.g., to lie more comfortably, to drink something, etc.

Neuropsychology/objectification. Observation by nursing staff and family.

Severity. Mild: simplest instructions for elementary motor skills are followed.

Specifications
- stupor, depressive,
- catatonic—often also negativism, e.g., resistance when opening the eyes,

Neuroscientific/cognitive neuroscientific models: akinetic mutism (exclude neurological lesions in the diencephalon or in the "supplementary motor area").

Inhibition of Drive
Definition. Experience of difficulty in starting an action or initiating a motor act. The person may feel that the limbs appear heavier than before.

Example

A person experiences that he cannot bring himselve to do things he considers extremely important—as if they are blocked. In some cases, one can observe that the person abandons attempts to act, i.e., he muster the effort but immediately give up again.

In contrast to loss of interest, the person experiences a inhibition of an action that interests him. ◀

Position in psychopathology. AMDP 81.

Related terms. Inhibition as a personality trait, in relation to social anxiety

Psychopathological interactions. Lack of physical freshness, fatigue, increased reaction to negative stimuli, interference from anxiety impulses.

Differential diagnostic distinctions:
- Personality trait: inhibition as general anxiety or shyness, expressed in overly cautious behavior,
- Simulation, aggravation.

Self-/other persons' judgment. Question about a peculiar feeling of inhibition of movements, more effort in daily activities, other persons' judgment necessary.

Interview for rating. Exploration of the person's previous daily drive and the current reduction in these domains. Relation to premorbid level, especially important if predominantly only subjective drive inhibition and not also obviously objective drive reduction is present.

Neuropsychology/objectification. Behavioral observation is not sensitive enough for slight retardation, but useful as objectification—characteristic: attempts to act are made but abandoned. Observation during neuropsychological examination tasks.

Severity. Mild to severely distressing.

Pathognomonic for: Depression.

Personality influences. The question is not answered to what extent inhibition as a personality trait interacts.

Conceptual problems of the feature. Questionably reliably diagnosable item, as it is often difficult to convey by language and apparently not easily accessible to introspection.

Neuroscientific/cognitive neuroscientific models: Dissociation in the motivational and executive-motor area: the decision to act can be made, but the motor action cannot be initiated: Possible is the experience of elementary motor problems in depression as heavy limbs, "sticking of the foot sole to the ground" and difficulties in climbing stairs, which were not previously experienced—not yet sufficiently investigated.

Mutism
Definition. Reduced amount of speech activity and speech acts.

Example

A person no longer speaks—but otherwise behaves inconspicuously.

Specific drive poverty reduction in the speech area can be assumed on the one hand; mutism can also occur for other reasons (exploration of specific environmental influences). ◀

Position in psychopathology. AMDP 87.

Related terms: Taciturn, reticent.

Psychopathological interactions. Delusion-induced muteness (prohibition to speak), anxiety and emotional exceptional situation—stress situation, dissociation, not fully conscious resistance attitude.

Differential Diagnostic Distinctions:
- consciously intended refusal to speak in a situation where a statement, e.g., in court, is to be made,
- aphasia,
- dysarthria/anarthria (laborious attempts to speak).

Self-/other persons' judgment. Other persons' judgment.

Interview for Rating. Interview attempt in writing, history taken from other persons.

Neuropsychology/objectification:
Observation of speech behavior:

1. Spontaneously little to no speech production,
2. Responses terse to none, normal articulation, quieter than usual?
3. Necessary communications (longer observation and history taken from other persons) terse to none.

Severity: Terse to mute.

Specifications:
- see lack of drive—Specifications,
- in conflict situations, with histrionic personality,
- depression: speech acts in the sense of taking care of one's own affairs are neglected.
- Writing as a substitute strategy possible?

Neuroscientific/cognitive neuroscientific models: S. lack of drive.

Specification:
- somatic,
- social.

Ambivalent/ambitendent
Definition. Opposing evaluations, emotions, or action tendencies are activated, which contradict each other, so that no action occurs; the person feels torn between two feelings or action tendencies.

Example

A patient disagrees with being admitted to a psychiatric clinic but does not leave the ward; he explains that he cannot accept being in the clinic but feels, for example, safer than on the street and in his apartment.

- A woman experiences severe feelings of hatred towards a man but feels strong affection for him and is sexually attracted (ambivalent). ◀

Position in Psychopathology. AMDP 75.

Related Terms. Decision, action conflict.

Differential Diagnostic Distinctions:
Inhibition of decision-making (thought and drive inhibition) in depression—an indecisiveness that also affects decisions without alternatives
- planned phase of decision-making—like in a "brainstorming" exercise,
- unconscious conflictual, which can be suspected, but the person cannot say anything about it.

Interview for Rating. When asking about a person's feelings or actions, inquire whether opposing feelings or tendencies are also experienced.

Severity. Mild and occasional decision delay and conflictual in decisions up to complete blockage or inability to decide in practically all areas.

Specifications:
- two values or two sensations are in conflict (ambivalent),
- two intentions to act are in conflict—referred to as ambitendent. In this context, so-called displacement activities are also observed (a concept from behavioral research).

Personality influences. Conscientious personality, which has scruples about overlooking minor inconsistencies.

Neuroscientific/cognitive neuroscientific models
1. An action cannot be realized due to a
   - manifest conflict of action on the motivational level
   - or an executive disorder—e.g., with insufficient inhibition of the "inferior" action option.
2. Tendencies that do not have to be conscious, which have developed in the person and which affect concrete decisions in the sense of ambivalence/ambitendence. The investigator can infer them from the overall situation; he will try to address and clarify them with the person, for example.

Features with increased drive

Increased Drive

Definition. The amount of targeted activities and the energy invested in one's own activities are increased; the dynamics in behavior are heightened. Full drive kicks in with offers and opportunities.

Example

A person is in a state of increased action readiness, it is noticeable that he is full of energy and constantly show initiative. He assert himmselve in many small matters, but also in far-reaching goals that he pursues with commitment. In the case of resistance to his interests, he may react aggressively. ◀

Position in psychopathology. AMDP 82.

Related terms. Part of the manic syndrome, overmotivated, enthusiasm.

Psychopathological interactions. Flight of ideas, pressure of thoughts, emotional level such as aggressiveness, agitation, curiosity, interest; grandiosity, missionary tasks, etc.

Differential diagnostic distinctions:
- Motor restlessness (concerns untargeted activity); perseverations,
- erethic state of excitement (organic mental disorders),
- Actionism in emergency situations,
- healthy engagement in one's own affairs, pursued with full dynamism,
- disturbed control in the drive domain—colloquially: "not being able to get one's affairs in order"—with disorganization and planning disorder being more prominent (see below),
- Agitation, e.g., in agitated depression,
- Delusional thoughts that demand activity (potentially difficult differentiation of delusion-driven actions in megalomania from pure drive disorder)—in mania and schizomanic states, however, both are often present.

Self-/other person's judgment. Other person's judgment.

Interview for rating. Question about plans, history taken from other persons (e.g., also concerning the premorbid level).

Neuropsychology/objectification. Interview behavior, behavioral observation.

Severity. Slight increase in actions compared to the premorbid level, which is still situationally appropriate, and where a steerability by the surrounding people can be found, up to excessive drive with strong, unrestrained activism and disturbance of the concerns of one's own person and others through situationally inappropriate activities, in which the person can no longer be influenced by fellow human beings.

Specifications:
1. Domains
   - Social activity (AMDP 93),—professional (related to plans).
2. Source of action motivation
   - Appetence-driven, sexual, food, etc.
   - Plan-driven, realistic, unrealistic, delusional.

Personality influences. Habitual variance in action dynamics; in bipolar disorders more frequently also higher premorbid drive level; narcissistic person with self-obligation to be active.

Conceptual problems of the feature. Increase in drive is not necessarily accompanied by disorganization, however, the two features often occur together—see below disturbance of control in the drive domain. In the increase in drive, the energy invested in one or usually several activities is in the foreground.

Neuroscientific/cognitive neuroscientific models Heterogeneous feature:

1. As in drive poverty with a different direction:
   - Action threshold lowered, considerations are less integrated into action

planning—in the sense of boundaries that are respected,
- In part:. Illusion of attributing the initiative to act to oneself: the person, who apparently no longer has control over the action strands, states that he is enforcing the many intentions to act.

2. Expression of grandiose ideas, overvalued idea of grandeur, grandiosity, megalomania ,
3. social disinhibition—loss of the usual caution and detachment.

Logorrhoea
Definition. Increased amount of verbal expressions. Increased communication through speech. Increase in drive in the speech area.

Example

Patient speaks incessantly, is difficult to interrupt. ◀

Position in psychopathology. AMDP 88.

Psychopathological interactions: See drive disorder, transition to manic thought disorder with loss of control over verbal expressions (with confusingly many associative cross-references, which, however, are not clearly integrated into the thought context for the conversation partner).

Differential diagnostic distinctions:
- repetitive requests for help in agitated depression (patient also wants to achieve attention against resistance),
- Perseveration, stereotypy
- Distinction (quantitative) from usual talkativeness.

Self-/other persons's judgment. Other persons's judgment.

Neuropsychology/objectification. Observation of interview behavior and spontaneous behavior in communication situations—feature: increased amount of verbal expressions.

Severity. Slightly increased amount of speech utterances up to uninterruptibility—degree of resulting communication restriction.

Specifications:
- emotional tension situation with communication intention,
- self-talk without communication intention,
- disinhibition of initiating contact.

Neuroscientific/cognitive neuroscientific models
Like increased drive (see there).

Disturbed control in the drive domain
Definition. Disturbance of control of the multitude of actions that are initiated, especially in several more complex action chains; it is evident that problems arise due to the lack of control and coordination of the many action approaches, which are incessantly newly initiated—appearing thoughtless towards others.

Example

A patient initiates a series of actions that he cannot complete. Everything remains unfinished. Not even simple everyday tasks are completed; instead, the patient, apparently thoughtlessly, starts the next activity. ◀

Position in psychopathology. In AMDP additional item "disorganised"; in severe mania and in some schizophrenic episodes, an important feature of behavior description.

Psychopathological interaction. Increased drive, impulsivity

Differential diagnostic distinctions. Disorganization—executive control disturbed: not just errors in the execution of complex action sequences (with working memory disorder, etc.), so not the disordered sequence of an action, but the lack of overview and completion of several started actions is central here; impulsivity; arrogance with no need to care about the execution of actions.

Self-/other persons' judgment. Other persons' judgment.

Interview for rating. Questions about disruptive factors in executing complex projects, history taken from other persons.

Neuropsychology/objectification. Behavioral observation (also in comparison to the premorbid situation).

Severity. Mild control disorder with increased drive, where not all actions are controlled, up to severe control disorder, where actions and arguments are only started and none are completed.

Further characterization:
- predominant increase in drive that exceeds the control capacity of action sequences.

Specifications:
Area: social contacts:

- thereby only initiating contact with many people, only starting social relationships and projects with the relationship persons.

Conceptual problems of the feature. Not easy to distinguish whether the need for control is not seen by the person, or cannot be exercised.

Neuroscientific/cognitive neuroscientific models
1. Executive disorder as a frontal lobe deficit is revealed by the drive disorder,
2. Increased drive or too strong motivators in relation to the control possibility or execution of control of actions,
3. Monitoring of actions, action planning, and resources (including time) is missing or not applied,
4. hypothetically, a dedifferentiation of premotor integration can be assumed, i.e., of control influences necessary for correct selection of actions, possibly due to the failure of functioning computational units in neural networks.

Disinhibition
Definition. Actions that were otherwise suppressed (due to negative consequences) and could be controlled by the person are carried out. The person initiates actions with problematic effects that impair the environment, other people, or their own interests.

Example

- A patient does not maintain the culturally required distance from other people, swears inappropriately, and is sexually harassing in words and concrete attempts at approach.
- A patient interacts with other people as if he were very familiar and he were friends with them—he does not respect personal space, touches them familiarly (e.g., by patting on the shoulder), and interacts too personally with them. When asked about his behavior, he states that he wants to approach the person and shows the behavior even though he knows he does not know them—behavior without distance.
- In a trivial argument, a patient grabs the partner's arm and twists it violently, causing the partner severe pain and leading to legal consequences—this is clear to the person, but he does not consider the possible consequences of his own action. ◄

Domains: usually not all domains are equally affected, such as shopping (especially online), eating, drinking, alcohol/drug consumption, negative social gestures (especially on social media), sexual behavior, etc.

Position in Psychopathology. In AMDP additional symptom "impulsive". Central term for frontotemporal dementias and organic personality disorder.

Area-specific: Impulsivity with, for example, control disorder limited to shopping or eating behavior.

Psychopathological Interactions. Disturbed insight into possible consequences of actions, irresponsible behaviors, impulsivity. Lack of control ability possibly due to fatigue.

Differential Diagnostic Distinctions:
Behavior is explainable by

a) Forensic psychiatric disorder with criminality and/or personality disorder with affect-poor, empathy-disturbed, narcissistic type, distinction from consciously and deliberately unscrupulously reckless behavior,
b) Judgment disorder,
c) Mania with arrogance, not having to pay attention to consequences—e.g., due to grandiose ideas ,
d) Delusion-induced misconduct, where the delusion explains why the person, for example, violates social conventions.

Further Characterization. Control disorder with known – but not included in action planning – negative consequences of actions.

Self-/other persons' judgment. Other persons' judgment.

Interview for Rating. Self-assessment of impulse control, examples, follow-up questions on behavioral problems.

Neuropsychology/objectification
Behavioral observation—characteristic: disturbance of the concerns of other people or the environment and observing the confrontation with this fact, with the effects of one's own behavior as an example of misconduct (to distinguish from consciously and deliberately unscrupulously reckless behavior),

- False positive reactions, e.g., in tests of the Go/no-go type,
- Testing the sequence of 1 or 2 taps (random order), which should be tapped back under the instruction that, if 2 taps occur, the patient should not tap. It is observed that the person cannot suppress the tendency to tap in response.

Severity. Mild—as isolated consequence-free transgressions to severe—with social untenability due to continuous serious assaults on fellow human beings.

Specifications:
- Lack of control over intentions related to needs,
  a) habitual control in more automatic actions is bypassed by the patient or
  b) bypassing conscious control in more complex actions with decision-making possibilities,
- Lack of consideration for others and possible consequences,
- Impulsivity increased with lowered action threshold.

Personality influences. Variance in impulsivity.

Neuroscientific/cognitive neuroscientific models
1. Disruption of action control—disruption of retrieval or integration of control information learned in upbringing,
   - Disruption of the integration of knowledge and insight into action planning as a frontal lobe disorder,
2. Disruption of elements of action control such as mechanisms that mediate anticipatory anxiety or fear of shame,
   - Control is exercised through anxiety about negative consequences (disconnection of the amygdala-orbitofrontal cortex connection, Reischies et al. 1988),
   - anxiolytic medication acts paradoxically disinhibiting: If behavior control is mainly achieved through anxiety, anxiolytic medication acts paradoxically disinhibiting,
3. Judgment disorder (insight into negative consequences weakened), this represents an additional factor—cannot explain the behavior alone,
4. Increased drive dynamics (hormonal disorder) which overstrain control mechanisms,

5. Impulsivity increased (transition to increased drive),
6. Action thresholds are lowered,
   - Stimulus–response channels are uninhibitedly activated (triggered by too many environmental stimuli),
   - Disruption of the "filter" that activates planning and situation-appropriate action schemes, inhibits others.

Motor Restlessness
Definition. Inappropriate increase in non-goal-directed movements.

Example

A patient incessantly walks around the room, repeatedly fiddles in his pocket without necessity, etc. Usually, it is an increase in various undirected movements. ◀

Position in psychopathology. AMDP 83.

Related terms. Fidgeting, undirected agitated behavior.

Psychopathological interactions. agitation, arousal, anxiety, aggression—possibly hallucinations.

Differential diagnostic distinctions: Difference to increased drive: In that case, increased targeted actions; perseveration—refers to pathologically repeated, but primarily intentional movements; hyperkinesias; epileptic seizure; logorrhea.

Self-/other persons's judgment. Prezdominantly other persons's judgment, self-evaluation is possible.

Interview for Rating. History taken from other persons.

Neuropsychology/objectification. Behavioral observation and observing the person's engagement with increased movements.

Severity. Mild increase in the movement of individual extremities to severe increase in non-specific movements of the entire body, which severely impairs social behavior.

Occurs in many psychiatric syndromes: affective exceptional situations, fidgeting in delirium, agitation and increased drive in mania.

Neuroscientific/cognitive neuroscientific models
1. Emotional tension (interest, agitation, aggression, etc.) increases motor displacement activity (concept of behavioral research),
2. Disturbance of motor activation, dopaminergic, noradrenergic tone, or receptor activation increases—see stereotypies.
3. Increase in motor activity with emaciation (see Sachdev and Kruk 1996).

Psychopathological features in the domain of psychomotor skills and dyskinesias
These are hyperkinesias or unusual movements, often in the facial, gestural, and linguistic areas and in hand motor skills, which appear socially inappropriate.

Dyskinesias or parakinesia represent a group of psychomotor disorders listed in the AMDP as a complex group of features that cannot be uniformly described.

Socially accepted gestures have developed from natural psychic expressions in cultural development, with national and regional peculiarities, into a canon, i.e., many other movements are considered socially inappropriate, frowned upon, obscene, cheeky, etc. Other movements are simply unusual and carry no particular or generally understandable meaning. In mental illnesses, unusual and taboo movements can occur.

Histrionic
Definition. The behavior seems to want to present something to others—partly with overly strong or seemingly fake emphasis, or the behavior appears tendentious, aimed at a specific reaction from the people present. Behavior seeking attention.

The behavior represents, for example, a role, an affect or pain. It is directly aimed at attracting the attention of others through speech or affective expression, or through the manner of execution.

What is presented is often not fully comprehensible to others, it appears fake, exaggerated.

Example

- A patient immediately gains attention by dragging himself to the caregivers, bent over in pain and loudly moaning, to request a painkiller.
- A patient presents herself as a noble lady who has experienced something terrible.
- A person behaves exaggeratedly, being emotional but superficially fake, and is only satisfied when he has gained the attention of others.
- A person embellishes and aggravates his symptoms, presenting them as a severe ailment. ◀

Position in psychopathology. AMDP 86.

Related terms. Theatrically.

Psychopathological interactions. Simulation, where conscious intent is assumed to create the impression of suffering from the illness. Concept of "secondary gain".

Differential Diagnostic Distinctions:

- "Splitting," acting behavior, which plays the involved persons off against each other—often containing passages of theatrical behavior,
- manipulative behavior,
- possibly explainable by cultural and familial background and from the experience (e.g., having always received support only in this way)
- formerly also referred to as "profile neurosis," the attitude of having to engage in "image engineering" in all social situations to make a career or gain influence,
- agitated behavior in depression, which openly demands attention—a plea for help.

Further Characterization. Often a discrepancy between the apparent goal of action and what is achieved, which is excessively efficient only in terms of the attention of others.

Self-/Other Persons' Judgment. Other persons' judgment.

Neuropsychology/Objectification. Behavioral observation and questioning, observing the engagement with the presented material.

Severity. Mild tendencies towards self-presentation to severe impairment of communication through continuous, all-encompassing efforts to present oneself.

Specifications:

- Aggravation: Tendency to distort answers in the interview for a goal—both consciously (simulation) and unconsciously
- Enjoyment of self-presentation.

Personality Influences. Histrionic personality.

Conceptual Problems of the Feature:

- Spectrum from fully conscious simulation to unconscious expressive behavior,
- cultural differences in illness behavior and appeal behavior.

Neuroscientific/Cognitive Neuroscientific Models

1. Development of the joy in being the center of attention,
2. Behavioral strategy that has proven successful for the person in development. A person experiences the need to emphasize and embellish the disorder because they believe they will not be treated appropriately otherwise, or they have had the experience of achieving goals more or faster this way (consider cultural peculiarities).

Tic
Definition: Involuntary, brief movement of a muscle group that occurs uncontrollably.

Example

Twitching in the shoulder, clearing the throat—can be temporarily suppressed by a person, but resumes when voluntary suppression wanes. ◀

Psychopathological Interactions. Arousal.

Differential Diagnostic Distinctions. Myoclonus.

Interview for Rating. Complaints about involuntary movements, history taken from other persons, checking the intention.

Specifications. Tic disorder, multiple tics in Tourette syndrome.

Suggestibility
Definition: The person is unusually easily influenced by other people—regarding perception, emotional attitude, adoption of beliefs, or execution of an action.

In this process, the controlled integration of conscious contents into the person's values and complex identity, which could effect a demarcation and control of the suggested movements and contents, is apparently not performed or bypassed.

- Relationship to hypnotizability.
- Marked in delirium: task to read aloud is given, but a blank sheet of paper is handed over.

Utilization behavior
Definition. Touching, grasping objects within reach without being prompted to do so, and without any discernible intention that led the person to grasp—the person apparently does not want to do anything with the object, i.e., possess or use it.

Example

A patient reaches for the things on the table in front of him, touches them. ◀

Neuropsychology/objectification. Bring a hand close to the patient's palm and observe whether he grasps or touches the hand. Repeat after he has received the instruction not to touch the hand. Similarly with objects lying on the table in front of the patient.

Group of catatonic movement disorders
A series of movement disorders has been observed in specific mental illnesses, predominantly in schizophrenia, and characterized as catatonic movement disorders. catalepsy, flexibilitas cerea, negativism etc. have been described as specific catatonic symptoms. Catatonic stupor is among the already described features—as well as mutism and motor restlessness, which are also mentioned as catatonic symptoms. Thus, it is a heterogeneous group of movements or elementary behavior disorders—in addition to the mentioned features: fidgeting, blinking, staring, stereotypies, iterations, mutism, verbigeration, grimacing, mannerism, pseudo-expressive movements, perseveration, counteracting, positivism, etc. Certainly, these features are not typical symptoms of schizophrenia. If catatonia is seen as a special form of schizophrenic disorders, one argument becomes clear: the disturbance of dopaminergic functions in schizophrenia could affect the motor effects of the transmitter dopamine in catatonia. For example, stereotypy in the behavior of animals after an increase in dopamine release has been known for a long time.

Stereotypy
Definition. Repeated complex movements or verbal expressions that are inappropriate to the situation.

Occurring continuously or for a certain period.

Example

A patient always says "tan, tan, tan"—he suffers from severe global aphasia. Or a patient repeatedly says a word that initially made sense (verbigeration). ◀

Psychopathological interactions. Arousal.

Differential diagnostic distinctions. Perseveration (previously meaningful expression becomes meaningless through repetition).

Interview for rating. Interview, also history taken from other persons.

Neuropsychology/objectification. Behavioral observation, spontaneous speech rating of the Aachen Aphasia Test.

Severity. Duration, degree of social disability due to stereotypies.

Specifications:
- Extremity motor skills,
- Speech.

Catalepsy
Definition. Remaining in unusual body postures or extremity positions, which are spontaneously assumed or induced by other people, e.g., the examiner.

Example

A patient stands like a mime, motionless, as if frozen in a certain posture with a slightly outstretched arm. The posture signals no request, and he does not make contact with other people, e.g., through eye movements. ◀

Related terms. postural stereotype.

Further characterization. Abnormal susceptibility of the will.

Interview for rating. As far as possible, an interview with a psychopathological examination should be conducted and a history from other persons should be obtained.

Behavioral observation, examination of muscle tone, observation of dealing with the postural disorder.

Pathognomonic for: Catatonic schizophrenia.

Conceptual problems of the feature. Due to the abnormal susceptibility of the will in this feature, it is only seemingly a motor symptom, which, however, requires a more complex explanatory model.

Flexibilitas cerea
Definition. The extremities have a moderately increased muscle tone and can be passively brought into a position by another person, in which they then remain.

Example

A patient allows the movements of the extremities, with increased tone causing specific postures of the extremities to be maintained longer than without the "waxy" increase in tone. ◀

Related terms. Waxy flexibility.

Psychopathological interactions: command automatism related to actions with significantly increased suggestibility.

Differential diagnostic distinctions: Spastic increase in tone
- Rigidity: lead-pipe-like, e.g., in malignant neuroleptic syndrome,
- postural stereotype.

Neuropsychology/objectification. Inducing various postures, muscle tone, observation of dealing with the postural disorder.

Command automatism
Definition. Performing movements following a command, even if they are nonsensical—if the person communicates, he says he did not intend the movements.

Example

A patient follows every command without question, delay, or sign of distancing. ◀

Related terms. Flexibilitas cerea—related to posture , echolalia .

Neuropsychology/objectification. Observation of dealing with the action.

Pathognomonic for: Catatonia.

Negativism
Definition. When the examiner requests a specific movement, the movement opposite to the request is performed.

Example

A patient lies unresponsive in bed and is examined. When asked to open their eyes and when attempting to open the eyelids with hands to assess the light reaction of the eyes, the person (without being dazzled) squeezes them shut. ◀

Differential diagnostic distinctions. Stupor.

Neuropsychology/objectification. Behavioral observation, observation of dealing with the action.

Pathognomonic for: Catatonia.

Mannered/bizarre
Definition. In both speech and mimetic-gestural expressive behavior, peculiarities that repeat themselves occur—like a particular strange style, often characterizable as weirdness. It can also rarely occur in non-gestural extremity movements, facial movements, or body posture.

Example

- A patient speaks in a stilted manner, in a style not adapted to the listeners and the expressed content.
- A patient repeatedly stretches their fingers in a sequence that makes no sense and appears like a nonsensical habit.
- A patient sits in a condescending pose that does not fit his situation in front of the examiner and in the company of fellow patients.
- Bizarre: completely inappropriate actions/movements that are so eccentric that they cause astonishment.
- Bizarre can also be the clothing, completely unusual in fashion and appearance, and therefore causing astonishment. ◀

Position in psychopathology. AMDP 85.

Related terms. Inappropriate grandiosity, extravagance.

Psychopathological interactions. In some cases, there is a feeling of being watched and displaying behavior in front of (non-present) people.

Differential diagnostic distinctions:
- histrionic with expressive character in front of spectators (mannered behavior also occurs without spectators),
- compulsive action.

Self-/other persons' judgment. other persons' judgment.

Neuropsychology/objectification. Behavioral observation and observation of engagement with movement.

Severity. From slight or marginal noticeable, rarely occurring to socially unacceptable in its bizarreness and due to repulsive aspects.

Pathognomonic for: Schizophrenia.

Specifications:
- predominantly mannered,
- predominantly bizarre.

Neuroscientific/cognitive neuroscientific model concepts
1. A kind of autistic theatricality, in which the person is convinced to behave according to the imagined situation or the delusional belief of being watched, or without regard to the possible astonishment of the observers,
2. Megalomania-triggered—pretentious,
3. A person develops an idiosyncratic behavioral/speech style that is maintained independently of the environment—shaped by an idiosyncratic world of ideas and not adapteded by feedback from the environment.

References

Bell EC, Willson MC, Wilman AH et al (2005) Differential effects of chronic lithium and valproate on brain activation in healthy volunteers. Hum Psychopharmacol 20:415–424

Berridge KC, Robinson TE (1998) What is the role of dopamine in reward: hedonic impact, reward learning, or incentive salience? Brain Res Rev 28:309–369

Berrios GE, Gili M (1995) Abulia and impulsiveness revisited: a conceptual history. Acta Psychiatr Scand 92:161–167

Cummings JL (1993) Frontal-subcortical circuits and human behavior. Arch Neurol 50:873–880

Danek A (2005) Kognitive Neurologie und Neuropsychologie. In: Förstl H (Ed) Frontalhirn, Funktionen und Erkrankungen, 2. edn. Springer, Berlin Heidelberg New York Tokio

O'Doherty J, Kringelbach ML, Rolls ET et al (2001) Abstract reward and punishment representations in the human orbitofrontal cortex. Nat Neurosci 4:95–102

Förstl H, Sahakian B (1991) A psychiatric presentation of abulia—three cases of left frontal lobe ischaemia and atrophy. J R Soc Med 84:89–91

Frijda NH (1986) The emotions. Cambridge Univ Press, Cambridge

Haggard P, Clark S, Kalogeras J (2002) Voluntary action and conscious awareness. Nat Neurosci 5:382–385

Houk JC, Adams JL, Barto AG (1995) A model of how the basal ganglia generate and use neural signals that predict reinforcement. In: Houk JC, Davis JL, Beiser DG (Eds) Models of information processing in the basal ganglia. MIT Press, Cambridge, pp 249–270

Jenkins LH, Brooks DJ, Nixon PD et al (1994) Motor sequence learning: A study with positron emission tomography. J Neurosci 14:3775–3790

Klages W (1967) Der menschliche Antrieb. Thieme, Stuttgart

Libet B, Gleason CE, Wright EW, Pearl DK (1983) Time of conscious intention to act in relation to onset of cerebral activity (readinesspotential): the unconscious initiation of a freely voluntary act. Brain 106:623–642

Lorenz K (1963) Das sogenannte Böse. Zur Naturgeschichte der Aggression. Borotha-Schoeler, Wien

Marschner A, Mell T, Wartenburger I et al (2005) Reward-based decision-making and aging. Brain Res Bull 67:382–390

Middleton FA, Strick PL (2000) A revised neuroanatomy of frontal-subcortical circuits. In: Lichter DG, Cummings JL (Eds) Frontal-subcortical circuits in psychiatric and neurological disorders. Guilford Press, New York, pp 44–58

Montague PR, Hyman SE, Cohen JD (2004) Computational roles for dopamine in behavioural control. Nature 431:760–777

Mushiake H, Masahiko L, Tanji J (1991) Neuronal activity in the primate premoteor, supplementary, and precentral motor cortex during visually guided and internally determined sequential movements. J Neurophysiol 66:705–718

Reischies FM, Baum K, Bräu H et al (1988) Cerebral magnetic resonance imaging findings in multiple sclerosis—relation to disturbance of affect, drive, and cognition. Arch Neurol 45:1114–1116

Reischies FM (1999) Pattern of disturbance of different ventral frontal functions in organic depression. In: McGinty JF (Ed) Advancing from the ventral striatum to the extended amygdala. Ann N Y Acad Sci 877: 775–780

Reischies FM (2005) Psychopathologie. In: Förstl H (Ed) Frontalhirn, Funktionen und Erkrankungen, 2.

edn. Springer, Berlin Heidelberg New York Tokio, pp 83–101
Reischies FM, Hartikainen J, Berghöfer AM (2002) Initial triple therapy of acute mania, adding lithium and valproate to neuroleptics. Pharmacopsychiatry 35:244–246
Reischies FM (1999b) Pattern of disturbance of different ventral frontal functions in organic depression. Ann N Y Acad Sci 877:775–780
Rolls ET (1999) The brain and emotion. Oxford Univ Press, Oxford
Rolls ET (2000) The orbitofrontal cortex and reward. Cereb Cortex 10:284–294
Sachdev P, Kruk J (1996) Restlessness: the anatomy of a neuropsychiatric symptom. Aust N Z J Psychiatry 30:38–53
Schultz W (2004) Neural coding of basic reward terms of animal learning theory, game theory, microeconomics and behavioural ecology. Curr Opin Neurobiol 14:139–147
Shima K, Tanji J (1998) Role for cingulate motor area cells in voluntary movement selection based on reward. Science 282:1335–1338
Shipley BA, Deary IJ, Tan J (2002) Efficiency of temporal order discrimination as an indicator of bradyphrenia in Parkinson's disease: the inspection time loop task. Neuropsychologia 40(8):1488–1493
Sims A (2003) Symptoms in the mind, 3rd edn. Saunders Elsevier, Amsterdam
Smith PL, Ratcliff R (2004) Psychology and neurobiology of simple decisions. Trends Neurosci 27:161–168
Tanji J, Shima K, Matsuzaka Y (2002) Reward-based planning of motor selection in the rostral cingulate motor area. Adv Exp Med Biol 508:417–423
Thorpe SJ, Rolls ET, Maddison S (1983) The orbitofrontal cortex: neuronal activity in the behaving monkey. Exp Brain Res 49:93–115
Tremblay L, Schultz W (1999) Relative reward preference in primate orbitofrontal cortex. Nature 398:704–708
Usher M, McClelland JL (2001) The time course of perceptual choice: the leaky, competing accumulator model. Psychol Rev 108:550–592
Vogeley K, May M, Ritzl A et al (2004) Neural correlates of first-person perspective as one constituent of human self-consciousness. J Cogn Neurosci 16:817–827
Yazawa S, Ikeda A, Kunieda T et al (2000) Human presupplementary motor area is active before voluntary movement: subdural recording of Bereitschaftspotential from medial frontal cortex. Exp Brain Res 131:165–177

Consciousness 8

Contents

8.1 Introduction

Consciousness is still a mysterious phenomenon that can only be outlined in this chapter. The goal is to explain consciousness disorders. But can consciousness disorders be understood without knowing what consciousness is? How would human consciousness be explained to an intelligent computer or a "Martian"—certainly an unsolvable task at the moment. "consciousness is the perception of what is going on in the soul" (Locke 1690). Is there an inner perception,

F. M. Reischies, *Psychopathology*, https://doi.org/10.1007/978-3-662-70293-2_8

so to speak, an inward-directed eye? And: Who perceives there?

Additionally, for psychopathology, consciousness seems to be involved in almost everything in the human psyche. Hughlin Jackson (1932) believed that a person's voluntary, attentively performed decision could not be represented without reference to consciousness. Will is "a name invented by humans for various aspects of the ever-present and yet ever-changing ultimate and highest mental state, which in its totality constitutes what we call consciousness."

In this section, this comprehensive topic must be narrowed down to the question of consciousness disorders. How can we understand the psychopathological states that are, for example, referred to as somnolence or coma? On the one hand, our explanation of consciousness disorders depends on the neuroscientific models of consciousness. On the other hand, we can hope that the experience of the psychopathological investigation of consciousness disorders might also help to shed a little more light on the mysterious phenomenon.

The concept of consciousness is often overloaded with claims—from anthropology, philosophy, etc.—for example, it is supposed to clarify self-consciousness, conscious responsible decision, animal consciousness, and more. In this section, beyond the explanation of sensory consciousness and also consciousness in actions (see perception and action), only a still to be defined everyday consciousness will be discussed. The varieties of reflective consciousness will be omitted here, i.e., only the everyday relevant areas that appear disturbed in psychiatric syndromes will be referred to.

Example

A 50-year-old woman is admitted because she had seen men in her apartment for days (who were not there) and because her behavior seemed strange to the neighbors. She reports incoherently about the experiences of the last few days, seems not to remember properly. Additionally, she does not understand questions or does not understand them immediately. The questions seem to "not reach" her. She appears inattentive, "fidgety." She is apparently awake but seems retarded and not focussed on any conversation topic. She gives the impression that everything is new to her, or unfamiliar ("wondering"). Neuropsychological examination procedures reveal concentration, memory, and orientation disorders. Serum analysis indicates a high suspicion of acute kidney failure. ◀

Conceptual Image of the Stage of Consciousness
Many clinicians imagine the concept of consciousness as a stage. It corresponds to the "Cartesian theater". On it are the potentially conscious contents of various kinds. Through a door, the more or less predictable events of the environment enter. They appear when it is time, according to the logic of the external world. On the other hand, we can actively let ideas appear or reactivate them at any time—the ideas appear as if through another door of the stage set. The "imagining" corresponds to the recall from the stores of world knowledge or our personal—episodic life experience. Attention, moreover, can make something light up like in a spotlight. Attention phenomena, which are generally associated with consciousness, are already discussed in Chap. 4. Consciousness corresponds in the image initially to what the observer experiences on the stage. To the images and messages of external events and the ideas and associations appear emotions, etc.—almost like colorations of the stage lighting, colored fogging, or theater music to make it vivid.

In everyday life, the observer has the feeling of having the situation under control, because he is not just an idle observer. He is on the one hand a spectator of what the world presents to him, on the other hand, director, lighting technician, and playwright at the same time—thus an actor who calls up ideas and memories like figures or flashbacks, turns away, can shape what he sees, like the painter his canvas. There are further manipulations, such as opening the newspaper, where the observer, through the sensorimotor feedback, as with every eye movement, has the feeling of exact control of the events.

Initially, the clinician develops a rough sketch of consciousness disorders, which ties in with what has just been outlined. In the theater image, a clouding of consciousness would be imagined as a darkening on the stage. Not only the constant background lighting but also the spotlight, which symbolizes attention, illuminates the wrong object and no longer sharply, but with a broad light cone.

If one transfers the conceptual image to the clouding of consciousness, it is initially obvious to assume that the person in a clouding of consciousness is no longer sure of the events on the stage. There are also misperceptions that are surprising and further unsettle the person. More importantly, however, is that they can no longer call up the right ideas about the events. The person can no longer cope with the events. In addition, inappropriate ideas, associations, and memories "step through the wrong doors" unbidden. The imagined events appear on the stage through the door actually reserved for real events. The scene gets out of control for the observer, who feels like a co-director.

All this causes the experiencing person an inability to recognize what is "going on", what the case is. In this context, something that cannot be represented in the image is important: The person who experiences and thinks he is directing forgets the events on the stage and does not form a predictive model of the processes. This is the case because the inner monitor, the recording in the person's information processing, is disturbed.

The last aspect already suggests: We need to rethink consciousness: The theater-spectator conceptual image is wrong. There is no independent observer, no playwright, or director. There is also no lighting technician. The consciousness disorders may perhaps bring us closer to what is wrong with the image.

In this chapter, insights into the disorder of two aspects of consciousness are presented:

1. Clouding of consciousness in the spectrum from clear wakefulness to coma and
2. Change in the subjective quality of conscious experience, as it occurs in trance and dissociative states.

Example

A mother suddenly appears strangely changed to the family. The family initially noticed that she does not respond in the usual way to someone who addresses or questions her. The facial expressions or gestures of the person addressing her seem to have no effect. When one hands her an object, she reacts very slowly and with delay. No paralysis is noticeable, no flaccid muscles. The mother walks around the apartment as usual. She can also have breakfast in the usual way, although generally retarded. On the other hand, the family notices that she no longer manages to give full attention to those who engage with her, even when, as usual, one tries to achieve the greatest extent of her attention. The turning of attention to the events in the surroundings is also reduced. For example, the mother does not look at the door when a person enters. In conversation, it is further noticeable that the mother cannot engage with the conversation topic as one knew her to, she does not think along, she does not visualize the addressed situation. She appears fleeting. She does not fully manage to engage in the respective conversation topic, like a person who is abruptly awakened from deep sleep, only gradually achieving full clarity about the situation. ◀

Stream of Consciousness

The conceptual figure of the "stream of consciousness", which in turn has much to do with thinking (Chap. 10), leads just as astray as that of the theater. For it suggests a horizontally linked occurrence in time. The course of consciousness contents is said to be horizontally linked like the associative chains of thinking. However, this image for thinking is also grossly simplified.

User Interface on the Computer
Let us turn to the analogy of brain and computer, for it might be advantageous to think of consciousness as a user interface of a computer program. The user interface shows the user a "frame" at a time. The user interface of a computer program determines how one moves from one frame to another through a choice (an input or clicking a box), in which different images are seen. In each new frame, there are action options for further decision-making. Consciousness and the emerging thoughts could thus be imagined more like a user interface of our brain-computer, for processes are running beneath the surface that we investigate in neuroscience but cannot experience. These processes determine the progression of what is experienceable on the "surface" for the person. In a certain way, we are thus dealing again with a stage, albeit the changing stage of the user interface of a computer.

8.2 Definitions

What are we talking about when we talk about consciousness and what can be reliably stated, what can be investigated? We will consider the subfunctions of consciousness, such as attention, monitoring, etc. Additionally, we are dealing with domains of conscious experience, such as conscious seeing, hearing, feeling, remembering, thinking, and acting, etc. There are several approaches to representing consciousness, which will be presented below.

8.2.1 Conscious Perception, Conscious Memory

The first approach arises from the contrast between conscious and unconscious mental processes. We first consider sensory consciousness. The majority of processes in the CNS occur obligatorily or optionally unconsciously. Helmholtz's unconscious inferences in the information processing of perception are already described in the corresponding chapter. Language processing also occurs automatically. Fodor (1983) postulated a modularity of mental functions; according to which, for example, the language module is to be imagined as an apparatus primarily isolated from other functions, into which consciousness components have no access. As an example, he cites that we cannot help but think of the word "apple" when seeing an apple. Merkel (1885) had already published early time measurements, which he measured for simple reactions—distinguishing between a conscious reaction and an unconscious one, which occurs much faster.

The contrast between conscious and unconscious mental processes that can be investigated includes, for example, conscious vs. unconscious perception, conscious vs. unconscious recall from memory, conscious vs. unconscious memory of an encoding situation, conscious vs. unconscious attention direction, and conscious vs. unconscious control of movement (planning and monitoring of execution). These distinctions can be experimentally investigated to determine what underlies the difference, which different mental functions and brain activations are involved (Crick and Koch, 2003, Koch 2005). Results from this approach will be described further below.

8.2.2 Components of Consciousness

The second approach to consciousness is based on the description of the various aspects and prerequisites of consciousness. Many authors have presented systems of consciousness functions, they have postulated components of consciousness. These are hypothetical consciousness components, which in many cases have not yet been clearly assigned to neuroscientific processes.

Consciousness apparently requires that several brain systems are active—the activation of at least some or even all of the following functions:

1. attention, wakefulness,
2. subjective motor control, sensorimotor feedback
3. activated self-model,
4. activated environmental model, monitoring of the environment,
5. actor role as the subject of experiencing the consequences of actions, e.g., already with eye movements,
6. subjective quality of perception (e.g., in the conscious seeing of colors),
7. mood functions—emotional readiness to feel, to experience.

The components are indicated as necessary but are probably not sufficient for consciousness—moreover, it is still unclear what processes lie behind all these components. Do all functions need to be active simultaneously? Are there not inattentive states of consciousness: Are there times of automatic actions, or those in which the person only feels like losing motor control, etc.? Let us consider the possibly necessary components individually:

Attention Clinically, disturbances of consciousness, at least the clouding of consciousness, are always associated with a disturbance of attention. Consciousness is only assumed when there is sufficiently high vigilance and intentionality to expose oneself to the respective situation (Chap. 4 attention). The question is whether attention must be focussed. There is likely a state of consciousness with free-floating attention.

A disturbance of working memory with the monitoring of what the situation entails is also practically always present.

Self-model Metzinger postulates the activation of the self-model as critical for consciousness (Metzinger 2001). The self-model can be understood as part of the monitoring system with a representation of experiences that relate to one's own "self".

If the self-model is not activated, automated, i.e., non-consciously controlled functions occur. This is the case in dissociative states. However, this can also occur in everyday life, during routine actions, i.e., non-pathological states (Dennett 1991).

Communicability Presumably, communicability is important for human consciousness. The activation of the semantic system and language module has enabled the communication of conscious mental processes to the group in evolutionary development: The advantage of consciously occurring perception, conscious thought processes, attention, and movement planning was that they could be discussed within the group. Actions could thus be socio-culturally controlled, co-determined, and shaped in communication.

The metaphor of consciousness as a blackboard in the team room (Baars 1988, 2002) is helpful for several reasons: Consciousness is thus compared to a blackboard for a work team on which various coworkers write their notes about the processes they have completed so that all team members can see them and continue to work with them. On the one hand, it is meant to suggest that the entries in consciousness arise from processes in the brains of the various workers that are not visible on the board. In the brain, this corresponds to the different modules such as those of visual, auditory object recognition, memory, imagination, language, etc. The blackboard image also has the communication aspect. In the brain, the activities of many modules occur simultaneously, which the brain must coordinate itself. The content of consciousness is a milestone for the organization of mental activity in one's own brain. The content that is currently attentively and consciously experienced organizes attention to the associated topics and thus concentrated processing (Chap. 4 attention) and also further information processing. This leads to the impression of the stream of consciousness. In the communicative aspect of consciousness, it plays only a subordinate role that the experienced is not communicable in all qualities. Possibly, the inexpressible qualities of conscious experience are just a peculiarity of the system that played no role evolutionarily.

Control

The role of the actor and action readiness (tight feedback in sensorimotor loops:)

Every person has psychomotor-perceptive feedback at every moment—even with fine movements of the body or eyes. This applies to sensory feedback from the extremities, but also from the environment, such as when touching the book. When moving the eyes and head, the retinal image changes. The motor activity initiated by the CNS is fed back sensorily and can be processed by the CNS in a controlling manner. It serves as confirmation that everything is proceeding as expected. When we feel with a long stick, we have the sensation of touch at the tip of the stick—"we feel at the tip of the stick." For self-perception as an actor, these feedback loops are important.

In addition to the sensorimotor feedback loops, there are also feedbacks from attentional shifts. They lead to changes in perception. This can be achieved with eye, head, and trunk movements—but also without moving the eyes, for example, to a peripheral area in the visual field or acoustically in the room as the "cocktail party phenomenon".

Activation of the environmental model

At this point, a complex circumstance must be pointed out. We do not perceive that we have a skin touch when we, for example, bump into the shelf from which we want to take something. It is an expected feedback. The expectation of feedback from the environment is a highly complex performance of the brain. The expected feedback depends both on my body extension and the movement of the hand as well as on my knowledge of where the shelf board is. The expectation thus has a component from the self-image and a component from the model of the environment. In Fig. 8.1, this is illustrated for the different levels of eye movement, limb movement, and social action such as speaking. At this point, it is important to emphasize how the model of one's own body, but also of one's own social role and action repertoire, and on the other hand, the model of the environment and fellow humans, is necessary for our actions (Chap. 6.2 Disturbance of executive functions). Is the self- and environmental model necessary for consciousness? The answer is yes, but it is not sufficient for consciousness.

However, if we encounter something unexpected during a routine action, e.g., an automated attempt to take something from the shelf, we are alerted. For example, something is sticky, or the shelf board is too far forward, etc. Then the situation suddenly becomes conscious to us. We switch to the conscious mode. This also allows us to talk about it, we call out "Something is sticky!" or "The board is shifted and can fall down!" to point out socially relevant news to fellows.

A person with a clouding of consciousness is said to be "not quite present," meaning that the person cannot communicate news, as in the last example of unexpected feedback when reaching into the shelf. Because the person is disturbed in the fundamental functions and cannot notice that something is not quite in its place, etc. A person with a clouding of consciousness has not activated their environmental model and self-model, or it does not work; the expectations of the feedback from the environment are not processed within the large neuronal network, or the comparison operations of the feedback with the expectations do not take place. The person appears to the people around them as absent, "not quite in the situation," or "does not know what is going on" (Sect. 8.3.2).

Updating of the environmental model

The environmental model includes, if it is to be accurate at all times, the respective updating. The CNS must register every change in the environment and adjust the environmental model accordingly. This is referred to as monitoring. This is necessary for the knowledge of what is currently the case, for the awareness of the environment, which has been included as a criterion for consciousness disturbances in the international classifications of psychiatric diseases. The monitoring of environmental changes is a function of working memory. The image of the flight radar metaphorically illustrates what happens;

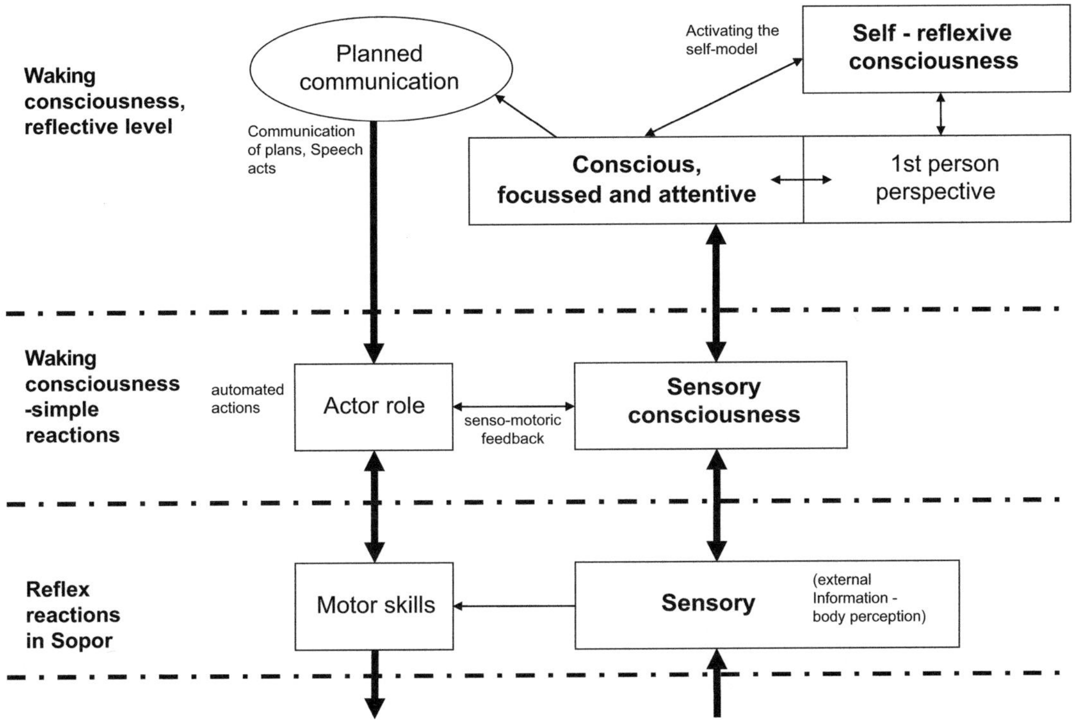

Fig. 8.1 Sensory consciousness is to be separated from reflexive consciousness. A sensory consciousness is generated by the sensorimotor feedback during movements of the limbs as well as the eyes. This is also to be expected in animals of higher developmental stages ("I am sitting on a chair and see trees and a street"). The second level of consciousness is reflexive consciousness ("I am aware that I am sitting here on the chair and looking around because I came here and am waiting for a friend who promised to come"). The activation of the self- and environmental model, combined with the integration of plans and memories, allows for a more comprehensive overview of the situation, which can also be communicated.

it is helpful for clarifying the awareness of the environment. The radar screen is updated with the currently measured positions of nearby aircrafts. Objects that reflect the radar beam appear on it. The image is updated with each pass of the directional beam. Objects such as aircraft or ships remain in place on the screen until the location data is corrected in a subsequent update (or, in the case of an aircraft crash, until it disappears from the screen). Monitoring represents the intermediate storage of situational and positional data that must be maintained before each new capture for the update. This is a metaphor for a central CNS function: situational orientation, which is available not only for the field of vision but also for oneself and all objects in the space.

Actor role as the subject of experience
The subject acts at all times, even if only with the eyes and the exact trunk position, and expects consequences from actions. Important beyond the sensorimotor feedback, is this especially in every decision-making process. It is assumed that in evolution there is a training of basic neural networks for behavioral adaptation through negative valence (Reischies 2021). Specifically, the sensorimotor and reward feedbacks of the person as an actor discussed above may coordinate the conscious experience of the person. It is experienced by oneself as the "central". Damasio (1999) aptly characterized the process as "from movie in the brain to brain in the movie".

Quality of experience
Subjective quality of consciousness: While model concepts already exist for the other components of consciousness, this is not yet the case for conscious experience. How does the complex subjective experience of perception, thinking, and memory, as well as the feeling of what is currently happening, come about? Philosophers call the subjectively experienced qualities, such as colors, qualia. How can I experience a quality like harmony, a shape? Psychophysics can explain to some extent how intensely a person perceives something, see, for example, Fechner's law. In other words: Perceptual qualities of some elementary physical properties are, within certain limits, reducible to neuroscience. But this does not apply to many other components of conscious experience.

Emotions have, compared to the experiential qualities of sensory impressions, a much higher significance in psychopathology. They can be noticed in the monitoring of mental processes, or they can remain unnoticed. Here it is important to characterize the monitoring of emotions as a function of consciousness.

Consciousness and valence perception
The personal experience represents, according to what has been stated so far, a unique moment for the person with their life history and situation. The person is familiar with and attuned to the situation to varying degrees; there is a basic mood regarding valence—more or less positive, more or less negative—and an emotional readiness to feel. This is to be distinguished from the possibly simultaneously existing emotions or affects (Chap. 11 emotion/affect).

Thinking Is thinking a necessary component of consciousness? Could it be that animals cannot have consciousness because they cannot think in a linguistic sense? When a person converses with others about a topic, the person will check the conversation content to see if he has knowledge or experiences available or not. If a person with impaired consciousness has a disturbed overview, recall of these contents, people refer to the person as someone "with whom one cannot converse."

Although animals cannot think in a linguistic sense, they apparently visualize spatial solution steps in test tasks.

This example can be used to discuss the psychopathological picture of an awake person with severe dementia or an apallic syndrome. Caregivers observe sleeping and waking. But is the person more than awake, is she also conscious? She looks around, acts with simple hand movements, can, albeit not very precisely controlled, take in food. The person seems to be able to feel pain, hunger, etc.—has a readiness for sensation and experience. Consciousness may be present. But thinking is presumably extinguished. Perhaps one could speak of a severe impoverishment of consciousness functions.

The presentation of the postulated components of consciousness suggests some conclusions:

1. Elements of consciousness and partial disruptability:
   - consciousness is a functional state of a system with many subsystems,
   - this explains that a number of constraints presuppositions for the state of consciousness must be met,
   - this may also explain the susceptibility of the state of consciousness, as can be seen from the variety of delirium causes.

   The individual subsystems of consciousness functions can be variably disturbed, i.e., different syndrome patterns result, in which individual functions are more or less disturbed. In delirium, patterns of changes in attention, individual subjective symptoms, and drowsiness are observed, which are noticed by others.
2. The conscious person experiences sensory qualities such as colors and harmonies, so-called qualia—e.g., in seeing, hearing—and sensory-motor feedback in every action. These give the individual an impression of reliable, ever-repeating constancy and homogeneity—this impression is overlaid across the various components and subprocesses

like a cloak. Thus, only subjectively do people have a homogeneous conscious experience; it is their experience. Apparently, people also hold on to this when individual elements such as vigilance, attention and working memory etc. are disturbed—they say they experience as before.

Conclusion

For clear wakeful consciousness, various functional systems must be intact and interconnected (see Reischies et al. 2003):

1. Constraints such as vigilance and activation of episodic memory, especially with checking the "familiarity" of each situation and situation-specific memories,
2. Control of focal attention in the global workspace (Dehaene and Naccache 2001),
3. close feedback in the sensory-motor systems of eye movement and the somatosensory system,
4. activation and updating of the self- and environmental model.

So far, we have drawn a picture of a living being that (1) is active in its environment—in its familiar actor role. It is (2) attentive and constantly receives information about the environment and its own body, which it compares with its self- and environmental model (it can reliably retrieve information about its body position in relation to the objects in the environment, visible or not (3)). Especially when it acts, the (4) continuous feedback—sensory-motor feedback has an important task: the living being experiences itself in close integration—with predictable and unpredictable sensory impressions about (5) the consequences of actions—from the latter it can initiate behavioral adaptation.

Distinguishable from this is the control over mental activities, thinking, remembering, emotions. In contrast to the sensorimotor close feedback, these show a lower degree of immediacy. If I give myself the task of imagining the picture of my grandmother, then probably one of her images will appear after a certain latency. If I want to think about a matter like tax payment, this usually succeeds. But emotions, e.g., anger, are difficult to summon; possibly, I can stimulate them through specific memories, music, or film scenes. The termination of tasks is a consideration in this context: I can erase an imagined picture with a new imagination, usually a thought as well, but emotions usually color the mood longer and are difficult to erase with new emotions. These last arguments concerned the arbitrary change. The consciousness provides a kind of monitoring for this: the imagination of the grandmother, the tax payment, the feeling of anger.

Based on the presented information, we come to a model conception of the functions of consciousness, (1) as a monitoring, according to the metaphor of the radar screen, on which the current voluntary activities of the person (the actor) and everything that has gained enough attention resources to cross the threshold to be depicted on the monitoring screen are recorded, for example, everything that is reported as an alarm by the emergency circuits and can possibly trigger anxiety. A query about the skin contact of clothing can be arbitrary. (2) The monitoring, the status information, is available in the CNS, i.e., the activities of the person are carried out accordingly or—in case of an alarm—stopped. The information is also available for reflective mental activities. This is the point where the psychopathological examination starts when the sick person is asked if they feel awake, etc. So far, no instance, no neural structure has been identified to which the status information would be fed back and which would fulfill the conceptual function of a "perceiver" or a "theatergoer".

8.2.3 Concepts of "Unconscious"

Consciousness and awareness of something: The term "conscious" can mean "being conscious" on the one hand and "being aware that" on the other hand (in English "conscious" and "being aware of something", directed at a mental content). Especially with thoughts and knowledge, we say "I am aware of that" and mean that we consider a fact—e.g., in a negotiation. Here, we separate the terms into "awareness of something" and "being wakeful conscious".

Unconscious is usually not used as "not being conscious", but only in the way that a person, for example, was not aware of an action.

This presentation is not the place to comprehensively present the unconscious as a concept. What is important for psychopathology is the non-conscious control. "Unconscious" as a concept of psychoanalysis is presented in the specialized textbooks of psychoanalysis. Here, it should only be emphasized that many phenomena can be characterized by a gradation regarding the relationship to focussed wakefulness.

Phenomena are:

- obligatorily unconscious—such as the brain's language processes,
- unconscious but in principle capable of being conscious (including dissociated content),
- automated processes (routine), accessible to conscious attention,
- temporarily escaping conscious control, somewhat like a short monitoring lapse,
- conscious but without focussing attention on it; processed with moderately increased arousal (Koch 2005; "short-lived coalitions"),
- fully conscious.

In psychopathology, potentially conscious but not activated content plays a significant role. Mechanisms for distinguishing from only partially and potentially conscious mental content are (Fig. 8.2):

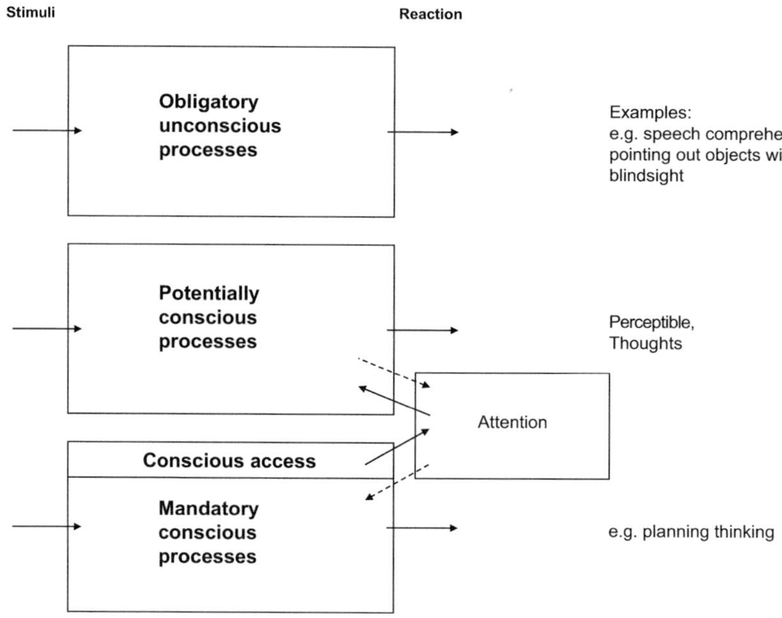

Fig. 8.2 Most processes in the brain are obligatorily unconscious. Top: Many processes run automatically. For example, people with cortical blindness can point to objects they do not consciously see ("blindsight"). This process runs obligatorily unconsciously (Weiskrantz 1986). Middle: Other processes can become conscious when attention is directed to them. An example is reading or speaking. Bottom: Certain processes, such as planning, can only occur consciously.

- actively ignoring or paying attention to something else, distracting oneself,
- not remembering it again,
- blocking associations in the thought process, mostly by actively, voluntarily recalling other content,
- inactivating an entire area—i.e., also trying to block contexts of the topic and never highlighting them with attention.

8.3 Clinic

Disorders of consciousness are found on the one hand in brain damage syndromes, for example in delirium, in the reduction of the functions of clear wakefulness with sopor and coma and dissociative states (as can be observed in histrionic or borderline personality disorders).

First, the disorders with a reduction of the functions of clear wakefulness must be delineated. Here, the term vigilance is often used, which, however, is not clearly defined. The essential difference between a tired person who is awakened and a person with a so-called quantitative consciousness disorder is that the tired person, once awakened, does not have significant and persistent disturbances in cognitive performance, whereas a person with somnolence after awakening will show the symptoms of their organic brain disorder, usually disturbances in cognitive performance such as memory impairment, disorientation.

Accordingly, we have at least three distinct domains of disturbance of consciousness:

1. The clouding of consciousness or the disturbance of the awareness of the environment
   1a. somnolence-coma type—with somnolence, sopor, coma
   1b. delirium type with so-called qualitative disturbances of consciousness
2. the narrowing of consciousness or the restriction to automated actions and
3. the subjective side of expanded consciousness as in trance states.

In disturbances of everyday consciousness, the involved processes can disintegrate, making the partial components of the functional bundle that enables consciousness recognizable. An example is the disturbance of attention, which is noticeable to the interviewer. The "absence" of a person is also noticeable. It must be distinguished from intended withdrawal from the conversation partner or pre-existing autism, etc.

Clinical Phenomena:
- sudden slowing down,
- reduced attention to the environment and altered, inexplicable attention-accompanying movements,
- reduced responsiveness, reactivity,
- the person appears "absent," "dazed," less capable of experiencing
- robotic, unresponsive behavior.

8.3.1 Disturbances of Consciousness and Awareness of the Environment

In delirium, consciousness is characteristically disturbed, primarily in the sense of clouding of consciousness. This can also be mild or go unnoticed, as defined for the so called "transient syndromes" (Wieck 1967). Confusional states are nowadays often described without reference to disturbances of consciousness. Disturbances of consciousness in mild delirium can be minor, and it remains unclear whether they are undetectable or absent (Fig. 8.3).

Dissociation
In the complex clinical pictures of personality disorders such as borderline personality disorder—but also in isolation—dissociation can occur (see below, disturbance of integration of experience). Actions and mental processes such as perception, etc., which usually

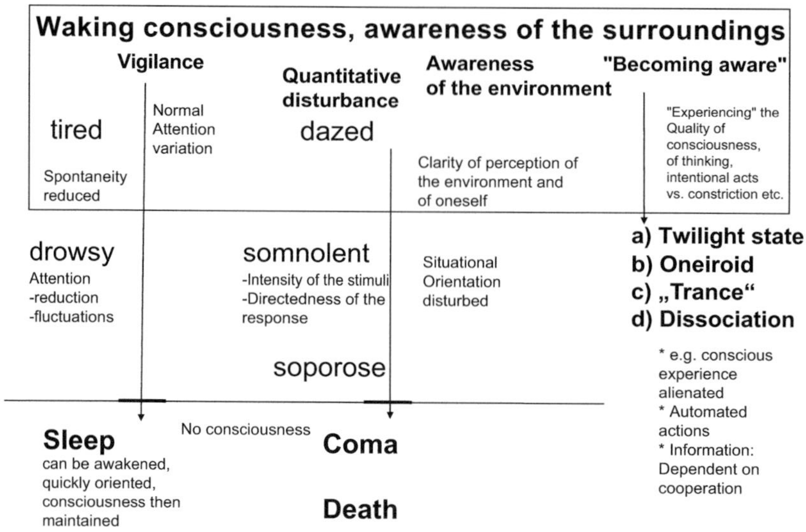

Fig. 8.3 Taxonomy of disturbances of consciousness. Clear wakefulness can decrease towards sleep (usually referred to as vigilance variation) on the one hand, and towards coma on the other, with the transitions of somnolence and stupor. The decrease towards coma is characterized by additional disturbances of cognitive functions. This includes a disturbance of awareness of the environment, memory, and other impairments. A disturbance of cognitive functions is also observed in delirium. A third change in wakefulness occurs, for example, in dissociative states: The person experiences that all processes happen automatically, feeling as if they are standing beside themselves. Another disturbance of consciousness is observed in trance, where perceptions and actions are experienced as strangely altered.

occur consciously, are carried out automatically. In dissociative states, routine processes run unconsciously and automatically, colloquially described by individuals as being “on autopilot.” Observers might overlook the state. However, it can happen that the dissociating person does not perform actions consciously, thus having no access to the normally freely accessible becoming aware of perceptions, actions, memories, etc. The dissociative state is presumably not uniformly describable (Jureidini 2004). It often leads to subjective psychological disturbances related to derealization, such as feeling “like in a movie,” “standing beside myself,” or “watching myself from the ceiling, from the floor above.”

Dissociation is a widespread feature, which in a mild and fleeting version is also reported by healthy individuals in stressful situations. The non-experience of negative emotions during dissociation could be an indication of the evolutionary significance of this state of experience.

Twilight State

In epileptic twilight states, similar features to those in dissociation can be observed, although information about this state is less well investigated. Patients seem to be fixated on something as if spellbound, so they perform everything else automatically. However, the focus of consciousness usually cannot be specified, and it is possible that they have subjectively trance-like experiences.

8.3.2 Severe disturbances of awareness of the environment/transition into coma

Clouding of consciousness, somnolence-coma type

Usually, disturbances of consciousness are discussed as syndromes in the transition to coma. Undoubtedly, they also play a central diagnostic role there.

Somnolence and coma: The disturbance of consciousness in brain injuries, for example, an acute traumatic brain injury, is also referred to as clouding of consciousness. It is classified among the so-called quantitative disturbances of consciousness, as a reduction of consciousness. These stand in contrast to the so-called qualitative disturbances such as those of the delirium type (also in delirium quantitative gradations are clinically relevant).

Usually, a gradation of clouding of consciousness is made for the somnolence-coma type:

- »Drowsiness«,
- somnolence,
- sopor,
- coma.

Somnolence is diagnostically to be differentiated from sleep phenomena. In somnolence, firstly, the awareness of the environment and secondly, the awareness of one's own person and one's own mental processes are disturbed. Somnolence can be seen as a complex concept.

For the disturbance of consciousness in brain injury syndromes, a central feature is the disturbance of the subjective side of consciousness. However, this is not easily verifiable in many states of somnolence. The subjective side of clouding of consciousness is not reliable in the psychopathological examination. For this reason, a change, an operationalization of the disturbance of consciousness, was made in the diagnostic classification systems. Disturbance of consciousness has been reduced to a disturbance of the »awareness of the environment«. This entails a narrowing of the feature. This solution was chosen to obtain a clinically more manageable conceptual tool for diagnostics. The awareness of the environment can clinically be easier testable.

In the investigation of traumatic brain injuries in sports, an attempt is made to document orientation, speech and possible drowsiness immediately, already "at the sidelines". In the clinic, the complex investigation focused on neuropsychological examination procedures is used, the Glasgow Coma Scale.

8.3.3 Disturbance of areas of consciousness

Subjectively, there are domains of consciousness: consciously seeing, hearing, but also consciously remembering and feeling. However, there is apparently no domain-specific clouding of consciousness, i.e., for example, no clouding only in the visual domain. Clouding of consciousness is regularly supramodal.

However, several psychiatric syndromes show deficits only in one of the domains of consciousness. Patients cannot experience anything in certain domains whereas others perceive something, i.e., they become aware of a sensation. An example is alexithymia. It is a disorder in which an emotion does not reach consciousness. The reasons for this condition cannot be further elaborated here.

A second example is the loss of the sense of illness, where a patient does not consciously experience that he shows signs of an illness, which are quite obvious to others. In this case, it is usually a perceptual disorder related to the self-model, as discussed above. Since this is deficient, it leads to misperception, i.e., the signs of illness are not perceived by the patient.

8.4 Diagnostics

Diagnostic features of clouding of consciousness

The two types of disturbances of consciousness, the somnolence-coma type and the delirium type, are associated with deficits in neuropsychological examination procedures. The formal test conditions are mostly very unsatisfactory. However, the immediate examination of an athlete after traumatic brain injury, e.g., at the sidelines, see above, is very valuable: The coach can find out whether the player was dazed or even somnolent at the time after the accident, whether he could speak, and when asked about the date and place, whether he was oriented and whether he responded promptly, etc.

An attempt is made to compile objective features of clouding of consciousness.

1. The reactivity is reduced—the person does not respond to stimuli from others, the interview, or facial, gestural, or prosodic stimuli to the usual extent. Example: The conversation partner hands over an object, and the patient reacts very slowly to the shown item (neurological impairments, e.g., visual impairment, agnosia, are excluded—this also applies to the other symptoms).
2. The person reacts with a delay. The latency of the response is higher than expected. This refers to a general, not solely motor, slowing down.
3. Disturbance of the full attention,
   a) Full attention is not given interpersonally, even with appropriate attempts to gain the greatest extent of attention. Example: The patient does not devote full attention to explaining or questioning during the life history, which can also be recognized by attention-accompanying movements.
   b) The attention to events in the environment is reduced. Example: The person does not look at the door when someone enters (considering possible sensory limitations).
4. Disturbance of the awareness of the situation or the interview topic,
   a) Slowing down: The awareness of the situation or the interview topic is not achieved promptly—for example, as if abruptly awakened from deep sleep, the prompt clarity about the situation is not yet given (again excluding neurological disorders, such as aphasia).
   b) Incompleteness: The awareness of the situation or the interview topic is not fully achieved, for example, as with a person abruptly awakened from deep sleep, who only partially understands the situation.

When listing the features, it is already noticeable that each feature must be psychopathologically examined for alternative explanations: Dissociative states, catatonic or stuporous states in schizophrenia and depression, pronounced intellectual disability, severe reduction of the general condition, and neurological neuropsychological disorders, etc., can simulate a disturbance of the awareness of the environment and attention. A sum score was tested for these features as a rating of the mild disturbance of the awareness of the environment for the diagnosis of delirium. In this rating, rating points are assigned for each feature: 0 not; 0.5 very slight, questionably present; 1 definitely present; 2 strongly present. Minimum 0, maximum 12 points. An initial application (Reischies et al. 2004) on 92 patients with delirium syndromes of various causes showed a median of 6 points (mean 6.6, standard deviation 3.1 points), and the score showed a close correlation to encephalographic changes in delirium (Reischies et al. 2005).

More importantly, the features of the awareness of the environment, as characterized above, correlate with the neuropsychological disorders of patients with various forms of delirium. This is not the case for the other features of delirium, such as vigilance disorders, emotional disorders, or hallucinations.

Furthermore, the reduction of

a) attention-related movements should be noted (eyes, head, fingers, hand, etc.), e.g., spontaneous pointing with the hand, looking, etc., occurs less frequently (this feature is especially noticeable to close relatives, history taken from other persons);
b) Inadequacy of attention-related movements in the respective situation. Example: The target of a movement is not understandable to the examiner (not caused by ataxia or hyperkinesis).

Regarding possible change in conscious experience (see below), the person must be asked about their experience of conscious perception in the psychopathological interview. The subjective assessment of clouding of consciousness is unreliable. For example, acutely schizophrenic patients report altered perception, but they generally do not exhibit clouding of consciousness.

The same applies to patients with histrionic personality disorders. Because patients with clouding of consciousness cannot provide reliable information about the changes in themselves, it is plausible to assume that the consciousness disorder itself is not consciously perceived. The diaphanous nature of consciousness has been emphasized (Berrios 1996; Metzinger 2001), i.e., the investigators postulate that humans look at the world through the processes of consciousness functions as if through a transparent film; they do not perceive the consciousness functions.

In psychophysics, the subjective quality of perceptions (such as how bright a stimulus appears, how loud, etc.) is very precisely examined. However, only special, trained, and reliable individuals are active in the investigations. The experiences from psychophysical studies cannot be transferred to patients with psychiatric disorders. Furthermore, the information in psychophysics refers to conscious sensory perception, about which the best information can be provided, but not to the conditions in consciousness disorders.

8.5 Neuroscience

In neuroscience, work is being done on explaining the "last mystery" of consciousness (e.g., Zeman 2001; Koch 2005). The ambitious research in this field leads to some hasty conclusions, i.e., the phenomenon is explained by this or that mechanism. The models still largely rely on speculative generalizations, etc. The neuroscientific models of consciousness are criticized from two sides. On one side are critics with arguments that the individual quality of consciousness can never be reduced to neural mechanisms. On the other side, it must be examined for psychopathology whether the described mechanisms are sufficient to explain the clinical diversity.

As, for example, Ramachandran (2004) and other neuroscientists and neurophilosophers have suggested, there is a first agreement that we must assume a series of neurophysiological mechanisms for consciousness. These, it is hoped, will explain a large part of the phenomena of consciousness.

Since the phenomenon of consciousness cannot be directly examined, approaches are chosen that were described at the beginning of the section to illustrate the phenomenon of consciousness. What are the differences between conscious and unconscious types of perceptions, conscious and unconscious memories from memory, conscious and unconscious actions, etc.—these differences can be examined in humans using neuroscientific methods.

8.5.1 Consciousness as system state of human information processing: Marginal factors

Central to the consideration of the neuroscience of consciousness disorders is that several functional systems, some of which are discussed in other chapters, must be intact for consciousness (Ramachandran 2004):

- sufficient vigilance and attentiveness—attention for domains such as conscious seeing, hearing, feeling, remembering, reacting,
- working memory for monitoring ongoing processes—"I am aware that xyz have happened or are happening,"
- retrieval for the recall of essential information for the respective situation—"I am aware that I have already experienced this situation on day x at place y," "The situation is familiar to me."

In the following, a comparison of conscious and unconscious information processing will be considered neuroscientifically for each domain.

8.5.2 Conscious Perception

One research approach is the search for neurophysiological correlates of conscious perception (Koch 2005). The phenomena of changed conscious experience, which, for example, include reflexive processes of the activated self-concept, are explicitly excluded (Damasio 1999).

8.5.3 Masking

A subsequent stimulus can achieve that the first stimulus is processed unconsciously, it does not appear in consciousness. These phenomena have long been studied, where, for example, the subsequent stimuli disturb the conscious perception of the preceding stimulus, the "backward masking." These are special perceptual situations that represent artificial contexts for perception. However, they can provide us with clues regarding the physiology of conscious perception. Recent results show something surprising: The masked stimulus can apparently trigger cortical processing, which is referred to as masking priming because it shows lasting effects and is also detectable in electrophysiological studies (Dehaene et al. 1998a, b, 2001). Despite the continued cortical processing, the stimulus is not conscious. So, researchers have asked, what are the necessary prerequisites for the becoming aware of the perception of a stimulus?

A first answer can be given by the investigation of the cortical traces of subliminal stimuli. A subliminal somatosensory stimulation, which did not have the strength to come to consciousness when attention was directed to the body part, is apparently associated with inhibitory cortex activation (Blankenburg et al. 2003). This result shows that cortical processing of stimuli does not necessarily ensure that they are consciously perceived. Cortical inhibition apparently can push the stimuli below the perception threshold. There was criticism of the experimental-psychological investigation of the perception threshold; because it can lead to a confounding of the criteria for stimulus detection and the criteria for conscious perception. In other words: The stimulus processing in terms of detection, i.e., the question of when a person detects a stimulus, could have a different threshold than conscious perception (Haase and Fisk 2004).

8.5.4 Dual task

Further investigations are those in which several things are to be perceived simultaneously. An object is shown in the foreground and attention is directed to it, and additionally, image elements are visible, but attention is not focused on them. However, these are used for testing. The question is whether the brain regions that usually take over the special stimulus processing are also active in this presentation without focused attention on these objects. An investigation used evoked EEG potentials. Clear EEG dipoles were found in the face-processing brain region even with subliminal presentation of faces (Hoshiyama et al. 2003). The faces were not consciously perceived. The results indicate that it has not yet been proven how the awareness of perception depends on the activation or non-activation of a special stimulus-processing brain region, because these are also active in unconscious processing.

8.5.5 Blindsight

Unconscious perceptions have also been studied in brain injuries with visual field restrictions (Weiskrantz 1986). The neuropsychology of unconscious perception in lesions of the primary sensory region in the cortex will not be discussed in detail here. Nevertheless, this finding should be mentioned because it can explain a crucial circumstance in the field of consciousness mechanisms: In patients with occipital brain lesions, it was observed that although they cannot consciously see, they are able to indicate the position of an object in certain situations; in other words, they point with their finger to an object they say they do not see. They cannot identify it either; they can only say that something is there.

There are traces of sensory processing that take place outside the damaged cortical brain regions. The sensory information is processed on a rudimentary "map" in the superior colliculi, which is the common explanation of these phenomena. From there, the motor cortex can receive information about the position of an object. These rudimentary functions are sufficient for certain visual functions after occipital lesions, but not for conscious perception.

Usually, the functions of localization and conscious seeing are coupled. In the case of the specific lesion, however, they fall apart. The effect is that the function of pointing is still preserved, but conscious access does not succeed. Normally, we can consciously devote ourselves to the localization of objects because we activate the consciousness-capable visual perception. We attribute the conscious pointing to the location of a seen object to conscious perception, although unconscious processes are responsible for it.

This necessitates the distinction between:

- obligatorily unconscious processes in the brain and the
- potentially unconscious processes, such as in visual perception.
- To be distinguished from these are
- obligatorily conscious processes such as planning and critical and productive thinking and communicating.

8.5.6 Active becoming aware

How does active becoming aware succeed, how can a person direct attention to the environment so that they consciously perceive what is otherwise processed automatically? This happens with "mindfulness". Apparently, for conscious processes like planning thinking and potentially conscious processes like perceiving the environment, a bidirectional activation pathway needs to be described and explained. On the one hand, the environment can gain attention, where the value assignment and "meaning" of an identified object are crucial—thus, the attentional resources that an object can bind to itself are important for this fate of further processing. On the other hand, a person can become aware of something in the process of planning or creative designing. A process is activated because it has gained meaning in the planning process that it did not have before. This is mediated through attention, which can be controlled like an intelligent filter. We can imagine that in a mindfulness exercise, for example, attention is first directed through thought processes to visual perception, then to auditory perception, and then to somatosensory perception. In doing so, sensory impressions come to consciousness that were overlooked, unheard, or neglected in the realm of feeling.

Conscious versus unconscious somatosensory perception

A peculiarity of somatosensory perception is that we process massive unconscious stimulation daily through our clothing, shoes, or seating, etc., unconsciously. Only rarely does somatosensory perception become conscious to us.

8.5.7 Conscious and Unconscious Emotion

The triggering of emotion is described in Chap. 11. Unconscious emotions are a clinically familiar phenomenon (e.g., when a person becomes enraged, and others have to inform them that they are being aggressive). Studies have shown that unconscious activations of central emotional processing through features, such as facial expressions in empathetic emotions, are possible through masking emotional faces by immediately presenting neutral stimuli (Whalen et al. 1998) afterwards.

However, it is a mystery what the difference is between these activations of central emotional functional units in unconscious emotional activation and those in conscious emotion. The fact that many emotions are habitually not or not sufficiently consciously processed, as in alexithymia, still seems insufficiently explained.

8.5.8 Conscious Recall from Memory

Implicit encoding and retrieval, i.e., unconscious storage and recall of memory contents, has been investigated in recent years.

1. An example of unconscious learning of memory contents is Hebb's learning. The task is to repeat random sequences. In Hebb's learning, one sequence repeats itself in random sequences over and over again; the improvement through repetitions is measured, whereby the repetitions are not consciously noticed by the subject. It is a special situation in which the learning is explicit. Only in the retrieval of the repeated sequences is the special situation of repetition implicit and thus the specific learning progress.
2. In other tasks, both encoding and recall from memory remain implicit. Examples are word completion tasks, letter gaps that need to be filled, such as t_m_t_. If the word "tomato" was mentioned shortly before in another context, the persistent cortex activity can contribute to a faster and more secure solution of the task.
3. This is to be distinguished from incidental learning, where encoding does not occur consciously, but recall from memory is explicit. An example of this is the recognition of words that previously had to be identified in a word-nonword decision, without the subjects being aware that the words would need to be remembered later. This essentially involves normal retrieval processes, only the storage did not have the quality of "wanting to remember."

What do studies show about differences in critical brain areas in conscious and unconscious retrieval from episodic memory? We can remember parts of the situation, such as that a certain person was present, but without recalling the entire situation. In conscious recall of a situation, the hippocampus was activated in functional imaging studies (Wheeler and Buckner 2004), whereas in retrieval processes from memory where conscious recall of the episode was not achieved, the hippocampus was not involved (Eldridge et al. 2000). Conscious recall activates additional regions that are involved, for example, in the visual processing of the remembered objects (Wheeler and Buckner 2004). These results are consistent with the model that in conscious recall of a situation, the visuospatial relationships are also retrieved, namely the spatiotemporal episode.

Procedural learning, such as learning to handle tools skillfully, can also occur unconsciously. Conscious learning of a motor skill and unconscious procedural learning were contrasted. Common areas were found to be activated, but additional areas were also activated during conscious learning (Willingham et al. 2002).

The dissociation of conscious recall and unconscious retrieval processes can go so far that a learning process can be demonstrated in the EEG using N 400 potentials (Sect. 9.4.11), which, however, does not manifest itself in the conscious response, the reproduction of the memory content. The response can be incorrect, although the N 400 potentials indicate that information processing in certain brain areas or networks was correct. This result was found in patients with memory disorders. In certain disorders, the conscious decision about memory contents can apparently be incorrect because it is based on the information processing of impaired brain areas, and the person apparently cannot rely on more efficient information processing.

8.5.9 Conscious vs. Unconscious Action

In physiology books, a distinction is made between the extrapyramidal and the pyramidal motor systems, with the extrapyramidal motor system being characterized as unconscious, automated motor function. However, a skilled pianist can certainly play his piece both automatically and consciously, even though he masters it "extrapyramidally." It is certainly correct that new, not yet mastered movements are initially performed and learned under conscious control before they can potentially run automatically. How do automated unconscious actions differ from conscious actions?

In a task to beat a rhythm, the rhythm of the given pattern was varied: cortical activation could be detected in the ventral medial prefrontal cortex more during unconscious slight rhythm adaptations, whereas only extensive, conscious adaptations showed activation in the dorsolateral prefrontal cortex (Stephan et al. 2002). The result is consistent with the assumption that the dorsolateral prefrontal cortex is active in executive functions that become conscious. In this sense, results that show a dissociation between short-term reward-dependent actions, which are subject to orbitofrontal control, and delayed rewarded actions, which are more attentive/conscious and associated with dorsolateral prefrontal activation, are to be interpreted (McClure et al. 2004).

Conclusion

Regarding the studies comparing conscious and unconscious information processing, it cannot yet be said whether the state of consciousness of mental activity depends on the activity of certain brain regions, even if the results show that conscious information processing is associated with the activation of certain brain structures. It can be summarized that more brain regions are active during conscious processes. The dorsolateral prefrontal region, which is crucial for working memory functions, seems to be involved in many cases where complex conscious actions are required. This is consistent with the idea of the activation of self- and environmental models in controlled actions, as presented in the introduction, and also with the activity of regions for working memory and monitoring.

8.5.10 Minimal Neural Events for the Awareness of a Perception?

Koch (2005) explicitly sought neural correlates for conscious processes in the brain. It should be mentioned that there is a fierce debate on this research question. According to Fodor (1983) and Ryle (1969), research on this is misguided. Fodor doubts such questions beyond the hard-wired neurons in the modules of the mind (such as language processing) because access to all information of all interconnected cells occurs, making it a global network. Ryle, on the other hand, and with him many humanities scholars, reject this research because it represents a category error to seek a neural correlate for a quality of a percept, which is a subjective event—subjective experience and neural activity are fundamentally incompatible categories. The quality of conscious sensation can never be reduced to processes in a neural functional system. The question remains open, as metabolic (pharmacological, toxic, etc.) changes in the quality of sensations can be observed.

In distinguishing between (1) a conscious perception—for example, my sock on my left foot—and (2) normally unconscious stimulus processing, not all neurons in the brain are involved. Why should the neurons of the acoustic representation of pitch be involved in this distinction? Fodor would argue that these neurons belong to a module, that of acoustic identification, and thus are not available for free associative connections. The discussion of these positions makes it clear: presumably, many neurons in many neuron groups will be involved in distinguishing between conscious and unconscious stimulus processing. The crucial question will be whether this is the desired outcome and whether a cerebral system of becoming aware of perceptions, memories, feelings, etc., emerges. The question is also to what extent this cerebral functional system is closely connected with the attention system. Additionally, there are specific neuron groups that are involved with monitoring, the self-model, etc. It is to be suspected that we are not dealing with a single neural network for conscious perception, but with several neural networks (which are connected with focused attention, the self-model, and monitoring).

8.5.11 Self-Generated Focus of Consciousness

Another area of neuroscientific research on consciousness phenomena concerns the becoming aware of mental contents, whether they are thoughts or sensory impressions. In recent decades, the concept of self-generation of the attention focus in neural networks has emerged, Chap. 4 attention. The image of the beam of consciousness as a spotlight in the Cartesian Theater, which Jaspers (1942) cites in his psychopathology, does not capture the physiological functions. For there is presumably no "pointer function" in the brain that could activate certain specific contents or locations. At most, the thalamic activation of occipitoparietal regions can be understood as such a roughly topically specific activation (Mesulam 2000). However, large parts of a brain region are presumably activated, and a sharp point-like activation of contents cannot occur through this.

Neuroscience has assumed the development of a focus in the neural network, with the activation maximum defining this focus. This activation maximum is determined by the current or just past contents that are currently activated.

Neurons form a workspace (global work space) into which all specialized modules pass their information—such as object identification, linguistic processing, spatial analysis, memory retrieval, etc. In this workspace, the activity will always take on a certain maximum (7 Chap. 4 attention). Through functions of working memory, a mental content can remain activated for a longer time if a task is associated with it for the person (7 Chap. 10 thinking; see Reischies et al. 2003; according to Dehaene et al. 1998a).

The activity maximum in the neural network is also not to be imagined as a local maximum that could be localized on the cortex, but as a distributed one, i.e., an activation of contents and their connections that are represented in different places in the network.

With regard to the attention network, it is now less assumed to be a pointer, but rather an automatic activation of relevant contents and action readiness in response to the "input" of a stimulus or a situation (Chap. 4 attention). The basal ganglia can activate specific cortical addresses via a programmable filter in the functional context of the frontal loops (Mega and Cummings 1994) and thus activate or preactivate the recall of stored contents. However, this is not to be characterized as a "spotlight," but as a complex filter, as used in computers to read out memory.

8.5.12 Sensory-Motor Feedback

Sensory-motor feedback and experience of being the actor: Motor actions of the person are accompanied by changes in perception. Since the CNS plans the movement, it can predict the effect. This is likely to occur through neural networks that are well-suited for calculating simple input-output transformations. If the feedback comes through the sensory system, a comparison between the calculated and actual feedback can take place.

A physiological example is the recognition of figures in the visual field when the person turns their gaze. This occurs inferotemporally by relating the motor commands for eye movements to the perceived displacements of the figures in the visual field. Desimone was able to identify recognition neurons that work inhibitory (Desimone et al. 1995). This could correspond with the postulated deletion of expectation and feedback information according to the concept of "corollary discharge" and the efference copy by von Holst (Holst and Mittelstaedt 1950). Comparable processes are assumed for hand or body motor skills with somatosensory feedback.

The consequence is that the CNS receives expected feedback in practically all movements.

We can assume that the effects of a person's own actions have been predicted, are compared with the feedback, and are usually confirmed. This alignment of action intention with changes in sensory information after the action also confirms the person's self-concept as an actor every second. This is likely to contribute to the phenomenal characteristic of the person's consciousness.

Unfamiliarity

A disruption of the described closed-loop processes has significant effects. Perplexity occurs as an affective reaction in many patients with consciousness disorders (see example in Chap. 8.1). Why does what they experience no longer seem familiar to them, why do they no longer understand? Perception occurs in the interaction of bottom-up and top-down processes (Chap. 2 Perception). In the constructivist interpretation of this fact, it is assumed that the person builds expectations of environmental stimuli that make perception more efficient (predictive coding). If people with a consciousness disorder now have a disruption in the elaboration of expectations and imaginations, i.e., can no longer form top-down expectations or form false expectations, they are disturbed in their perception of the environment. They are often surprised in their understanding of what the environment shows. This leads to perception and especially comprehension disorders.

Not only elementary closed-loop processes of sensory-motor feedback (see above) are meant here. The above also applies to the more complex expectation brought to action situations. Frontal lobe functions are assumed for the top-down processes (Reischies 2004, 2005). A consequence of this is: An acute disruption of the biochemical properties of the transmission of information between nerve cells will lead to a collapse of prediction in the neural networks. This can, for example, lead to thought disorders, as seen in acute psychoses (Hoffman 1987). It can also lead to changes in the processes of predicting motor effects. The model of "catastrophic interference" (McClelland et al. 1995) has been introduced for a collapse in the computational quality of neural networks when the transmission weights at individual nodes change. This can be the case in acute consciousness disorder when biochemical disruptions lead to a disruption of synaptic information processing.

There can also be a dysfunction of the mediotemporal system of familiarity, which can transmit the signal of familiarity, or more so, the alarm signal of the violation of familiarity. If there is a disruption in this system, alarm and, example, anxiety are triggered incorrectly.

8.5.13 Summary

The interaction of the functional systems for the state of consciousness is not yet nearly clarified. One can state:

1. Attention functions, both sustained unfocussed and phasic focussed, are necessary to ensure consciousness and also to be able to actively and flexibly change it. Attention functions are presumably also involved in the active "becoming aware of …". Attention resources can be bound by certain percepts that have learned significance for the person and thus lead to a becoming aware of the sensory information.
2. Monitoring functions enable an overview of the various recent processes and the overall state. Disturbances affect the awareness of the environment and situational orientation; the patient no longer knows what is happening. Monitoring is to be explained as one of the many aspects of working memory.
3. This monitoring of what is currently happening is part of the self- and environmental model, namely the current part that is maintained by working memory. There are also parts that originate from the knowledge store and parts that come from episodic memory.
4. In addition, the person always experiences themselves as the actor of movements and receives current pre-calculated somatosensory feedback, such as calculated changes in the retinal images after eye movements .

5. Memory functions: On the one hand, recognizing the environment as familiar, known surroundings is important. Retrieval functions are necessary to establish the respective references of the current situation to past episodes and semantic or knowledge aspects.
6. Priming processes in selecting the attentively perceived environmental parts (Chap. 4 attention). Psychological "structures" play a role here, learned, trained, and innate mechanisms that guide selection in an individual and temporary manner. Recently, a function of neural networks that predict the next steps has played an increasing role in the discussion. They prime, so to speak, the more efficient processing of the next upcoming processes.

Demented patients are awake, but they can no longer relate the currently perceived environment to their previous experiences and their knowledge. If they then lose the current monitoring, they no longer know "what is going on" and are often diagnosed as delirious. This can occur in addition to the pre-damage of critical brain structures and thus explain why demented patients particularly often develop a delirium. The diverse functions of standard wakeful conscious state are only partially present in dementia and "thin out" as the disease progresses.

Studies of functional imaging on differences between conscious and unconscious mental events yield the following picture: In conscious mental processes, more brain regions are active than in unconscious ones. So far, no universally valid consciousness region has been found, i.e., a region that is always active when a percept becomes conscious. It could therefore be that no specific brain region has to be active always when perception, memory, or action is consciously performed.

Are sub-functions of consciousness associated with the activation of specific brain regions? Certain brain regions could be involved in specific conscious processes, such as the hippocampus in conscious remembering (Eldridge et al. 2000) or the dorsolateral prefrontal cortex in conscious corrective movements. This raises the question of whether these regions, which are involved in many functions, must exceed a threshold of activation for the consciousness of the process to be achieved.

The data are consistent with various assumptions about the consciousness of mental functions:

- with the assumption of the necessity of attention in conscious mental functions,
- with models of an activation of special monitoring and control and special distributed networks—"global workspace" (Dehaene and Naccache 2001),
- with models that assume the activation of the self- and environmental model (see Reischies et al. 2003).

The data are consistent with the assumption of a normal state of consciousness, one could say standard consciousness, that people have in attentive wakefulness; it does not require focussed attention.

Important for this assumption is that there cannot be at one time multiple levels or a variation in the quantity of consciousness, at least: We could not know anything about it, could not recognize it. We cannot, as with color blindness, resort to Ishihara plates to relate our experience of colors to that of other people. A specialist might try to diagnose an attention deficit syndrome that relates to this unfocussed attention, but only by the presence of a behavioral syndrome.

From this standard consciousness, the activation of (laborious) focussing succeeds, for example, for the obligatorily conscious processes of planning or intentional communication. The quality of focussed attention can be examined (Chap. 4 attention).

It is speculated that this standard consciousness is related to the evolution of social communication. A member of the social group must be in standard consciousness and be able to communicate. In standard consciousness, the activation of controlled actions or plans, about which the members of the group can be informed, succeeds. In human society, accountability in this state also plays a role. Each group member can provide feedback on past actions and their reasons.

8.6 Psychopathological Symptomes of the Consciousness Domain

Clouding of Consciousness—somnolence -Type
Definition: Reduction of wakefulness with impairment of cognitive functions such as orientation, memory, and slowing, etc. Quantitative gradation with drowsiness, somnolence, sopor and coma.

Example

A young man is found motionless on the sidewalk. During examination by paramedics, he can state his name but cannot provide any information about the cause of his condition. After a brief response, he seems to fall back into an unconscious state. Upon repeated questioning, he says he has no pain and shows no pain reactions when being moved onto a stretcher, where he again seems to fall asleep. A state following an epileptic grand mal seizure is diagnosed. ◄

Position in Psychopathology. AMDP 1.

Related Terms. Quantitative clouding of consciousness.

Psychopathological Interactions. Fatigue, reduction in drive (akinetic mutism)

Differential diagnostic distinctions:

- Fatigue, severe sleep deficit
- Apathy
- Loss of drive in stupor

Increasing loss of communication in progressive cerebrovascular damage, e.g., beginning global aphasia, intoxication

Further Characterization. Quantitative aspect of the feature:

Drowsiness as a slight restriction of clear wakefulness, which can partly be registered by the person.

Somnolence describes a state in which the person seems to be dozing off, appearing sleepy. Cognitive performance impairments are usually diagnosable in this state. An attempt at a psychopathological interview may show the inexplicability of the apparent fatigue. The person can report a difference from previously experienced fatigue.

Sopor is called a difficulty in waking up a person who immediately falls back into the previous state of apparent sleep after the awakening attempt.

A state in which the person is not arousable is called coma. Further gradations of coma severity can be achieved using electroencephalographic or imaging examinations.

Self-/other persons's judgment: other persons's judgment

Neuropsychology/objectification
- Gradation according to the neuropsychological feature list Glasgow Coma Scale: reaction to awakening stimuli, speech, memory, orientation, etc.

Severity :
Mild impairment recognizable in some cases by drowsiness. Moderate impairment with characteristic awakening reaction up to coma

Specifications:
Etiological special forms—obligation to diagnostic clarification of life-threatening causes, neurological examination of persons with impaired consciousness.

Neuroscientific/cognitive neuroscientific model concepts

Damage in the centrencephalic system in the upper brainstem with disturbance of the activating systems.

Various other acute brain injuries possible—whereby the disturbance in the centrencephalic system only dominates the clinical appearance—see Fig. 8.3

Clouding of consciousness—delirium type
Definition: Disintegration of consciousness functions with disturbances in the areas of attention, orientation, episodic memory, targeted actions, and affects. Hallucinations and delusional misjudgments may occur. The person is unable to become aware of the current facts of their own person and surroundings, and the examiners suspect an altered experience of the environment.

An important specification concerns the activity level—hyperactive and hypoactive delirium syndrome.

Example

- An older man, previously healthy, is found in bed in the morning, makes no effort to get up, seems not to register the visit, and no longer reacts as usual; asked what is wrong, he says "nothing special," appears perplexed and uninvolved. Diagnosis: Hypoactive delirium with beginning pneumonia.
- A woman who was able to do her work without any problems a few days ago is suddenly unsure about what is "going on," no longer knows what situation she is in. She walks around restlessly and aimlessly and asks obvious questions that can be explained by the situation. She has clearly lost control over her actions and the understanding of perceptions of the environment—her actions show that she is not clear about what is happening. Diagnosis: hyperactive delirium in alcohol withdrawal. ◀

Position in psychopathology. AMDP 2—compared with the general concept of consciousness disorder limitation with regard to the concept of "disorder of awareness of the environment" required for delirium:awareness of the environment.

Related terms. Qualitative clouding of consciousness.

Psychopathological interactions. Fatigue, drive reduction, disturbance of general information processing in dementia and other brain function disorders, disturbance of working memory.

Differential diagnostic distinctions:
- dissociation,
- perplexity in a completely unfamiliar environment

Further characterization. Consciousness as general monitoring of everything that is happening mentally is impaired by many types of information processing disorders, but not in a psychopathologically specific way. Therefore, operationalization is necessary:

The person is disturbed in following what is happening around and with him—the model of the current situation is only partially activated or no longer available.

Awareness of oneself and the environment is disturbed: The person cannot become aware of the current facts of their own person and surroundings—in mild form recognizable as a delay in the awareness of the interview topic.

Self-/other person's judgment. Other person's judgment.

Interview for rating. Pay attention to the promptness and completeness of the awareness of interview topics, adequacy of attention-related movements to the environment.

- try to find out what imagination the person has of the situation he is currently in.

Neuropsychology/objectification
- Behavioral observation in the interview situation, reaction to approach to the person,

attention-related movements that show whether the person is surprised by self-evident things,
- neuropsychological examination usually not possible—a testing could prove a multidimensional disorder of cognitive processing, but it must be clarified to what extent this cannot be explained by other simultaneously occurring (e.g., in case of acute brain damage) or pre-existing (dementia) disorders.
- Tests that examine working memory or executive functions. In contrast, overlearned and routine functions such as elementary sequence recitations, etc., are often undisturbed or only slightly disturbed (Reischies et al. 2007).

Severity: Beginning with slight impairment, in some cases recognizable by a bahavior described as "not quite present," "clouded": reduced reactivity, slight unplannedness and lack of overview in everyday life, up to noticeably lost control over actions, lost classification of perceptions of the environment—slight uncertainty and errors in situational assessment up to completely missing situational orientation with misjudgment of the nature and concrete design of the current (examination) situation and, according to external anamnesis, also other situations.

Pathognomonic for: delirium.

Specifications

According to the activity level: In hyperactive delirium, there is an obligation to protect the person from dangers they can no longer detect. In hypoactive delirium, there is a risk of overlooking an underlying disease requiring treatment, such as pneumonia.

Partial syndrome: Confusion without many other psychopathological features of this symptom—questionable to diagnose as a form of delirium (DD: transient amnestic syndrome)

Course: sudden onset often during alcohol withdrawal

Conceptual problems of the feature. Awareness of the environment has so far mostly been confounded with situational orientation. In the classification systems, the diagnosis of delirium requires the disturbance of awareness of the environment. The disturbance of awareness of the environment is presented here as a characteristic of the clouding of consciousness of the delirium type.

Neuroscientific/cognitive neuroscientific

Model concepts

1. Monitoring function disturbed,
2. attention to the environment usually also disturbed, on the one hand reduced orientation of intentionality to the environment, possibly active withdrawal (e.g., from anxiety and perplexity)
3. disturbed free access to potential contents of consciousness,
4. models of the self as well as the environment are disturbed.

Narrowed consciousness

Definition: An awake person can not be distracted by usual sensory stimuli, seems absent or fixated on a content of consciousness.

It cannot be clarified due to the inaccessibility whether a content of consciousness remains effective for a longer period or whether the person currently has no activated content of consciousness.

Example

- A patient suddenly begins to act automatically, as if in a dream, does not respond to the addressing of a topic, the eye movements are predominantly fixed straight ahead or on the ground and do not turn to new objects in the environment; the patient also does not turn to newly arriving persons.
- A patient is unable to speak after a severe motorcycle accident; he stares ahead and cannot be distracted by anything. ◀

Position in psychopathology. AMDP 3

Related terms. dissociation, "shock."

Psychopathological interactions.
narrowing of attention, of thinking; brooding, derealization, agitation.

Differential Diagnostic Distinctions. Thought narrowing—narrowing is limited to thinking, narrowed thinking is contained in narrowed consciousness but also occurs without narrowing of consciousness itself—attention can still be distracted by stimuli,

- not voluntarily, e.g., in meditation,
- the focus of consciousness can possibly be experienced by the person after the end of the state, there is no amnestic gap, as in delirium and epileptic twilight states.

Further Characterization:

- Image: the beam of consciousness captures (if at all) only a small part of the stage, a single actor, whom the spotlight operator automatically follows, regardless of which actors on the stage are main characters or what important situations are,
- disturbance of the direction of attention leads to unresponsiveness to distracting environmental stimuli,
- the narrowing of consciousness results in a failure to integrate all aspects of one's own person and situation.

Self-/other person's judgment. Other person's judgment.

Interview for Rating. Is the person responsive? In a narrowed state of consciousness, a cautious attempt to distract with (pleasant) stimuli. After the end of the state: Did the person perceive the entire situation, e.g., after a traumatic event.

Neuropsychology/objectification. Behavioral observation of eye movements and attention-related movements of the extremities or trunk.

Severity. Limited to absent reaction to environmental stimuli. Difficulty in gaining attention.

Specifications: • Attention narrowing,
- Trance-like state,
- Dissociative stupor.

Personality Influences. Hypnotizability.

Conceptual Problems of the Feature
- Stupor and dissociative disorder of the integration of experiences—unpleasantly experienced but not specifically with anxiety,
- the question of whether there are subtypes cannot be easily decided: epileptic narrowed consciousness without agitation as an attention-flexibility disorder, excitement, anxiety, derealization type, hysterical dissociation,
- question, whether dissociation as in stage fright and being beside oneself in exams, state in combat situations should be included,
- possibly a milder form, from which one can still easily jump out.

Neuroscientific/cognitive neuroscientific models
1. Distraction of attention impossible, recall of associations and memories does not succeed unrestrained,
2. the execution of automatic movements dominates mental activity; therefore, it is not possible to respond flexibly to the environment; the person does not "act" or is occupied with automated actions,
3. emotional-cognitive complexes of fundamental importance to the person bind attention (question whether it can be a consequence of a predominant affect, such as anxiety, which suppresses all thoughts, memories, and distractions),
4. Disposition to hypnosis, dissociation,
5. Person has experienced that in these states unbearable contents can be repressed,
6. self-model and environmental model are inactive, only focal aspects, which do not have to be related to the concrete situation, reach consciousness—described as an integration disorder,

7. Drive without control by the "supervisory attentional system" (see Bob 2003).
8. The narrowing of attention can be conceptualized as a disorder in the ability to disengage from one feature and focus on a new topic.

Disorder of integration of experience—dissociation
Definition: This disorder is described as part of the reaction in acute stress reactions:

The integration (1) of memories of previous similar events or episodes addressed in the situation, (2) the awareness of one's own identity and person, (3) the clear conscious perception of immediate sensory perception of the environment, and (4) the control of movements no longer succeeds.

- In acute stress reactions and in states of dissociative stupor, the above-mentioned integration no longer succeeds.
- Interview of the subjective side of the conspicuous behavior.
- Highly complex feature, pathognomonic for dissociative disorder, mentioned as a criterion in ICD-10.

Alteration of conscious experience
Definition: State of subjectively altered conscious experience—the person becomes aware that he experiences the internal and external situation as changed.

Example

- A person reports dreamlike unreal, altered experience.
- A patient reports an overjoyed experience, in which everything seemed easy to him— and everything appeared more intense, brighter than usual. ◀

Position in psychopathology. AMDP 4.

Related terms. Intoxication, delusional enlightenment experiences, meditation states can lead to expanded consciousness, trance, revelation experiences, Eureka experiences.

Psychopathological interactions. Delusion, hallucination, illusion,

- close relationships with intense emotions, e.g., joy, euphoria,
- depressed mood when a sudden catastrophic event occurs that worsens the perspective (but then usually dissociation).

Differential diagnostic distinctions:
- dissociation, in which there is also a narrowing of consciousness,
- Affect that occurs in an event significant to the person; also affect that occurs in a delusional experience, e.g., having received a message from God.
- Ecstatic experience

Further characterization. Conscious perception of an altered self-/environmental awareness, which may be accompanied by an intense emotion.

Self-/other persons's judgment. Other persons's judgment with information about introspections.

Interview for rating. Question about a change in experience, about the feeling; is the patient in joyful agitation?

Neuropsychology/objectification. Behavioral observation—attention-related movements such as turning towards somebody do not occur or are altered (not mandatory),

- emotional reactions that are not explainable.

Severity. In order to be considered a symptom, the feature must lead to a change in cognitive or communicative functions; up to an excited exceptional state that hinders interaction with the patient.

Personality influences. Esoteric and schizotypal features.

Neuroscientific/cognitive neuroscientific models

1. self-model and/or environmental model is perceived as not fitting, possibly reorganized,
2. intense emotions affect consciousness functions—in the sense of disturbing or altering.
3. Metabolic disorder of the neural systems for subjective quality of sensation, the qualia.

References

Baars BJ (1988) A cognitive theory of consciousness. Cambridge Univ Press, Cambridge

Baars BJ (2002) The conscious access hypothesis: origins and recent ecidence. Trends Cogn Sci 6:47–52

Berrios GE (1996) The history of mental symptoms. Cambridge Univ Press, Cambridge

Blankenburg F, Taskin B, Ruben J et al (2003) Imperceptible stimuli and sensory processing impediment. Science 299:1864

Bob P (2003) Dissociation and neuroscience: history and new perspectives. Int J Neurosci 113:903–914

Crick F, Koch C (2003) A framework for consciousness. Nat Neurosci 6(2):119–126

Dehaene S, Naccache L (2001) Towards a cognitive neuroscience of consciousness: basic evidence and a workspace framework. Cognition 79:1–37

Dehaene S, Kerszberg M, Changeux JP (1998a) A neuronal model of a global workspace in effortful cognitive tasks. Proc Natl Acad Sci U S A 95:14529–14534

Dehaene S, Naccache L, Le Clec' H et al (1998b) Imaging unconscious semantic priming. Nature 395:597–600

Damasio AR (1999) The feeling of what happens: Body and emotion in the making of consciousness. Harcourt Brace, New York

Dennett D (1991) Consciousness explained. Little Brown, Boston

Desimone R, Miller EK, Chelazzi L, Lüschow A (1995) Multiple memory systems in the visual cortex. In: Gazzaniga MS (Ed) The cognitive neurosciences. Bradford, Cambridge, pp 475–486

Eldridge LL, Knowlton BJ, Furmanski CS (2000) Remembering episodes: a selective role for the hippocampus during retrieval. Nat Neurosci 3:1149–1152

Fodor JA (1983) The modularity of mind. MIT Press, Cambridge

Haase SJ, Fisk GD (2004) Valid distinctions between conscious and unconscious perception? Percept Psychophys 66:868–871

Hoffman RE (1987) Computer simulations of neural information processing and the schizophrenia-mania dichotomy. Arch Gen Psychiatry 44:178–188

von Holst E, Mittelstaedt H (1950) Das Reafferenzprinzip. Naturwissenschaften 37:464–476

Hoshiyama M, Kakigi R, Watanabe S et al (2003) Brain responses for the subconscious recognition of faces. Neurosci Res 46:435–442

Jackson JH (1932) Selected writings. Taylor, London

Jaspers K (1942) Allgemeines Psychopathologie, 5. edn. Springer, Berlin

Jureidini J (2004) Does dissociation offer a useful explanation for psychopathology? Psychopathology 37:259–265

Koch C (2005) Bewusstsein—ein neurobiologisches Rätsel. Spektrum—Elsevier, München (englische Originalausgabe 2004)

Locke J (1690) An essay concerning humane understanding. Basset, London

McClelland JL, McNaughton BL, O'Reilly RC (1995) Why there are complementary learning systems in the hippocampus and neocortex: insights from the successes and failures of connectionist models of learning and memory. Psychol Rev 102:419–457

McClure SM, Laibson DI, Loewenstein G, Cohen JD (2004) Separate neural systems value immediate and delayed monetary rewards. Science 306:503–507

Mega MS, Cummings JL (1994) Frontal-subcortical circuits and neuropsychiatric disorders. J Neuropsych Clin Neurosci 6:358–370

Merkel J (1885) Über die zeitlichen Verhältnisse der Willenstätigkeit. Philosophische Studien 2:73–127

Mesulam MM (2000) Principles of behavioral and cognitive neurology. Oxford Univ Press, Oxford

Metzinger R (2001) Bewusstsein. Mentis Verlag, Paderborn

Ramachandran VS (2004) A brief tour of human consciousness. Pi Press, New York

Reischies FM (2005) Psychopathologie. In: Förstl H (Ed) Frontalhirn, Funktionen und Erkrankungen, 2. edn. Springer, Berlin Heidelberg New York Tokio, pp 83–101

Reischies FM, Diefenbacher A, Reichwaldt W (2003) Delir. In: Arolt V, Diefenbacher A (Eds) Psychiatrie in der klinischen Medizin. Springer, Berlin Heidelberg New York Tokio, pp 259–284

Reischies FM, Neuhaus AH, Hansen ML et al (2005) Electrophysiological and neuropsychological analysis of a delirious state—the role of the anterior cingulate gyrus. Psych Res 138(2):171–181

Reischies FM, Gabriel A, Zerhoch N, Neuhaus F (2007) Investigations on psychopathologischal and neuropsychological symptoms of delirium. Z. Gerontopsychol Psychiatr 20:141–149

Reischies FM (2021). Leid Erleben—ein Fundament der Psychopathologie. Pabst Scientific Publishers

Ryle G (1969) Der Begriff des Geistes. Reclam, Stuttgart

Stephan KM, Thaut MH, Wunderlich G et al (2002) Conscious and subconscious sensorimotor

synchronization—prefrontal cortex and the influence of awareness. Neuroimage 15:345–352
Weiskrantz L (1986) Blindsight. Oxford Univ Press, Oxford
Whalen PJ, Rauch SL, Etcoff NL et al (1998) Masked presentations of emotional facial expressions modulate amygdala activity without explicit knowledge. J Neurosci 18:411–418
Wheeler ME, Buckner RL (2004) Functional-anatomic correlates of remembering and knowing. Neuroimage 21:1337–1349
Wieck HH (1967) Lehrbuch der Psychiatrie. Schattauer, Stuttgart
Willingham DB, Salidis J, Gabrieli JD (2002) Direct comparison of neural systems mediating conscious and unconscious skill learning. J Neurophysiol 88:1451–1460

Language

9

Contents

9.1 Introduction

Aphasia is referred to as a disorder of acquired language, i.e., a language disorder occurs due to an illness after a person has acquired the language in childhood, as native language. The language system trained in childhood in the brain is damaged, for example, due to a stroke. This results in a multitude of striking symptoms. In this context, aphasia is not described in detail as it is in neurolinguistic text books (Stemmer and Whitaker 1998), but only the aspects required for psychopathological examination.

Example

A 78-year-old woman was brought to the psychiatric clinic. It was learned that she lives alone. The reason for admission was that she had apparently suffered from severe anxiety in recent nights, calling the family and the police. During the examination, the patient seemingly avoided every question.

F. M. Reischies, *Psychopathology*, https://doi.org/10.1007/978-3-662-70293-2_9

She spoke in clichés. The pronunciation was practically flawless and in an inconspicuous speech melody. At first glance, she seemed to be an older woman who communicated fluently in everyday speech. Facial expressions and gestures matched the statements. The examiners were initially unsure why the patient could not make precise statements about her life and recent events. However, it became clear in the further course of the examination that she did not properly understand the questions. She showed deficits in neuropsychological examination procedures, such as being unable to list word sequences like the months, and upon closer listening, some semantic paraphasias became apparent, i.e., she used some contextually incorrect words. The diagnosis was a severe language disorder in dementia, also referred to as "empty speech", i.e., it consisted of contentless clichés. ◄

In representations of psychopathology, a section for language disorders is usually missing. Language disorders are to be assigned to cognitive symptoms—they occur as part of brain damage syndromes and brain degeneration syndromes and in severe schizophrenic psychoses—for example, paragrammatism, glossolalia in schizophasia, neologisms and specific comprehension disorders .

Disorders in the areas of speaking, language, and thinking (listed):

Disorders of speaking: Dysarthria, dysprosody (disorder of speech melody), of speech sound

Disorders of language: Paraphasias (phoneme sequence in the word), lexical errors (word choice), grammatical errors (sentence level).

Disorders of thinking: Formal thought disorders, content-related thought disorders.

Can we separate the disorder of language from that of thinking? We attempt to clarify this question in these sections on language and thinking. Formal thought disorders have close relationships to the cognitive functions underlying language and are partly attributable to cognitive features following brain damage or brain dysfunction.

Aphasia was formerly also referred to as brain tool disorder. The term indicates that a person can loose the ability to communicate via the "tool" language system. Disorders of speaking occur in neurological diseases, but also in intoxications, which are very common in psychiatric patients. This also applies to grammatical errors that occur in dementias and—less frequently in schizophasia. Psychiatrists must be able to diagnose all symptoms of dementia.

One of the striking characteristics of most language disorders is that the language use suddenly no longer function naturally for the person. People are used to simply starting to speak. For example, a person stands in front of a picture and the task is to describe to someone standing at a distance what can be seen on it. The person will simply start speaking. This situation changes mostly when an aphasic disorder occurs. This disorder becomes noticeable to the affected person. One could say the user interface of language communication, which otherwise goes unnoticed, suddenly appears unfamiliar.

In this section, errors affecting the language system are considered—they appear in (1) the words (lexicon), (2) the rules of sentence formation (grammar), and (3) the segments and pronunciation of words—(phonemes, articulation). The neuroscientific mechanisms of word comprehension differ from those of word finding for speech production.

9.1.1 Language Comprehension

Disorder of Word Comprehension

When a spoken word is to be understood, the phonemes of the word must first be discriminated—for example, whether there was an "c" or "s" (e.g., cereal or serial). Disorders of the phoneme level of language predominantly occur in brain damage syndromes, such as ischemic strokes in the language region. If a phoneme could not be understood exactly, the analysis of the word and also that of the level of Sentence Comprehension helps, if in the above example both a word with "c" or "s" was possible. This works like modern handwriting recognition in a computer, where a plausible word is selected from the possible words based on the context, thus compensating for recognition inaccuracies. The hierarchical linguistic levels of language comprehension are intertwined in the processes of language comprehension—the phoneme discrimination includes the lexical processes up to the pragmatic understanding of the situational context of language communication. Grammar as well provides a framework for understanding the sequence of words.

It is assumed that an input lexicon is organized in the CNS, where on the one hand the phonematic specifications of a word are represented.

Disorder of Sentence Comprehension

In language comprehension, working memory plays a special role. As long as a sentence spoken by another person is not understood, the words remain in a working memory and can still be understood in a changed word meaning or another role in the sentence. The sentence "the policeman bites the dog" is difficult to understand in English, if the role of the dog as object has been meant: The unusual content is confusing (in English the grammatical word forms help identify subject and object)—the familiar roles of victim and perpetrator for that situation do not help (Heeschen 1980). After rearranging the sequences in the working memory and analyzing the syntactic roles, the actor-object relation can be understood.

Working memory is not only necessary for language comprehension to help with incorrectly identified phonemes but also for long complicated sentences, especially in German, a language in which, as joked abroad, the verb of the sentence always comes on the next page. The reference of demonstrative pronouns (this, that, etc.) to nouns in the last sentence also burdens the working memory.

In everyday communication, fewer errors occur in language comprehension than in speech production. But the difficulties in language comprehension can be illustrated. There is a game in german language to understand unusual sentences when they are spoken: "Abbots mow hay? Abbots do not mow hay, abbots pray." Rare words without semantic context are not easily understood. These examples illustrate that even healthy individuals make mistakes with unusual words and content. The usual auxiliary role of the respective higher hierarchical levels fails.

A process of parsing (the grammatical decomposition of the sentence) has been described, which is supposed to manage the assignment of the sequence of words in a sentence to the categories of understandable statements; that is, "who did something?", "what was done?", "with whom was something done?"

1. Individual words, or their grammatical word forms, give an initial indication of the role the word can play in the sentence, i.e., whether it could be the subject, object, etc. The sentence structure also provides clues. Thus, the perpetrator should usually be mentioned first and the victim second when forming a simple sentence.
2. Sentence parts are determined in their role (subject or object)—for example, subordinate clauses can represent what is the subject or object.

From these arguments, a consequence for language comprehension becomes clear: Apparently, several processing paths are pursued in parallel:

1. the identification of the word meaning and
2. the assignment of the grammatical role using an intermediate storage,
3. pragmatic classification of the sentence to be understood in a statement context (what is currently being discussed, what has already been said, what needs to be clarified, etc.),
4. finally, an assignment to a speech act of the conversation partner occurs. What is his intention? (Chap. 13 Delusion—content disorders). The results of the many subprocesses enable sentence comprehension. Intermediate solutions must be held in working memory for varying lengths of time.

9.1.2 Speech Production

Why is speech production particularly error-prone? Word-finding problems, for example, even appear in healthy individuals when they are tired or distracted. In addition to the selection of words, the complexity of organization in the planning and production of a sentence is considered here. In speech production, pronunciation is the final step. Ultimately, sequences of phonemes must be articulated. The final stages of speech production are related to motor skills and speech apraxia.

What happens at the beginning when a person has the intention to perform a speech act? For example, a person wants to get another person to close the window. The path from the intention of a speech act in a social situation, such as "I want to get him to close the window," to the spoken sentence is long and involves many subcomponents.

a) First, the speech act determines the topic of the utterance. In our example, it is about the window. Possible word-finding problems already begin here. In the neuroscientific section (see below), the explanation of retrieval of words in trained neural networks is demonstrated.

Around the topic "window," a series of word combinations and common sentences are available in the semantic system. It is based on elementary propositions of world knowledge, such as "windows protect against cold," possible adjectives and specifications, possible verbs like "close the window," "clean the window," etc. These relations, modeled in the neural network in Fig. 9.2, belong to semantics. Every person has a series of elementary propositions about things and situations that are related to properties, class memberships, and ownership.

The first word, the topic "window," must be held in the working memory. More information for the item in the working memory is added to the topic with further steps.

b) The next unit follows: "closing" (the window). The sentence: "Close the window" includes an addressee "you," who must be connected with the topic and the action "closing."
c) In the next step, the sentence form is determined, for example, the request, "Please close the window," with the grammar of sentence structure. The person asks a question, "Could you please close the window?" because they do not simply want to say, "You close the window now!" Thus, besides grammatical processing, it is also a communicative determination of the specific sentence type.
d) For the grammatical processing of the sentence, the subject, predicate, and object must be determined. Then, the grammar processing of the morphemes for the correct word form must be ensured. Throughout the entire process, the topic held in the working memory and the preliminary sentence forms can be repeatedly modified.
e) Finally, the phoneme-motor skills are activated, which control the articulation of the words. Additional to this the speech melody and accompanying gestures are activated, which can have a linguistically clarifying function.

From this sequence of steps for the production of a speech act intended to prompt a person to close the window, the complexity of the processes that implicitly occur daily becomes evident.

9.1.3 Classification According to Linguistic Criteria

Disorders of language can be classified according to linguistic criteria, such as disorders of word finding and word comprehension, disorders of sentence grammar and understanding of grammatical forms, and so on. However, this has not proven clinically useful. From aphasia, one can learn that although logical classifications of symptoms can be represented, they do not help in the neuroscientific explanation of the disorder. This circumstance can be illustrated as follows: Many language errors occur affecting the morphemes, for example, a patient makes an error in a word form when he starts to tell his medical history: "Well, the illness go like this. I…". Phonemes are wrong, the word form is wrong, and a grammatical error can be diagnosed in the sentence formation. Following this example, we do not seek the units for neuroscientific investigation of language errors in linguistic categories but describe the psychopathologically relevant facts in the categories of language comprehension and production.

9.2 Clinic

Patients with mental disorders exhibit language system disorders when the neural processes for language are disrupted, i.e., the neurophysiological organization of language comprehension and speech production is impaired. This leads to a diagnostic consequence: From the diagnosis of aphasic language disorders in the narrower sense, it can be concluded that these are not functional problems, but that there is a suspicion of a disorder of brain functional systems. This conclusion has far-reaching consequences, for example, in the subsequent necessary diagnostics of possible neurological diseases of the brain.

9.2.1 Language Comprehension Disorder

Spontaneously, hardly any patient will indicate that they did not understand what was just said. They will try to infer the meaning of what was said from the communicative context, from semantic standard relations. They may guess what might be meant. As a result, language comprehension disorders become less apparent in clinical everyday life. Therefore, during the interview, it must be observed whether questions need to be repeated, whether questions are not answered precisely, but only generally addressed.

If there are errors in language comprehension, the above-mentioned processes of language analysis are apparently disturbed. However, it should be checked whether a person also does not understand written language (if they have learned to write and read).

A test of language comprehension is carried out, for example, in the Aachen Aphasia Test (Huber et al. 1983). A language utterance must be assigned to a selection image. This test has hardly been conducted on psychiatric patients. Patients with dementia show difficulties here, but they may already be disturbed in the analysis of the images to be pointed at.

First, it must be clarified whether the person is hard of hearing: Are there acoustic problems (with particular attention to cerumen in older patients)? 1. phoneme discrimination faulty; 2. word identification unreliable, lexical problems; 3. working memory erased too quickly, sentence comprehension cannot be achieved in the next step through reanalysis of the sentence elements (disambiguation) in case of uncertainties; 4. identification of the grammatical role of words disturbed; 5. decoding of sentence meaning no longer possible; 6. assistance of semantic assignment from the context disturbed.

In addition, there are often attention problems that need to be considered in differential diagnosis.

Dedifferentiation

Usually, in psychiatric examination, it is not possible to differentiate the disorder of language comprehension at the phonematic, word, or syntax level, but rather diffuse language comprehension disorders are evident, affecting many levels of language processing simultaneously and are attributable to diffuse brain damage, as in dementias, delirium syndromes, or intoxications.

Understanding the speech act intention

Understanding the intention of an utterance can be disturbed, especially understanding indirect speech acts, i.e., speech acts with an intention that is not made explicit, for example, a request concealed for reasons of politeness. Understanding speech acts can be disturbed, a disorder in identifying the speech act intention of the communicating person. An example is the request to the partner to close the open window by saying, "I have a cold." Formally, the sentence is a description; in content, in the speaker's intention, however, it is a request (Bara et al. 1997).

Schizophrenic patients, persons with suspicion or paranoid delusion often do not understand the speaker's intention or reinterpret it—for example, in terms of their bias. This is possibly shaped by anxiety and projection of their own aggressiveness. Here, it cannot be considered as a language comprehension disorder.

9.2.2 Speech Production

Disturbance of Retrieval from the lexical storage—word-finding problems
In aphasia, there is an incorrect selection of words—semantic paraphasias, which are also referred to as verbal paraphasias. A patient says "The cook fries the pan," i.e., he chooses an incorrect word for an object. The incorrect words usually have relations to the correct word, in phonemic or semantic terms.

For the production of non-routine sentences, i.e., language describing new facts, many additional steps beyond the activation of the correct words must be carried out: In one step (1) the syntactic constraints of word choice must be worked out (word class, etc.), (2) at the level of sentence structure rules, the order of the words is determined, (3) at the level of individual words, word endings are specified according to grammar, etc. (morpheme level). In aphasia, the brain regions responsible for this are disturbed. In fluent aphasia, Wernicke's aphasia, a characteristic type of error occurs: patients use incorrect endings and intertwine sentences, etc. In non-fluent aphasia, another type of error, agrammatism, is observed, where omissions predominate, particularly affecting endings and grammatical words. In severe cases, a telegram style results.

At the level of motor control and pronunciation of individual words, the phonemes of the word must be selected. In the clinic of aphasias, phonemic paraphasias are observed. A patient says instead of "known": "bone".

In some patients with brain damage, a disturbance of the motor control of articulation occurs; it may lead to verbal apraxia. The characteristics are described in the textbooks of neurolinguistics. The variety of symptoms in aphasias, the disturbance of acquired language, cannot be addressed here. In addition to the disturbances of spoken language, symptoms of written language also occur, such as alexia, agraphia. Special words have particular processing mechanisms, such as number words used in calculations (Dehaene et al. 2004).

Semantic disturbances
In schizophrenic thought disorders, a semantic disturbance is partly underlying. (see below; Chap. 10 thinking). The thinking is severely disturbed, and sentences are uttered that are not understandable (they may contain grammatical errors and neologisms.

The necessity of a differential diagnosis between aphasia and schizophrenic thought disorder should be briefly mentioned here, although the corresponding cases are clinically very rare. From the spontaneous speech findings, differential diagnostic considerations arise between the incoherent speech of a schizophrenic patient and the speech in jargon aphasia :

1. In jargon aphasia, so many phonemic or semantic paraphasias occur that the listener can no longer understand the content.
2. In schizophasia, unusual words accumulate. Patients partly play with sound combinations, resulting in a completely incomprehensible speech production (glossolalia). According to Kraepelin's report (1903) and own

experiences, a schizomanic component seems to play a role in this form of schizophasia. This may be related to the fluent speech production, which is only given in case of sufficient speech drive. Additionally, the disinhibition in the manic syndrome causes patients to produce a multitude of speech anomalies.

Disruption of Communication Behavior
First, violations of societal conventions of communication rules by patients must be considered. Especially individuals with mania violate the rules of conversation. Examples include: they talk too much and interrupt their conversation partners, do not answer questions—or respond with counter-questions. Violations of communication rules also occur in schizophrenic patients—on the one hand in the context of negativism in catatonic patients and autistic communication that do not address the conversation's history and what the partner has understood (see below, Theory of Mind). On the other hand, there is also incoherent answering, which refers to deviating from the conversation topic, even though the patient has understood the questions posed (see Thought Disorders, Chap. 10).

Many communication problems with individuals suffering from psychiatric symptoms are less related to the language system in the narrow sense than to the intention to speak. In depression, communication ceases due to a reduced drive to speak. Additionally, there are fears and insecurities (Reischies 1993).

The observation of speech behavior, the manner of expression, provides the examiner with clues about the patient's psychopathological condition. These clues are often implicitly evaluated, meaning the examiner does not consciously account for them. This applies not only to the level at which a patient produces language but also to the communication behavior, adherence to conversation rules, speech drive, and the rate of minor speech errors and comprehension problems, forming an implicit picture of the patient's language for the examiner.

9.3 Diagnostics

The systematic examination of language disorders still follows the Wernicke-Lichtheim diagram (Fig. 9.1). The various levels of disorder are tested with a series of task types:

The examination of language comprehension 1. at the word and 2. sentence level, 3. repetition, 4. describing the meaning, which the person has understood, as well as language comprehension disorder with preserved repetition (see Fig. 9.1), and 5. naming.

This includes the observation of articulation, speech fluency, paraphasias and grammatical errors in spontaneous speech. There are comprehensive aphasia tests, such as the Boston Diagnostic Aphasia Examination and the Aachen Aphasia Test. In the psychiatric clinic, this formalism is usually not followed, mostly for time reasons – the complete aphasia diagnosis takes many hours.

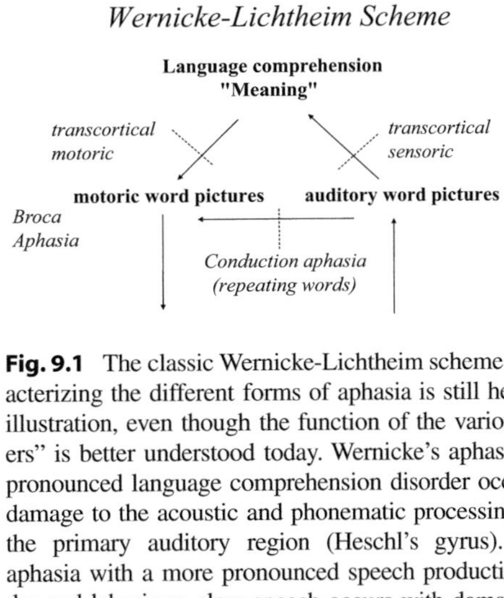

Fig. 9.1 The classic Wernicke-Lichtheim scheme for characterizing the different forms of aphasia is still helpful for illustration, even though the function of the various "centers" is better understood today. Wernicke's aphasia with a pronounced language comprehension disorder occurs with damage to the acoustic and phonematic processing around the primary auditory region (Heschl's gyrus). Broca's aphasia with a more pronounced speech production disorder and laborious, slow speech occurs with damage to the precentral regions in front of the motor representation of speech motor skills (Broca's area) as well as usually the underlying basal ganglia and white matter. Conduction aphasia with a prominent repetition disorder is caused by a disconnection syndrome due to lesions between Wernicke's and Broca's areas. In dementias, the type of transcortical sensory aphasia is observed, with language comprehension disorder while repetition is preserved (quasi as a preserved cortical reflex arc for repetition)

9.3.1 Testing Language Comprehension

Usually, a language comprehension disorder can be inferred with sufficient certainty from the course of the interview, for example, by the examiner paying close attention to whether the person understands the interview questions.

To confirm a suspicion of a language comprehension disorder, comprehension at the word level is examined. For example, the person is asked to point to things on a board after they have been named. Differential diagnosis may require distinguishing it from a hearing disorder.

Proverbs

Complex language comprehension is often tested by explaining proverbs. In this task, difficulties in understanding a situation on a pragmatic and metaphorical level become apparent. Types of errors include:

1. proverb not understood or misunderstood,
2. concrete exemplary paraphrases, i.e., explanations that do not reach the metaphorical level.

When explaining proverbs, propositional language is required, i.e., non-routine statement-making language. Many patients have not been accustomed to using more than communicative habitual phrases for a long time. They have difficulty describing an unfamiliar situation. Additionally, proverbs involve situations with metaphorical levels of meaning. A test was presented (Barth and Küfferle 2001) that tests the understanding of proverbs through multiple-choice questions. This bypasses the area of problems in speech production. However, the task is also successfully used in the diagnosis of schizophrenic thought disorders (see thought disorders). Explaining proverbs is an effective means of assessing both linguistic abilities and the differentiation of the person's cognitive abilities and education. If errors occur, it must be diagnosed in detail whether it is a language disorder or a lack of education, an intelligence disorder, or a thought disorder.

9.3.2 Speech Production—Spontaneous Speech in the Interview

For the assessment of speech production disorder in aphasia, the clinical evaluation of spontaneous speech in the interview is central. Almost all features of aphasia become apparent to the trained examiner in conversation: phonemic paraphasias are noted, grammatical errors, semantic problems (language comprehension see above), word-finding problems with paraphrases, etc.

Neuropsychological examination procedures for language comprehension and speech production disorders

1. Word finding:
   - Boston Naming Test (in the CERAD Neuropsychological Battery, Monsch 1997; Berres et al. 2000) as in spontaneous speech, certain types of errors occur: (1) repeated attempts ("it's on the tip of my tongue"); (2) paraphrases; (3) empty, clichéd language; (4) imprecise expressions; (5) long pauses.

   Differential diagnostic distinctions must be made from disorders of the level of drive, psychogenic mutism, etc., colloquial habits, and regional peculiarities. The person's level of education must also be taken into account.
2. Language comprehension: (1) observation in the interview; (2) explaining proverbs: comprehension and propositional language; (3) Token Test (showing square and round tokens in different colors—"please show me the red rectangle"); (3) repetition: long sentences, digit span, (4) word fluency—fluency—semantic: animals, e.g., for 1 min, letter fluency: initial letters, for 1 min each (e.g., for F, A, and S).

9.4 Neuroscience

In a first critical phase of language development, the child learns to distinguish the phonemes of the native language. The difficulties of people from Asia in learning to distinguish between "l" and "r" of European languages as adults are an argument for a critical phase of language learning, i.e., something that is not learned during this developmental phase of the child cannot be easily or at all caught up later.

Another critical phase concerns the learning of grammar. Here is an European example that adults with Polish as their native language repeatedly have the problems with the correct German sentence structure, even if they have been speaking German for many years.

From the analysis of localized brain lesions that lead to aphasias, it has been known since the late Nineteenth century (Broca, Wernicke) that there is a localization of the language-processing brain regions in the language-dominant hemisphere. The Wernicke region is located near the auditory region of the Heschl gyrus, and the Broca region is between the representation of the mouth and throat musculature or their motor control and the region in the frontal lobe necessary for the updating of working memory. This localization can explain the disorder in the organization of speech production in anterior lesions of the language areas.

Phoneme discrimination

Information processing for language is an example of modular information processing (Fodor 1983). Phoneme analysis occurs somewhat automatically, and we cannot help but think of an apple when "apple" is said. The automatic process provides us with the image of the apple and the appropriate associations, for which no attention is required and which cannot be consciously intervened in.

Humans have the remarkable ability to understand articulated sounds – adapted to the respective speaker. The difficulty initially lies in the continuum between p and b, between t and d, or between m and n on the acoustic level. For discrimination, a perceptual mechanism develops in childhood that assigns a "p" up to a certain threshold and then a "b". This is an example of unconscious perceptual decisions (Chap. 2 Perception—neuropsychological disorders). Analyses of neuronal mechanisms have shown that neurons apparently have exactly this activation characteristic.

9.4.1 Trained Neuronal Networks

An explanatory model for phenomena of word comprehension and speech production as well as the peculiarities of their disorder after brain lesions is provided by neuronal networks (Fig. 9.2). Neuronal networks could be used as models of language processing. An example is the network model by McClelland et al. 1995, other applications are discussed in Stemmer et al. 1998. Meanwhile, the success of large language models in artificial intelligence has confirmed the described approach (LeCun et al. 2015).

In the neuronal network tested by McClelland, words are provided as nodes, and it has been shown that a neuronal network can produce possible elementary sentences.

It is assumed that units representing input neurons are listed in the first column. This input includes nouns, and in another input row, elementary verbs such as "is a, can, has…". The second step of parallel processing in the neural network is the series of computing units called "hidden units". These neurons serve the neuronal network as an intermediate representation for calculating the output connections. They usually have no identifiable meaning. In the third step of simple neuronal networks, the output neurons are found, which are activated by the calculation of the input constellation. In the output row, there are nouns or verbs. The trained network can now find the word "bird" for a noun like "blackbird" and "is a". Or "A blackbird" and "has" is connected with "feathers".

Traditionally, considerations have been made for a semantic system on how word meanings are represented in the CNS. In this model, it is assumed that all feasable sentences could be stored in the connection strengths between neurons or neuronal ensembles that represent semantic units such as words. This involves the representation of semantic knowledge in the form of elementary

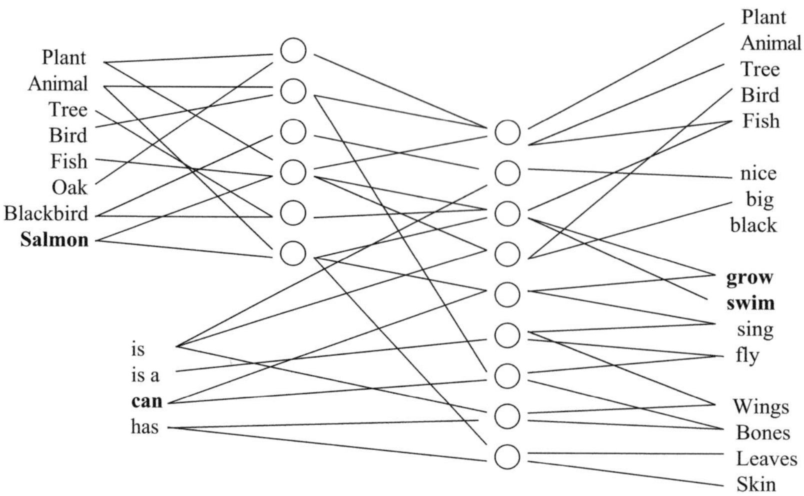

Fig. 9.2 Neural networks are used to explain language acquisition and linguistic processing (McClelland et al. 1995). The names (e.g., plant) and verbs (e.g., is) are connected with optional complements (e.g., plant) to form a valid sentence. The network is trained in many iterations, meaning the connection strengths between the nodes are reinforced when the network activates one of the possible sentence complements, e.g., "Salmon can swim." It has been shown that neural networks implicitly learn to map the regularities of language (e.g. grammar) and the environment or nature.

propositions, which are available to the person at any time. The sentences shown above represent such elementary propositions as "A blackbird is a bird" or "… can fly". From these semantic connections, the person can also generate more complex sentences.

The example network is particularly illustrative, but it is possible that other construction principles for connectivity between representations of the cortex are realized in the brain. Further research will have to clarify this. An argument for the shown network is the following finding: When a person is presented with a sentence word by word, but the sentence has an implausible conclusion, such as "A blackbird has gloves", a specific potential, an N400, is very consistently found in the electroencephalogram (EEG) (Kutas and Hillyard 1984). This is an example of the use of neuronal networks in language comprehension. The shown network connections are activated and generate a CNS signal when the plausible sentence connections that the network can anticipate do not occur.

9.4.2 Errors in Language Processing

How do semantic paraphasias, i.e., the selection of an incorrect word, occur? From the feature representations of a sememe, the lexical entry can be found. Thus, from "feathers, sings, flies, grows, bird, and color" (Fig. 9.2), a suggested word can be activated or further looked for. One explanation is based on the ability of neuronal networks to complete a missing element (principle of the blind spot in the visual field of an eye). From all the semantic properties listed above, the neuronal network completes: "blackbird."

Now, if one assumes that this network is damaged, errors in word finding occur. Depending on the degree of damage, statistically more or less incorrect words appear. In some forms of aphasia, patients suffer from massive verbal paraphasias. If damage is assumed in the specific neuronal networks trained for the rapid selection of words in speech production, the increase in the error probability can be explained. This is consistent with the clinical observation that in a disturbance in the language system, only an increase in the general number of errors in word finding is noticeable: Thus, it is not the case that individual words can no longer be found.

The errors mostly remain within the semantic context. This is consistent with the fact that in the neuronal network, the semantic environment is activated, and only an error in the selection of the critical word occurs.

Phonemic paraphasias can also be explained by errors in, however, other networks, namely neuronal networks of pronunciation planning. Phonemic paraphasias occur when the specific neural network trained for the selection of phonemes for word articulation, for the pronunciation of the word, is damaged. These neural networks are not overlapping but at least partially differently localized. This leads to syndrome dissociations: Some patients with a specific localization of strokes have more phonemic, others with different lesions have more semantic, verbal paraphasias (Fig. 9.3).

9.4.3 Dedifferentiation and Error Statistics

After strokes, the probability of producing an incorrect word or an incorrect phoneme increases. It is not as previously assumed that words are completely "forgotten." Then the lexicon would be incomplete. However, this does not correspond to the experience of brain damage syndromes. An important advantage of the neuronal network model is the property of "graceful degradation"—if a neural network is disturbed, for example, if an area of computing units fails, the complete performance does not fail, but the error rate increases. This corresponds to the clinical experience after strokes and in the development of dementia of the Alzheimer's type. In aphasias that occur after strokes, the error probability increases from nearly zero in healthy individuals to a percentage proportional to the extent of the network damage. This property of neuronal networks thus explains a characteristic of brain damage syndromes that is otherwise very difficult to understand.

9.4.4 Parallel Processing Paths in Language Comprehension and Hierarchical Processing Paths

Within approximately 1 second, the linguistic processing of acoustic stimuli, i.e., normal spoken language, seems to take place. It is currently assumed that several analysis paths are pursued in parallel. For instance, the word form must be determined and the word meaning identified, which occurs in the language-dominant hemisphere. In the other hemisphere, typically the right hemisphere, pitch is analyzed and, in conjunction with the context words, a prosody is perceived. Two aspects of pitch and volume are particularly important for the analysis of spoken language: phrasing, such as at the end of a sentence, and accent, e.g., to emphasize the actor and to clarify syntactic ambiguities.

Studies, especially by the research group Friederici et al. (2006), have shown that word form determination occurs before semantic analysis. Apparently, only when the word form is determined can the semantic analysis be completed—it proceeds "licensed" (Fig. 9.4).

9.4.5 Aphasic Errors and the Diagnosis of Brain Damage Symptoms

The occurrence of typical aphasic errors can serve as evidence for a brain damage syndrome and thus determine the type of further diagnostics. The aforementioned example explains that the occurrence of phonematic paraphasias can be taken as evidence of damage to specific brain regions. Specialized neural networks are disrupted, which are only activated in the process of language generation and thus cannot be subject to functional—in the sense of "meaning-related"—disorders. The disruption of neural networks, such as the shown semantic network, is used to explain schizophrenic thought disorders (Hoffman 1987; Spitzer 1993).

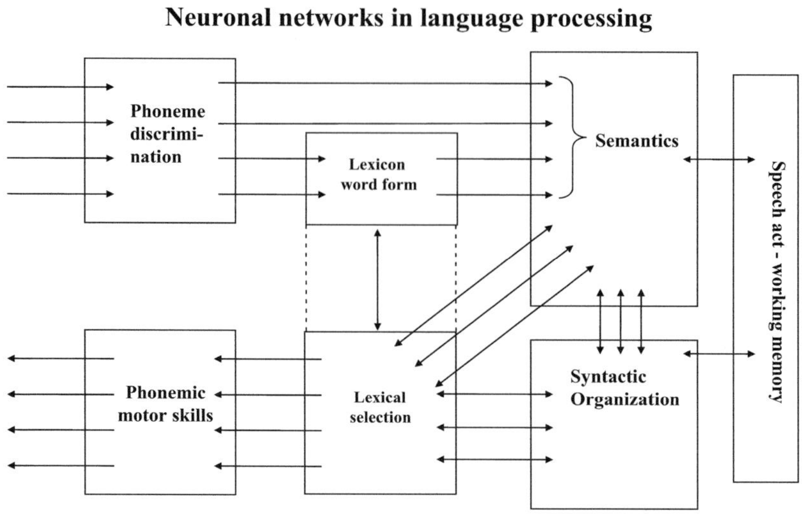

Fig. 9.3 Different trained neuronal networks are involved in information processing for language comprehension in the CNS (for phoneme and word identification). Additionally, there are neuronal networks for speech production (lexical selection, phoneme selection, etc.). Different neural networks are hierarchically structured in a CNS language system. If neural networks are damaged, the entire information processing does not fail, but only the error rate increases, for example, in the rate of phonemic or verbal paraphasias ("graceful degradation"). The impact of degenerative or toxic/metabolic processes on language functions can also be described by the neuronal network models.

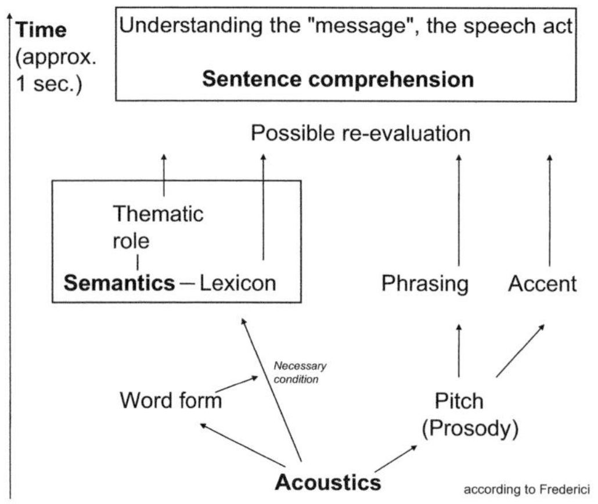

Fig. 9.4 A simple sentence can be decoded in approximately 1 second in the CNS, including phonematic information, word form, lexical unit, thematic role, and embedding in a communicative context. In parallel, especially for the last aspect of the communicative context, the course of pitch, the speech melody (prosody), and the emphasis are analyzed (Mod. after Friederici et al. 2006).

9.5 Psychopathological Symptoms of Language

Word-finding disorder

Definition: A person cannot find words in conversation that they have otherwise used; i.e., there is a delay or absence of the appropriate word intended by the person during word-finding.

The person may pause while speaking and wait to see if the word comes to mind, try to use descriptions "I mean a device for digging, for turning over soil," or apologize "I can't come up with it right now."

Example

An older woman has not been able to find words in fluent speech reliably for several weeks and describes them or says an incorrect word. She repeatedly interrupts a description of everyday events because she cannot find a word that certainly belongs to her active vocabulary. ◀

AMDP additional item
Word-finding problems usually also when writing.

Neuroscientific/cognitive neuroscientific models
Disorder of retrieval from the lexicon (trained neuronal network)

Self-/other person's judgment.
Other person's judgment; possibly complaints about the experienced effort to find usual words.

Aphasic speech production errors
Definition. Disorder of word and sentence production—in the sense of paraphasias or errors in the grammatical structure of speech utterances due to disturbances in syntactic language processing.

Example

- A man after a stroke speaks fluently, and the speech shows many errors in word choice: verbal paraphasias.
- A person speaks words in which individual or multiple phonemes are incorrect, phonematic paraphasias.
- A person forms syntactically incorrect sentences, e.g., sentence entanglements (A sentence starts correctly but is then completed by a second part of another sentence that does not fit grammatically and semantically).
- A person cannot repeat words. ◀

The errors usually also occur in written language.

Position in psychopathology. Not in AMDP.

Psychopathological interaction. Thought disorder, e.g., neologisms in schizophrenia, glossolalia in schizophasia.

Differential diagnostic distinctions. Developmental dysphasia with already disturbed early language development.

Further characterization. Disorder of the trained language system; the language functions were intact before the disorder, as they were acquired in child development.

Self-/other person's judgment. Other person's judgment.

Neuropsychology/objectification: Spontaneous speech disorder, disorder of naming and sentence formation (Aachener Aphasietest).

Severity. Individual errors that are hardly noticeable to complete inability to communicate.

Specifications. See presentation of neuropsychological syndromes.

Conceptual problems of the feature. Aphasia belongs to the so-called brain tool disorders, i.e., disorder of information processing that affects one of the "modules" of the mind (Fodor 1983), in which automated information processing takes place.

Word comprehension disorder
Definition: Disorder of the ability to understand simple language utterances, a word, a simple sentence about a concrete matter.

Example

Follow-up questions to a simple story that was told cannot be answered without a severe memory disorder being present.

It must be ensured that the person can hear the utterance correctly.

In the interview, it is observed that a person does not respond with a normally expected answer to a question or change in behavior after perceiving information, an instruction, or an explanation.

If the language system is disturbed, the disorder is usually also observed in reading. ◀

Position in psychopathology. Not in AMDP.

Differential diagnostic distinction: Autism, concentration disorders, distractedness due to phonemes.

Further characterization. Comprehension disorder.

Self-/other person's judgment. Other person's judgment.

Interview for rating. Observation in standard interview, history taken from other persons.

Neuropsychology/objectification. Appropriate responses to interview questions, short stories, pointing test, Aphasia test.

Severity. According to the grade of impairment of exploration.

Disorder of comprehension of sentences
Definition: A person cannot adequately process and grasp the meaning of more complex linguistic representations, although they understand simple words. They cannot comprehend the content of a longer sentence, a proverb, or a multipart request, i.e., they cannot behave accordingly.

Example

A man cannot understand explanations in the admission interview, and he explains a proverb incorrectly—i.e., he paraphrases the concrete statement. He identifies simple words correctly—e.g., in a pointing test. ◀

Position in psychopathology: AMDP 9.

Psychopathological interaction. Aphasia, intelligence, element of judgment disorder (see Chap. 15).

Differential diagnostic distinctions: Elementary word comprehension disorder or language comprehension disorder in aphasia, incoherent answering, triggered by another psychopathological disorder, autism, concentration disorders, resistance against the examination, distractedness by phonemes, intellectual disability (clarify through external anamnesis to what extent the person was able to solve similar tasks in the past). Acutely occurring clouding of consciousness.

Further characterization: Also occurs while reading—complex reading comprehension is disturbed.

Interview for rating: In general, sufficient indications already in an admission interview. Educational anamnesis.

Neuropsychology, objectification: Proverbs (several examples that the person knows—pay attention to the person's representation of the metaphorical level).

Severity: Minor without everyday consequences to unable to master the complex tasks of daily life (requires support).

Neuroscientific/cognitive neuroscientific models

1. weak input model: already incomplete activation of elementary concepts in language comprehension has a cumulative effect,
2. Problems with logical connections,
3. Disruption in subsystems, e.g., in working memory or in retrieval of associations and elementary propositions of the environmental model.

References

Bara BG, Tirassa M, Zettin M (1997) Neuropragmatics: neuropsychological constraints on formal theories of dialogue. Brain Lang 59:7–49

Barth A, Küfferle B (2001) Die Entwicklung eines Sprichworttests zur Erfassung konkretistischer Denkstörungen bei schizophrenen Patienten. Nervenarzt 72:853–858

Berres M, Monsch AU, Bernasconi F et al (2000) Normal ranges of neuropsychological tests for the diagnosis of Alzheimer's disease. Stud Health Technol Inform 77:195–199

Dehaene S, Molko N, Cohen L, Wilson AJ (2004) Arithmetic and the brain. Curr Opin Neurobiol 14:218–224

Fodor JA (1983) The modularity of mind. MIT Press, Cambridge

Friederici AD, Bahlmann J, Heim S (2006) The brain differentiates human and non-human grammars: functional localization and structural connectivity. Proc Natl Acad Sci U S A 103:2458–2463

Heeschen C (1980) Strategies of decoding actor-object-relations by aphasic patients. Cortex 16:5–19

Hoffman RE (1987) Computer simulations of neural information processing and the schizophrenia-mania dichotomy. Arch Gen Psychiatry 44:178–188

Huber W, Poeck K, Weniger D, Willmes K (1983) Der Aachener AphasieTest. Hogrefe, Göttingen

Kraepelin E (1903) Psychiatrie, 7. edn. Barth, Leipzig

Kutas M, Hillyard SA (1984) Brain potentials during reading reflect word expectancy and semantic assiation. Nature 307:161–163

LeCun Y, Bengio Y, Hinton G (2015) Deep Learning. Nature 521:436–444

McClelland JL, McNaughton BL, O'Reilly RC (1995) Why there are complementary learning systems in the hippocampus and neocortex: insight from the successes and failures of connectionist models of learning and memory. Psychol Rev 102:419–457

Monsch AU (1997) Neuropsychologische Untersuchung in der Beurteilung der Demenz. Schweiz Rundsch Med Prax 86:1340–1342

Reischies FM (1993) Pathology of language behaviour in affective psychoses. In: Blanken G, Dittmann J, Grimm H et al (Eds) Linguistic disorders and pathologies, Vol IX. Handbook of linguistic and communication science. De Gruyter, Berlin, pp 513–522

Spitzer M (1993) The psychopathology, neuropsychology and neurobiology of associative and working memory in schizophrenia. Eur Arch Psychiatr Clin Neurosci 243:57–70

Stemmer B, Whitaker HA (1998) Handbook of Neurolinguistik. Academic, New York

Thinking 10

Contents

10.1 Introduction

"The delay, the loss of time through thinking, I see as prudence"—Publius Syrus.

The word "thinking" has many meanings. First, we follow the description by Benson (Benson 1994); all processes that handle thought content should be considered as thinking. Thought content is mental content; it is capable of being conscious. In thinking with, words, they are semantic units, but beyond that, they are also figures, e.g., from intelligence tests, which a person can handle pictorially. When processing the thought content has taken place, the result is again available in the awareness of the thinking person—whether a figure is imagined again after a rotation or an argument is formulated with a new aspect. In this context, the consideration must be limited to verbal thought content.

F. M. Reischies, *Psychopathology*, https://doi.org/10.1007/978-3-662-70293-2_10

Psychopathology has described a variety of formal thought disorders from the psychopathological examination of mentally ill people. In psychology textbooks, the word thinking sometimes no longer appears. Most often, explanations of inferential thinking are found under the heading "Cognition." Cognitive neuroscience is dedicated to the formal logical functions of the brain. One problem with this is that statements about thinking can only be made that include consciousness (see above).

In many tests of mental performance, such as in intelligence tests, the person processes the task mentally and initially does not communicate. They do not perform any overt action during the task solution. At the end of the mental operations, there is a decision, which is either spoken or executed as an action. We have a mental task before us with a thinking-target (as Kraepelin already formulated, Kraepelin 1903). We infer from a correct answer that the person must have thought. It should be noted: The severity of thought disorders in psychopathology has different dimensions than the disturbance of thinking in cognitive science.

First, the target of thinking of the mental operation should be considered. One can examine the efficiency of thought processes by giving the patient a thinking task and evaluating whether and when the target of thinking is reached, the correct answer is given. Every question to the patient essentially represents a thinking task, and, in this regard, the type of answer and the latency can be assessed. The type and efficiency of processing a thought goal is a central object of psychopathological examination.

Thinking drive: The efficiency of thinking leads to the question of the drive or motivation to think. Why does a person think? Experiences with thought disorders in psychiatric conditions teach us that thinking is not taken for granted. In severe depression, a person reports not thinking at all. On the one hand, it is assumed that 1) in a depressive illness, thinking drive is reduced, the general drive level is greatly reduced, and for that reason, the person hardly thinks. This explanation is probably too short-sighted: 2) The necessity of an expectation of reward applies to the execution of any attentive mental process. In other words, the severely depressed person no longer thinks because their thinking leads to nothing. Additionally, they have uselessly circling negative thoughts in rumination and experience this as rather worsening negative feelings. (3) Thinking is avoided if it could lead to anxiety. For a person to think, the path must apparently be cleared beforehand—there must be thinking drive and specific motivation to think about the thinking-target . It is important to consider this level because it also includes avoidance attitudes, resistances, and even defense mechanisms or coping styles. These influencing factors may inhibit or divert thinking activity.

Many patients refuse to cooperate in the psychopathological examination, show resistance, especially when it comes to neuropsychological examination procedures. Why is a person motivated to think attentively in a conversation and an examination? Apparently, some people have a high motivation to solve even tricky thinking tasks in their free time. It could also be that they have a generally high drive level.

Introspection: Statements about subjective difficulties in thinking, which a patient expresses, must be evaluated very carefully. In this context, purely subjective thought disorders are not addressed. These are mostly the complex area of self-perception, introspection with its specific susceptibilities to error.

Thought Content

We had described thought content as mental content that is consciously processed; how can we describe it more closely?

- Semantic units (verbal thinking),
- Visual units: form/color/spatial aspects of an object (e.g., a traffic light),
- Others, e.g.: acoustic units: pitch/time/rhythm/motifs.

Source of Thinking Goals

- self-generated (a problem has been discovered),
- task from external (exam, job),
- routine (task learned, e.g., regular mental training with puzzle solving).

Thinking Processes

- transforming, controlling (processing a change),
- transformations (performing an operation on a thought object (e.g., dividing digits by 3, see intelligence tests),
- problem-solving, recall of various transformations until the final condition is met (intelligence tests).

Thought Result

- decision reason, action (giving an answer, multiple-choice marking; reaction sign, time measurement),
- knowledge (consequence is considered in future decisions),
- intermediate result (for complex thinking goals, planning).

Everyday-relevant thinking: The emphasis in this context should be on everyday and behaviorally relevant thinking. Characteristic disturbances of thinking, which help diagnose a psychiatric clinical syndrome, have psychopathological significance; these usually impair the everyday behavior of patients.

Everyday thinking is disturbed in many psychiatric conditions. We have already mentioned the ruminative thinking of severely depressed individuals. Their negative circular thoughts, rumination further worsen the mood.

For schizophrenic psychoses, the fundamental disturbances of thinking must be diagnosed and explained—especially those formal thought disorders that can have consequences in behavioral fault. Thinking is not performed efficiently or not at all. In psychopathology, it is generally not about the level of potential problem-solving captured by intelligence tests.

Also excluded is contemplative thinking, which can be characterized as aimless thinking (Singer 1993). We consider thinking that can be measured by the efficiency with which it reaches a thinking-target . Of course, people also think about nothing specific for long periods of the day, get distracted by stimuli, or string together ideas. However, there is no reliable information about this type of thinking for a psychopathological examination (see above, introspection).

Example

A woman wants to celebrate her 80th birthday and talks to an old friend. She has become slow in thinking. She thinks of inviting friend “x”. Then her thoughts jump to the birthday meal with the question of whether she want to cook the meal or if it should be ordered. She then considers going to a restaurant. This brings her to the aspect that a restaurant with many people could become very expensive. She asks her friend if she sees the matter differently. She then considers that she would rather leave the money in the account, “you never know.” She thinks about how many people she would have to invite. In doing so, she thinks of another friend. This friend loves to eat fish… Meandering, the ideas turn in slow circles. The lady is not able to organize the planning of the birthday party. Another example is shown in Fig. 10.1. ◄

Many researchers see behaviorally relevant thinking as probatory action. There are close relationships to executive functions (Chap. 6). In contrast to executive functions, which become evident in concrete actions, this is about the planning consideration of matters of life in the future.

In the psychopathological examination, the categories of speaking, language, and thinking must be distinguished, as symptoms from all three categories can occur (Lott et al. 2002). Especially in severe acute schizophrenic conditions, there can be a disturbance of language with lexical and grammatical errors as

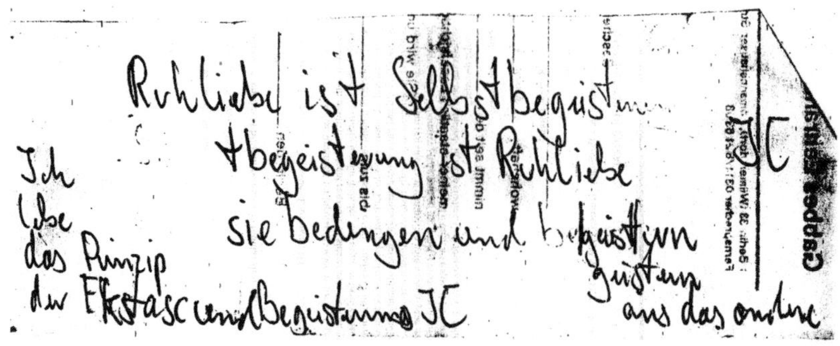

Fig. 10.1 Note of a schizophrenic patient as an example of a thought disorder: "Calm-love is self-enthusiasm; self-enthusiasm is calmlove. They require and inspire each other. I live the principle of ecstasy and enthusiasm."

well as a disturbance of formal thinking and thought content. Then, in many cases, a distinction will not be possible.

We can only touch upon the complex area of the question to what extent thinking occurs consciously. In everyday life, people are occupied with their tasks, which mostly require routine attentive thought processes; the individuals are clear-headed but are mostly not aware that they are thinking (in the sense of awareness, "awareness of something," see Chap. 8). Many severely depressed patients report that they immediately start brooding during breaks in activities, which they find tormenting. Other people do not notice that they are brooding during a break in activities and need to train themselves to register it.

Formal Thought Disorders

The thought processes depend on various neuroscientific mechanisms, such as recall from semantic memory, holding in working memory, activation of attention, execution of a trained transformation of the thought content, etc. (see below).

The variety of involved processes makes thinking susceptible to disorders. Accordingly, a multitude of psychopathological features of thinking have been distinguished. They can partly be traced back to disorders in the various neuroscientific mechanisms.

There is no simple definition for formal thought disorders. Formal thought disorders involve a disturbance of everyday thinking, which affects, for example, the

- efficiency of thinking, or its susceptibility for mistakes,
- the flow of thoughts (e.g., goal-directedness, brooding cycles, etc.),
- the speed, etc.

Contrast to Content-Related Thought Disorders

In this section, formal thought disorders are described, while content-related thought disorders are described in the chapter on Delusion. Griesinger separated formal from content-related thought disorders (1861), where for content-related thought disorders the following applies:

- Contents that are exaggerated or false, delusional thoughts, etc., another content-related category,
- specific contents that cause anxiety (Chap. 11, Sect. 11.5.2 and 11.5.5).

In formal thinking, the focus is not on the type and truth of thought contents but on the quality of the thought processes. It is not about the correctness or emotional consequences of specific thought contents.

Content-related thought disorders can disrupt everyday thought processes but do not necessarily have to; there is a certain dissociability of content-related and formal thought disorders, i.e., patients can have one but not the other disorder. For example, in a pure paranoid disorder, a content-related but usually no formal thought disorder is observed, and in some patients with disorganized schizophrenia, the opposite is true, strong formal without content-related thought disorders (i.e., without delusional thoughts).

Concept of Association Chains

As in other areas of psychopathology, popular concepts stand in opposition to the explanations of neuroscience. They were useful for the initial steps of psychopathological development but hinder progress. This includes the concept of association chains, which Sims (2003) uses to illustrate formal thought disorders. According to this, the course of thinking is determined by the content-related causal connection of thoughts. One idea should follow the next, etc. However, this is a course that only runs on the horizontal level. For the neuroscientific understanding of thinking, however, the nonlinear, multidimensional organization of thinking is crucial. The "thinking-target," as Kraepelin already called it, represents a particularly important instance. It distinguishes behaviorally relevant everyday thinking from contemplative associating. The target of thinking is held in working memory and serves the organization of retrieval for further elaboration in the course of subsequent thinking activity (see below).

In the notion of the stream of consciousness, the comparison with a computer's user interface was used. The stream of consciousness is determined in many aspects by the course of thinking. The image of a user interface of the brain is also useful for thinking. 1) We consciously experience a thought content. Without noticing it, 2) processes run beneath the surface of what is displayed on the computer screen, like calling up and editing one of the pages of an operating system or a file program. 3) Usually, we select something, like an operation, a transformation, etc.—that is, we press a key for this. However, we only experience the next step, namely, that 4) a new image appears with the result— another thought "occurs" to us, which was intended with the choice of transformation. This new thought content/screen content is part of the solution to the current thinking problem, or not. Thinking leads 6) to the thinking-target, or it continues. Otherwise, it is a new topic that now becomes the target of thinking. In summary, the experienced association chain can be explained as a product of the multidimensionally considered thinking processes (see Fig. 10.2).

Automatic Thoughts and Emotional Aspects

Everyone will have had the experience that practically at any time, but especially in quiet moments, thoughts appear from somewhere, which are referred to as automatic thoughts. Essential is that they were not intended to be thought by the person. Not necessarily rejected, but not actively retrieved, not intended, they suddenly appear ("it thinks me"). They play a significant role in psychiatry.

In everyday life, people often retrieve emotional connotations with a thought content, i.e., what valence an object, a person, a problem, etc., has. In part, emotions are also activated, at least fleetingly. The mental engagement with these emotional aspects of thought content sometimes takes up a large portion of time spent thinking.

10.1.1 Everyday Thinking

Everyday thinking, as already introduced above, is a thinking that is needed, for example, in conversations and in the organization of everyday life. Since many psychiatric disorders become apparent not only through a decline in efficiency in professional life but also in personal everyday life in one's own home, the focus of interest should be on this. In other words, the mental disorders treated in psychiatry are often accompanied by such a degree of formal thought disorders that everyday life without job requirements is significantly disrupted.

As already stated at the beginning, everyday thinking must be distinguished from specific thinking requirements. Everyday thinking thus stands in contrast to specific ways of thinking in academic professions, in tests, etc. In other

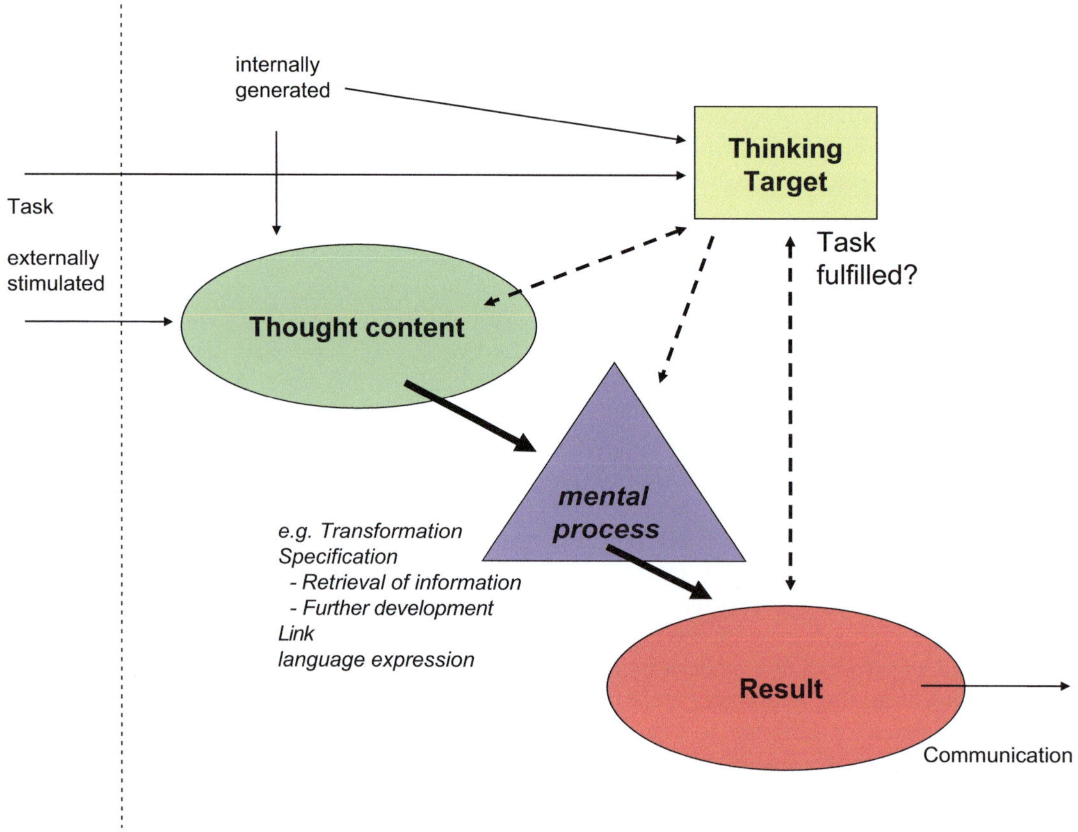

Fig. 10.2 Schema to illustrate psychopathological thought disorders. The focus is on the relationship between the development of thought contents, which are uttered by the patient, and thinking goals that are set by tasks or questions in the interview. It is therefore mainly not about general cognitive processes, as they are tested in intelligence tasks. Disorders in the thought process in psychopathological syndromes occur, for example, 1) when the thinking-target is lost or 2) the thought operations are disturbed, 3) the thought operations can no longer be sufficiently related to the target of thinking, or 4) drive disorders affect the thought process (further kinds of disturbance in the following text)

words, this is not about reporting on all the different ways of thinking that are necessary in various cognitive tests of problem-solving abilities or all possible job requirements.

1. Job requirements for thinking are highly variable, e.g., processing forms with reference to legal situations, assessing construction plans with reference to statics, etc. In specific thinking in academic professions, a multitude of disturbances of various intelligence components and memory are evident. The high variance refers to the types and levels of cognitive demands.
2. Mental exercises such as solving puzzles, or for example, chess.
3. Tests
   3.1 Intelligence tests with thinking tasks

From the above, one thing becomes clear: thinking is not equated with cognition in our context. It is about identifying the neuroscientific systems that lead to the failure of thinking functions in psychiatric disorders.

It was somewhat surprising that in severe depression (Reischies and Neu 2000) or in schizophrenic patients, many of the intelligence functions are not or only slightly impaired (Reischies and Mentzel 2001), but the patients fail in the most everyday tasks and show psychopathological formal thought disorders. Here, the reference to the difference between performances with one's own drive and externally motivated drive is helpful (see Chap. 7 Drive), because people with depression perform surprisingly well in test situations with externally motivated drive for thinking; however, they fail in everyday life tasks that require self-initiated thinking, planning, etc.

A sudden change in performance at work provides an indication of possible disturbances that may manifest in formal thinking. Of course, it already constitutes a serious disability if a top manager suffers a slight impairment in formal thinking after a disorder of cerebral blood flow. The emphasis on everyday relevance also aims to appropriately assess the impact of psychopathological disorders for each patient.

Specification of everyday thinking
If intelligence tests or certain job requirements demand processing thought content through specific mental transformations, this is rarely the case in everyday life.

In the following, we will focus on verbal thought processes that are related to the recall of knowledge about the thought content. Take the example of arithmetic, where a number is transformed by the mental operation "times 3", e.g. 12 * 3. This occurs in everyday life, but rarely.

A thought content focusses the attention on this specific content, on knowledge about this content. Properties (from the environmental model) and the associated action routines are retrieved for the thought content. This often already fulfills the target of thinking.

10.2 Functions of Thinking in Everyday Life

Thinking fulfills many functions in everyday life. Two exemplary functions are discussed in more detail below. One example deals with thought contents such as organizing everyday needs or putting actions in order, the other with everyday conversation about behavioral alternatives.

10.2.1 Organizing Everyday Needs

Internal stimuli occur throughout the day, such as the need to eat—a person considers whether it is worth going to a restaurant at that moment. Other topics include news of interest or the organization of sports activities ("how do I fit all this in today?"), and many more.

The example of addressing the need to eat can illustrate behaviorally relevant everyday thinking. Besides perceiving the need and recognizing the necessity of organization, evaluation plays a particularly important role in our context, which can be understood as the thinking-target.

It comes to the evaluation of:

- Conditions, options: e.g., is going out to eat now possible, allowed, personally favorable or unfavorable?
- Accidentals: e.g., can I go out to eat with person x today (possibly relationship aspects with this person), random special conditions in the specific situation, such as randomly perceivable new options.
- Recall of fulfillment possibilities: e.g., where can I eat well here? Knowledge of where it is possible,
- Evaluation.

In disturbances of behavior regarding the satisfaction of needs, of course, many other factors come into play, such as impulse control, memory disorders, etc.

Thinking disorders affect the described processes. Patients, for example, need prompts or impulse generation for eating, clothing, toilet, walks, and other everyday activities. Various causes can be considered for this. The person may have problems appreciating the context. For example, in a psychiatric ward: the conditions and rules on the ward must be recalled. In everyday home life, these are usually routine decisions, often regulated by time routines, for example.

Control of Attention Processes
Through thought processes, the control of the respective attention focus is effected. The recall of the next content in thinking determines where the person's attention is directed.

10.2.2 Conversation in Everyday Life

As a second area of everyday thinking, we consider the conversation about everyday circumstances as an example. As the thinking-target, there is usually a conversation topic or a question, i.e., a requirement posed by the conversation partner.

First, what the partner has said must be understood—language comprehension and the social understanding of the conversation partner's intention will not be considered here (Chap. 9 Language).

Central is the transformation of a partner's statement into a task, e.g., 1) knowledge query: "What is the new regulation on train fares?", 2) autobiographical information: "What is your name?", 3) recall of specifications: "What does buying the ticket mean for you?", 4) complex report with sequence "How was your vocational training?" Information from autobiographical, episodic memory or from the environmental model must be organized. 5) Valence-related evaluation "What do you think of …", sensation: "How strong is the pain and what kind?", 6) evaluation of a probability: "Will there be a tax demand?", 7) planning related to the person: "What are your plans for the future?".

10.3 Elements of Everyday Thinking

Selectively Activated Content
A thought content must first be selected. This selection and the storage of the thought content in working memory is considered by many researchers to be the central first steps of thinking: selection and working memory (working memory Chap. 6 and see neuroscience, e.g., Deco and Rolls 2005; Brown and Marsden 1988).

Step 1—Selection of a Thought Content
Alternative a. In the process of perception, semantic units are identified that are subjectively significant to the person. A content not only briefly appears in the stream of sensory influences but can be fixed as a target of thinking or initially as a thought content.

Alternative b. The thought content can also be primarily recalled in other ways, for example, through a question in conversation or a need and the evaluation of the conditions to satisfy the need (see also automatic thoughts).

Step 2—Fixation of a Thinking Goal
An important condition of everyday thinking, besides the recall or selection of a content, is the retention of the thought content in working memory. This makes a content a thought content, to which specifications can be added, such as knowledge, episodic memory with personal experience, etc. (Fig. 10.2). A function related to selective attention is necessary to avoid distraction from competing ideas.

Step 3—Selective Attention
Verbal thinking has been conceptualized in this context as a sequential handling of semantic units. In thinking, there is an interaction of many cognitive components. Particularly important for this is the organization of selective attention. Attention must be able to be directed to distant aspects during the thought process—for example, a person first thinks about the option of doing a renovation himself, then about the possibility of hiring a craftsman off the books, i.e., without tax registration; he directs his attention to legal and tax aspects.

Step 4—Updating of Working Memory
The specifications, properties of the thought content, or experiences added to the thought content modify the thought content. One can imagine this as certain sentences about the thought content first being activated , elementary propositions

about the thought content (Chap. 9 language). These activated statements about the thought content are initially kept in the buffer store. After mental operations, the buffer store of the thought content is refreshed or changed. This updating of the thought progress is subsumed under working memory functions. If a thinking-target is present, then the entry in working memory can be related to the target of thinking after the mental operations, with the question of whether the target of thinking has now been achieved.

Some people report that they always maintain a second level of thought in conversations, where associations, ideas, evaluations that do not need to enter into the conversation can be processed in parallel. To what extent such a practice leads to formal thought disorders in the case of a decompensation of cognitive abilities is not yet known in detail.

Conclusion
In everyday thinking, the selection from the many simultaneously incoming pieces of information, the retention of the thinking goal, the mental transformations and intermediate results, and the executive control over longer thought processes are crucial.

10.4 Clinic

Which subprocesses of thinking are affected in clinical thought disorders? Which disturbances of constraints have an impact?

A first example is a disturbance of thinking due to intense emotions or affects. Since antiquity, the necessity of the control of emotion for thinking has been emphasized. Thinking is restricted by agitation of affects because intense emotions, such as panic or anger, keep certain contents activated. Additionally, thinking is inefficient, for example, because intermediate storage is repeatedly erased. Thinking is not efficient in such a situation, and the "probatory action" cannot be successfully carried out (Chap. 11 emotion and affects).

In severe psychoses, in brain damage syndromes and regressive states, formal thought disorders usually have serious practical consequences for performance. Caregivers report, "Mr. X cannot manage a phone call." Another person in a clinic with an acute schizophrenic psychosis cannot take the bus to fetch something from his own apartment. This is because he cannot make the preparations, first to get a city map, second to get a bus ticket from the social worker, third to find the bus line, and fourth to be shown the bus stop, etc. There is a relationship to executive disorders.

Social workers know many people with mental illnesses who fail when applying for social benefits or conducting bank transactions. The abundance and complexity of bureaucratic information obligations play a role: Patients cannot make sense of being asked certain questions by the social welfare office. They cannot retrieve the contents addressed in questionnaires. Of course, disturbances that have nothing to do with thought disorders, such as language comprehension disorders, especially with cumbersome legal expressions, also play a role. For these reasons, psychiatric interviews pay attention to the ability to respond to questions and where the person's difficulties lie in answering questions.

Disturbance of selection and recall selectivity
Let us consider individual subprocesses of thinking: The selection of thought contents can already be impaired. If there is a target of thinking, for example, to apply for social assistance, it happens that a thought content not corresponding to this target of thinking is activated. In the incoherence of schizophrenic patients (see below), thought contents are expressed that are far removed from the semantic fields of the preceding contents—the thought sequence appears incomprehensible to the conversation partner.

Recall efficiency
Errors or failures in the retrieval of information.

For example, a person cannot think of anything on a topic or at least not the most important specification. Depressed patients complain that no thoughts come to mind at all. They feel they cannot keep up in conversations with their friends.

What must be retrieved in everyday thinking ?

Details of the current thought content must be retrieved for a question (such as applying for social assistance)—specifications, a specific selection of properties of the object that is currently relevant—for example, details about spatial conditions, color, etc., or assumptions about the duration of a process. These specifications are details retrieved when imagining the thought content in the context of the environmental model.

These specifications are partly in the form of elementary propositions about a thought content:"The pizza will cost about €8." These are experiences made in a situation.

Recall from semantic memory is tested, for example, through fluency tasks. In semantic fluency, as many words as possible should be found that belong to a semantic category such as "animals" or "clothing." This performance is objectively and subjectively impaired in many psychopathological syndromes: The number of retrieved words is low. In the thought inhibition of depressed patients, recall to thought goals does not succeed, which is subjectively experienced as tormenting. The slowing of thinking can in some cases be explained by a reduction in recall efficiency. In the disturbance of selectivity, incorrect mentions additionally occur.

Disturbance of Maintaining Thought Contents in Working Memory

In circumstantiality, the target of thinking is temporarily lost from the focus of attention, but in some cases, it can still be remembered—for example, if the interviewer's question is still retrievable, but other, "far-fetched" thought contents are already at the center of thinking.

In fluency tasks, which were discussed above, there is a deviation from the target of thinking, for example, naming different "animals." Details about a specific animal are told, precisely what came to the person's mind at that moment.

In schizophrenic psychoses, the disruption of a train of thought, the disruption of thought, is observed. This disturbance consists of the sudden loss of all information about the target of thinking, the previous course of thought. The feature of incoherence can be associated with a disturbance in maintaining a thinking goal in working memory.

In schizophrenia, there are peculiar problems with the subject's ability to influence, to control the thought process. This is a conceptually difficult area (see ego disturbances, Chap. 13). If someone cannot concentrate well, they feel they do not have complete control over their thoughts, losing control. A person with schizophrenia reports the experience of helpless attempts to influence his own thoughts. They also fail to perform an "interrupt," a stop of a train of thought; most people achieve this by voluntarily bringing another thought, an imagination, into the focus of attention (see below).

Other patients fail to direct their attention to distant contents. The direction of attention to a specific semantic area is disturbed: then an aspect cannot be sufficiently appreciated, for example, in the narrowing of thinking (see below). It is usually assumed initially that the association does not succeed. However, it is only partly a disturbance of retrieval from memory, but in certain cases also a disturbance of directing attention to another semantic field. Incidentally, it must be noted that we do not yet know exactly how attention to thought contents and how retrieval from memory are neurally organized. It may be that both processes have more in common than suggested by the categorical division of psychopathology. In other words, the two functions, on the one hand, the recall of mental contents and, on the other hand, the direction of focused attention as a process of an active filter, have close connections (Chap. 4 attention).

Often, the organization of directing attention to the various aspects of the problem is disturbed. The recall of a new association, a distant property of an object, simultaneously directs attention to this semantic field.

Attention can be fixed on a topic by emotional factors. Thinking cannot then be diverted from it. An example is the early phase of grief, in which practically all the time is spent thinking about the lost person. This is referred to as the phase of "grief work". In this process, rumination and narrowing of thinking occur.

Disturbance of the Organization of Thinking
Various thought disorders occur due to disturbances in the organization of thinking, which have already been mentioned: for example, disturbance of the complex processing of thinking goals, circumstantiality or flight of ideas. If no new thought contents are activated, it can lead to perseveration of thought contents, as seen in the thinking of demented persons.

Disturbance of the Evaluation of Options
A disturbance of the cognitive evaluation of options can be observed in situations where multiple options of action are available, and a decision must be made between them. The target of thinking is the evaluation—a disturbance can occur 1) in the repeated retrieval of the alternatives to be evaluated and 2) in the integration of the evaluation aspects accumulated in the various thought processes for one and the other decision alternative. In this process, the working memory must be updated with the status of the decision-making process according to the results of the evaluation processes. This thought function is often also impaired by emotional symptoms.

Disturbance in the decision
The decision between alternatives concerns several psychopathological areas—both the area of thinking and the formation of judgment and action preparation. Not only after a decision for one action is action readiness built up. Disturbances of these actually subsequent processes also affect the psychopathological areas of formal thinking. In Chap. 7 Drive, the neuronal processes of accumulators, which stand for one or the other action, are presented. These are closely linked to decisions. When one of the action options reaches the threshold, the corresponding action is initiated. Under time pressure, a decision is forced: When the time for the decision has come, the action options that come closest to the threshold will trigger the action.

For this reason, the problems of decision-making ability are usually separated from formal thought disorders. In decision-making—due to action readiness and motor implementation—influences of drive, as well as influences of motivation, or expectation of reward etc., are added.

From the thought processes result actions, judgments, but also emotions:

a) The action readiness, which is adapted to the environmental model of the person, can be disturbed. This has to do with thinking in relation to reward expectations.
b) Judgment; in judgment disorder, the integration of various aspects of the thinking goal can be disturbed (Chap. 14). This is the case, for example, in memory disorders, as the arguments can be forgotten during integration (Chap. 6 Working Memory).
c) Emotion or emotional mindset (affective-cognitive complexes, alexithymia) or attitude related to the person (splitting). Especially through emotional components: fixation on specific contents that have nothing to do with the thinking-target—directing attention repeatedly to a focus (rumination and content-related thought disorder).

10.5 Diagnostics

Colloquially, it is said: "I know now how he thinks" or "he doesn't think about that at all". In everyday knowledge of people, attention is paid to the thinking of conversation partners, colleagues, or superiors. Thinking reveals something about the possible hidden goals of the people a person is dealing with. People are interested in uncovering the unspoken intentions or ulterior motives of others. This is to be seen in connection with the "social brain"; the development of the brain takes place in the closest contact with family and other people. Paying attention to the thinking of others, their intentions, and ways of thinking is so self-evident that it requires effort to explicitly focus on it. In psychopathology, characteristics have been identified that can be diagnosed by paying attention to the thinking, the sequence of thoughts, and the so-called way of thinking of patients.

In the diagnostics of formal thought disorders, the efficiency of thinking is brought to the forefront. This corresponds in everyday life to observing how well a conversation partner can follow the argumentation and development of the conversation, or how quickly; People infer this from the reaction and response of the conversation partner (or also by paying attention to eye movements). In psychopathology, pathological characteristics of the course of thought processes are also of interest.

General Aspects

Thinking does not need to include overt behavior; it can take place without communication to fellow humans. "Thoughts are free" includes the decision about the expression of thoughts. The decision of the person to express their thoughts depends on the quality of the therapeutic alliance, i.e., it is connected with the success in the effort to build a trusting interpersonal relationship with the person. Only in a calm, open, trusting atmosphere between a person and the interviewer can an optimum exchange of the patient's information and the psychiatrist's advice and help take place. However, it remains safe to assume that much will not be communicated by an examined person.

Sometimes a facial expression or eye movement reveals that a thought expressed by the conversation partner at least touches the interest or fears of the patient.

If a person is not fully aware of their illness and refuses cooperation, formal tests of thinking components are often not feasible. Then, the only option is to assess thinking in the rudimentary communication between an interviewer and this person who refuses to make contact. It is conventional to then speak of "not assessable" in the findings.

From the above, it is clear: Formal thinking is indeed assessable in conversation, but not if the communication remains formulaic or the person evades. In some cases, some features can be assessed from brief statements. But a comprehensive and reliable assessment can only be made after longer conversations. The patient's ability to converse is psychopathologically crucial; an open conversation should be achieved as much as possible a) in the interview or b) in the free group conversation. In groups, e.g., psychoeducation-rounds, other thinking contents are often expressed than in the psychiatric diagnostic interview.

Relation to Target of Thinking

The formal thought disorder is mainly considered in relation to a target of thinking and the sequence of thoughts that are expressed (Kraepelin 1903).

Psychopathological Symptoms

In formal thinking, as shown above, disturbances of various neuropsychological functions are evident; in many cases, they appear exclusively or particularly prominently in thinking; for example, the disturbance of the control of thoughts by emotions or by a delusional topic, or the ability to abstract or retrieve knowledge.

Tasks

In addition to the biographical interview, the psychopathological examination pays attention to spontaneous responses, and tasks are given, e.g., the person is asked to formulate reports, for example, about school or professional developments, experiences, or assessments. This is supplemented by neuropsychological examination procedures.

The verbal fluency task ("verbal fluency") is usually seen as a specific language test, but it also tests thinking functions. As many words as possible should be named that belong to a certain category, e.g., animals, clothing items, or what can be bought in the supermarket. If the reader tries the task once, they will be convinced that it involves more than word finding: The execution also reveals details about the search process and its flexibility. Fluency must also be seen as a test of selection and working memory. We assume that the following processes are involved:

a) Selection of related items—the restriction to the search area must be implemented (animal fluency: zoo, farm, sea, etc.), with relation to executive planning disorders,
b) the selection criterion must be held in working memory
   - errors of deviating from the task, for example by saying sentences or making comments,
c) word finding.

Clinical Differentiation from Other Disorders Affecting Thinking
Some features must be differentiated from formal thought disorder, especially aphasia. This refers to the possibility of disturbance in the linguistic area: word finding, aphasic disorder of sentence formation, articulation disorder.

Furthermore, a lack of talent must be excluded. Disturbance of specific mental transformations, which are tested in intelligence tests, e.g., mathematical, semantic conceptual, logical, or spatial operations (e.g., mental rotation tasks). A variety of disorders can affect thinking, which must be counted among other cognitive operations and psychopathological areas.

10.6 Neuroscience

Cognition is not a human peculiarity. Cognitive processing and intelligence performance are studied neuroscientifically and in behavioral research in many species. Primates cannot communicate linguistically; they can only show via behavior that they want something and have "understood." However, the thinking considered in psychopathology is verbal thinking, and animals are not capable of this. This is also due to conscious and flexible attention, in which human thinking about mental content takes place. Primates have attention functions and probably also a sensory consciousness, but the level we consider also involves the awareness of the thought operation. An example is the symptom of thought chasing, the disturbance of thought control.

Computers surpass humans in performance in chess, a prime example of thinking games that require foresight in considering the next moves. They can generate texts about established knowledge. The technical models of cognitive processing will allow future conclusions about the disruptibility of this information processing in human mental disorders, particularly the disturbance of learning of neural networks (see below).

First, it must be asked how a model of thinking in the human brain can be imagined.

Human thinking does not require a special neurophysiological "thinking system" that other species do not possess. The peculiarity of human thinking is rather to be found in the complexity of semantic processing, knowledge, and episodic memory contents, as well as in the ability to draw on a differentiated environmental model to come to "reasonable" conclusions. In the modest scope of everyday life, this includes, for example, considering the private household, tasks and resources, and above all, financial reserves. Typically, a poor person includes environmental conditions in their everyday decisions.

One of the approaches to the neuroscience of thinking comes from neurology. Benson summarized some elementary aspects in his book "The Neurology of Thinking" (1994). In recent years, the individual mechanisms already mentioned above, which become effective in thinking, such as recall from semantic memory, working memory, etc., have been more closely investigated. The explicit investigation of thought processes has receded into the background. There are many reasons for this. First, the phenomenon of thinking has been divided into sub-aspects. Today, the research of executive functions and working memory particularly covers two aspects or areas of thinking. Another branch of research deals with the recall of semantic knowledge, which has already been discussed in the context of language. The domain of formal thought disorders leads in psychopathology to the collection of neuroscientific aspects of thinking, i.e., the fact that in the psychopathology of thought disorders, various functional disorders are revealed.

10.6.1 What Pathway

An important neuroscientific finding was that there is a special ventral stream of information processing (Ungerleider and Mishkin 1982). It has been called the "what pathway," in which objects are identified as semantic units, i.e., in the visual system, the shapes of objects and in the auditory system, the sound characteristics of objects and persons. They are cortically represented. This identification of objects is described in the first section on perception.

From there, not only can connections between object representations in the tertiary association areas be realized, but, for example, personal memories from episodic memory in the mediotemporal region and emotional qualities in the amygdala can also be processed.

10.6.2 Interaction of Bottom-Up and Top-Down Processes

Furthermore, neuroscience clearly showed that frontal control processes can steer information processing ("top down"). Thought processes must be organized, and disturbances of thinking often concern the lack of organization. In this process, cortical ensembles and entire brain areas must be activated or inhibited. This is necessary, for example, when concentrating on a sensory channel. This includes the activation or suppression of specific cortical-subcortical projection pathways through the frontal loops. It is a management of the course of information processing.

10.6.3 Activation of a Thought Content

In the first example, we will consider the activation of a content and then that of the combination of two contents. The example will be "taxi." Neuronal ensembles have been addressed, for example, by the perception of a taxi or a sign indicating a taxi stand. The expectation of reward, e.g., solving a transportation problem, drives the thinking activity. A semantic unit is active (taxi) and stored in the working memory, quasi in the monitor.

The activation of the semantic unit occurs effortlessly automatically. This happens in modules (Fodor 1983), such as the perception or language module: a) A semantic unit (sememe) is activated from perceptual elements, b) the lexical unit, the word "taxi," and c) a mental image of the typical taxi color, the taxi sign on the roof of a car from the image memory (image thesaurus), d) action schemes as habitual reaction patterns—such as hailing a taxi, e) episodic information—i.e., recent experiences with taxis, but also from movies, etc., f) emotional connotation (such as anxious concern that the money might not be enough).

It becomes clear that many properties are automatically called up with a semantic unit (Fig. 10.3).

Houk 2001 speaks of "partial thoughts" that are initially activated and require further processing. Pick had spoken in 1931 of not yet formulated, intuitive thoughts as the starting point of thinking and speaking processes. These would first be ordered before they could be expressed in a sentence.

First, entities closely related to the semantic unit, such as pictorial imagination, sound image, etc., are automatically activated, see above. A semantic unit will then activate a further semantic field around the unit (Chap. 9 Language). These are elementary propositions around the semantic unit: "A taxi is (too) expensive," "You have to wait for the taxi," or personal experiences "Taxi drivers are pushy these days." Many other statements about the semantic unit are ready, they are pre-activated. Thus, specifications are added to the already activated and in working memory held semantic units. For example, in the content-poor, formulaic language of dementia, only the in early years established sentence shells are expressed

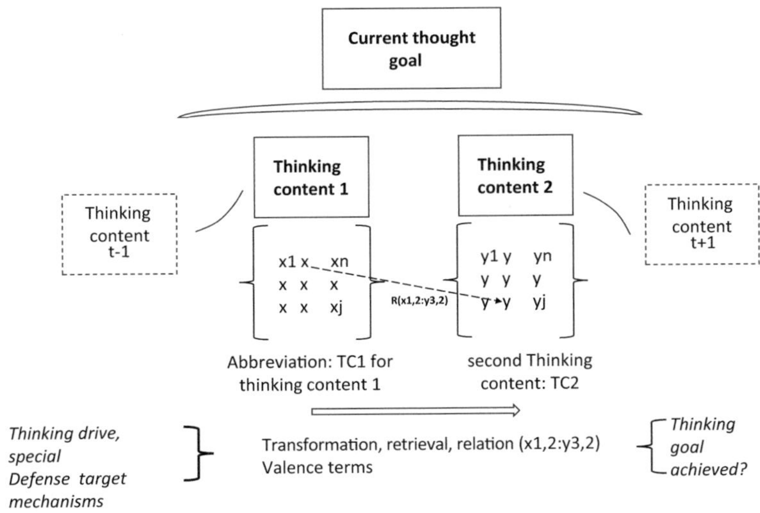

Fig. 10.3 Thinking processes that are specifically disturbed in psychopathological syndromes: Thinking processes that are relevant to everyday life and communicated in everyday situations involve the recall of associations, emotions, and intentions to a thinking-target. This recall can be insufficient or specifically restricted, e.g., by emotional contents or intentions that belong to anxiety, delusions, or compulsive symptoms. Thus, the complex processes in everyday thinking affect a range of symptoms from other psychopathological areas.

about a topic. Then the "facade" still appears well preserved.

However, specifications can also be retrieved in a special controlled process (see below).

10.6.4 Two Simultaneously Active Thought Contents

What happens with the activation of two thought contents, e.g., "the taxi" and "the payment"?

a) Let's assume the second content can be added as a specification by the first: "What about the taxi?" By the activation of taxi, the "payment" has been co-activated, i.e., information already belonging to the first content has been retrieved.
b) A second semantic unit can also be externally given as a thinking task, such as in a reflective essay, e.g., about "transport and costs," etc. The second word is not associated but given in the situation, for example, conversation partners. Here, the combination is the topic of thinking; e.g., "paying for the taxi"—as an unsolved problem, who pays, whether the money suffices, whether it will be reimbursed, how the receipt can be claimed for tax purposes, etc. The target of thinking "payment" prompts the second recall from environmental knowledge regarding properties and from episodic memory regarding personal experiences—paths for further thinking arise from the problems or contradictions in the properties and the semantic fields around the two semantic units. With two elements, logical, mathematical, or geometric operations can also occur.

10.6.5 Selective Activation and Becoming Aware of Thought Contents

The thought content can arise from internal stimuli such as hunger or pain or during the retrieval of other topics in the course of everyday thoughts (quasi-automatically). The person might exclaim, "That reminds me…".

The "becoming aware" that something is a relevant thought content is presented in Chap. 8 consciousness. Here it should only be noted that a content crosses an attention threshold, such as when becoming aware of a person in a crowd.

In a way that is not yet known, the threshold of conscious perception is crossed. Thus, the recognized person can become a content of conscious thinking. Now, 1) properties, specifications can be elaborated on, or 2) another thought content takes over again.

There is the model of thalamic activation, which theoretically can occur both in the process of information processing of the frontal loops and through the nonspecific activation of the reticular formation. People often experience arousal when an object becomes the thought content and interrupt their current actions or speech acts. The nonspecific activity of the reticular formation and the locus coeruleus could serve as an explanation for this (Ascending Activating system). However, the selectivity of the selection is a quality feature of thinking. General activation, nonspecific attention can interfere with selective retrieval processes.

10.6.6 Selective Activation of Thought Contents

First, the situation of simultaneous processing of thought contents should be addressed. The model of trained neural networks can serve as an explanation here. Neural networks model the simultaneous parallel processing of input information to a trained (successful) output information or response of the system. They are therefore suitable for explaining simultaneous information processing, as it often occurs in thinking.

A thought content has a context. The pattern of thought content and context triggers the activation of another thought content that is important to the person in that context (as in the last example "taxi" and "pay") or a pattern of thought contents activates a specific response at the output of the neural network that is advantageous for the organism (Fig. 9.2).

The principle of trainable activation of an output pattern given an input information is fundamental to many current CNS models of cortical functions (Rummelhart 1986; McClelland et al. 2003; Spitzer 1996).

The processes in a Parallel-Distributed-Processing model are particularly illustrative (Chap. 9 language; Fig. 9.2); this consists of three layers of network nodes, the "neurons", namely a layer of input and output neurons as well as at least one layer of neurons, which are referred to as "hidden units" and can be considered as a computational "layer"—today, training is done with more than one computational layer of neurons (deep learning, LeCun et al. 2015). The neurons, the network nodes, are each connected to all neurons of the next layer. The strength of the connection or efficiency with which the specific subsequent neuron is activated is subject to change through feedback during learning; this happens during the training of the network. The result of a training run is classified as correct or incorrect. If a correct output occurs, the currently active node connections are strengthened. Various algorithms can be applied for this. The simplest, the Hebb rule, has also been used. In many training sessions, one of the possible combinations of connectivity between the network nodes is established, leading to successful output given a specific input. The neuronal networks have remarkable properties, so they can implicitly learn rules etc. (Rummelhart and McClelland 1986; McClelland and Rogers 2003).

Hoffman was able to demonstrate that the disruption of information processing in neural networks is suitable for explaining thought disorders, as they occur in schizophrenia (Hoffman 1987). He used cortex models, in which each node is connected to every other node, so-called Hopfield models (see e.g., Spitzer 1996). The models are suitable for explaining thinking errors such as overgeneralization, i.e., a false conclusion based on insufficient information. In contrast, there is another type of neuronal network, which has already been introduced in Chap. 9 Language, the Parallel-Distributed-Processing model (McClelland and Patterson 2002), see above. For this type of neuronal network, the damage to the "hidden units," a computational layer between the input and output layers, can be considered, which has been proposed as a model for explaining schizophrenic thought disorders as a result of damage in certain brain regions of schizophrenic patients (see Reischies et al. 2001).

The information processing at each node can be varied in the computational model. This models a biochemical disruption of synaptic information transmission, connection strength, and feedback learning, as well as the cellular mechanisms of generating the action potential (for the output). Of course, neuronal networks are rough simplifications of the complex relationships of a group of the many millions of nerve cells in the human cortex. But even by modeling these essential input and output characteristics of a few node elements and their networking, important characteristics of human information processing could be explained.

In direction of attention, a cortical network of the Mesulam model has also been reported. This involves the cortical activation of an attention field upon the input of a sensory-detected object.

Usually, only an elementary 1:1 pre-activation has been assumed in cortical-cortical activation. But on the basis of the models of neuronal networks, it became clear that even in cortical-cortical activation, complex computational processes with the success of environmentally adapted selection and graduation of activation can be carried out.

Disruptions affect:

a) Neural networks: a lack of appropriate response, for example, due to inadequate processing of the addresses with which the network can call up associated content (in this case, the input information that leads to calling up the appropriate response),
b) a faulty selection in neural networks (leads to incorrect activations, see Hoffman 1987, models of schizophrenic thinking),
c) lack of control, a disinhibition of selection processes that are not stopped, e.g., in the case that each pattern of neuronal activity again becomes the address of a new association, which then generates further associations in the network. This can be used to explain thought pressure or flight of ideas.

Successive activation of Thought Contents

A thought content combined with a second thought content as well as with the context of the first thought content can exist as a sequence. If thought contents occur at different times, a simultaneous pattern can still be provided for thought processing in working memory. Examples are sequences of numbers that we hear sequentially but process as a whole number. In the cortex, the sequential inputs are represented in an ordered manner and held in working memory so that they can each serve as parallel input for processing in the thought process.

There are also specific temporal sequences in thinking. For example, habitual thought processes are known—comparable to work routines or daily routines of individuals as "quirks," etc. Ritual sequences of thought contents are used in meditations.

These are to be distinguished from causally conditioned sequences, i.e., sequences that only arise in the course of thinking and should therefore be situation-adapted. Thinking predicts in probatory action what will happen, for example, when an action is performed. The neural networks can be trained in everyday life in the manner described above. The cortical networks predict the usual sequence of events, and upon success, the necessary connections are strengthened. From the experience of a sequence of thoughts that was successful, the recall of usual everyday sequences can be enabled.

This learning of sequences is also accomplished through imitation. The role of imitation not only for motor but also for cognitive development can thus be explained (Subiaul et al. 2004). The role of mirror neurons for this sequence learning mechanism is to be assumed. Mirror neurons are active both when the subject performs the activity and when the subject sees another subject performing the movement (see Gottlieb 2002).

In the sequence models of neural networks, the initial state in the first pass becomes the input state for the activation of the next subsequent state. It is important to realize that a complex neural network can encode many different input-output patterns.

10.6.7 Frontal Loops

The cortical functionality includes the sequence of cortico-subcortical loops, which can process a sequence of thought contents or motor actions one after the other, i.e., in addition to the purely cortical network connections, the subcortical connections, especially the cortico-subcortical projection loops, the frontal loops, must be considered (see Chapter Drive, Fig. 7.4). Each neuron of the cortex regions is connected via the cortico-subcortical projection loops with the subcortical nuclei and back through the thalamus ultimately with itself—apparently especially also with the neighboring areas.

Special sequences that are trained, especially motor sequences, such as when playing a musical instrument, seem to involve these loops on the one hand and many other brain areas on the other. The encoding of sequences in the basal ganglia has been described (Houk 2001). The additional involvement of the cerebellum is not discussed in detail here.

For psychopathology, it is crucial: Sequential retrieval can be beyond control. In thought pressure and flight of ideas, but also in thought control disorder (see below disinhibition of thought content retrieval) and partly also in incoherence, uncontrolled retrieval processes in thinking can be diagnosed.

10.6.8 Selective

The quality of thinking is also related to the selectivity of the information held in working memory. Selectivity refers to the delineation of semantic fields, the specificity of what is retrieved for a topic. Here, the quality of training, education, and intelligence level play a role. If, as a rough example, as mentioned above, not "taxi" but a more general concept like "car" is processed as a topic, it cannot lead to fruitful ideas.

10.6.9 Working Memory in Thought Processes

A thought content must remain activated in working memory for the duration of the thought process. 1) The target of thinking in working memory must be successively compared with the processed thought contents—each time concerning the question of whether the target of thinking has been reached. 2) If it is about optimization (a best solution), the best result so far must also be held in working memory and updated gradually if necessary.

The results of a thought process must be stored again in working memory (see below). The demands on working memory are thus variably complex, depending on the type of thinking task. At the end of the thought process or when changing topics, working memory must be cleared. This will now be described in more detail.

Retention in Working Memory

A thought content, in the above example the object "taxi," is encoded as a semantic unit in the ensemble code sensorily, with its spatial information (parietal and dorsolateral prefrontal), as working memory (e.g., dorsolateral prefrontal) or evaluation (e.g., orbitofrontal), etc.

Predominantly in the dorsolateral prefrontal cortex, an activity that can evoke this representation is retained in working memory. This occurs (see Houk 2001) possibly a) through the activity held in frontal cortico-subcortical projection loops, the Frontal Loops; this could cause a continuation of cortical activation, b) through local cortical mechanisms (see Gao et al. 2001; Gao and Goldman-Rakic 2003), c) an important finding of neuroscience for these functions was the discovery of the sustained-activity neurons in the prefrontal cortex (Fuster 1990). Independent of the incoming information from the sensory channels, these neurons encode enduring processes. Whenever information should not be erased by the subsequent sensory impressions so that it can guide a later action, the brain must temporarily store it. This temporary storage occurs through the sustained activity of neurons. The sustained-activity neurons are predominantly found in the dorsolateral prefrontal cortex, in front of the precentral gyrus and above the Broca's speech region on the language-dominant side. However, this working memory function is not lateralized but should be seen as a bilateral function.

A model of this storage assumes that initially Frontal Loops are necessary to build a working memory, but subsequently, with automation, local cortical mechanisms take over the function. Many researchers currently assume support of working memory by the Frontal Loops (see above).

The disturbance of working memory is expressed in particular features of formal thought disorders:

1. For example, patients "lose the thread."
2. An evaluation of possible options occurs only after the thought process has ended. A disturbance of working memory will thus also affect judgment ability.

Specification of the Search for Mental Contents

In the course of thinking, information is added (such as the increasing elaboration of properties relevant to problem-solving), which further specifies the search. If a person is looking for another person in the crowd and only later remembers that the person being sought is wearing a red T-shirt, the search will become more efficient after this. The improvement of search processes also applies to a search in the lexical memory or knowledge store. The search will be more precise after the specification (essentially a more accurate address).

A function of the Frontal Loops is characterized as a gating mechanism, a gatekeeper function that primarily acts on the thalamus (Carlsson 2001; see Houk 2001). The cortex-activated dual inhibition ultimately activates the thalamus, which otherwise is under tonic inhibition by neurons of the pallidum. The very specific process controlled by the cortex, unlocking the gate of the thalamus to allow precisely specified sensory or other cortical activity to pass, can be seen as a programmable filter.

The concept of a filter is again connected with the neuronal networks. It is assumed that the frontal "loops" function is based on a neuronal network addressed by the cortex as input. It determines the output via the—relative to the cortical neurons—few neurons of the striatum, thus controlling the thalamus. The thalamus, in turn, controls the sensory input of the cortex. So, in addition to the cortical-cortical connections that can be described according to the model of neuronal networks, functions of the Frontal Loops are also characterized in the manner of neuronal networks (Reischies and Mentzel 2001). When a further specification is achieved in the course of the thought process, the filter can be reprogrammed in this way, and indeed more precisely.

Updating Working Memory

If a specification has resulted from a thought process (see above), we can now describe that neuronally a refinement of the new "address" has taken place, which can now, in turn, evoke new, more appropriate contents. In intelligence tasks, a transformation or a calculation may also have to be performed. A new thought process must be retained in working memory, which is described as "memory updating" (Oberauer 2005).

In our above example of the taxi, a sensory information might possibly be added to a thought content. Various taxis might have been sighted on the street and at a taxi stand. On the other hand, it might have been realized during the thought process that the person has too little money and can only use a taxi if they share it with others.

10.6.10 Integration of Various Information Sources

How does someone come to sufficient consideration of a thinking goal? In everyday life, considerations are usually interrupted. The information collected for the evaluation is integrated into an assessment (Sect. 10.1.1 everyday thinking; for example, searching for a place and opportunity to have lunch). The experience of having to think about something, such as taking money with you, can already train a series of points that one thinks about when organizing everyday matters.

As described in central motor control, it is assumed that neurons involved in action initiation exhibit a so called "random walk," i.e., a "random" course of membrane potential, meaning noise of unspecific information. However, this "random walk" shows a drift due to the integration of specific information, which, with sufficient input and integration, can lead to the triggering of a correct decision, an action (Chap. 7). Disturbances occur in hasty decisions, which can be observed in mania. On the other hand, anxieties can cause brooding, i.e., endless loops of consideration, because it is not certain whether everything necessary has been considered. These are thought disorders, as known from obsessive-compulsive disorders.

Access to all associated contents, knowledge, episodic experience etc.

Fodor distinguished between modular and non-modular information processing (Fodor 1983). Non-modular information processing, in contrast to modular information processing, has, in principle, access to all contents represented by a brain. This is only in principle the case. Restrictions of free access to all represented contents are in everyday thinking the result of the fact that the recall of thought contents is trained in neuronal networks and thus trained associations are called up for the individual person, i.e., only the learned specifications of a thinking goal. It is usually assumed that people's ways of thinking in everyday life go beyond the trained connections only exceptionally (see the exercise of "brainstorming" to overcome these trained thinking paths).

Access to certain knowledge or experience components may not function in certain cases. Wernicke (1906) used the term sejunction to indicate that certain accesses are not possible in psychiatric disorders. These are disconnection models. In psychoanalysis repression theories were presented. The omission of remembering certain experiences can result in a loss of automatic retrieval due to the lack of refreshment: the matter is not remembered, and over time, the content is forgotten.

On the other hand, an experience coupled with an emotion can be particularly frequently remembered and thus overwhelmingly present (see trauma memories). This can also lead to a distortion of balance in information processing, leading to fixed thought patterns. Thus, both a trained inactivation of retrieval from episodic memory can occur, as well as a conditioned over-retrieval, e.g., when a sad event is repeatedly thought of, and each time painful memories arise.

In the thinking style of histrionic personalities, the emotional side of the activation of various aspects of a question predominates. Emotional activations direct the retrieval of knowledge, but also information from episodic memory. Personal experiences with the topic gain the upper hand over the aspects that are kept by environmental knowledge, so to speak, in the paths of reason.

Consistency

In philosophical thinking, the highest value is placed on consistency. This is not the case in everyday thinking. Not only would all different aspects of a thinking goal have to be appreciated (see above); but additionally, all thoughts on the topic would have to be examined for contradictions. In the everyday experience of psychopathology, it becomes clear how many contradictory contents and beliefs coexist in a person's thinking. W. James is attributed with the statement that thinking is mostly just a rearrangement of prejudices. The contradictory statements often stem from the experience of different life situations. These thoughts are not later brought into connection with each other, and if this does happen, a false conclusion is not corrected. This is important for the discussion of content-related thought disorders (Chap. 13 Delusion).

Here, too, interactions with personality traits arise. The thinking style of histrionic personalities has already been mentioned. A person with an obsessive personality exhibits a particular thinking style, usually characterized by anxiety, aggression, and working memory disorders in the processing of thinking goals. Patients with obsessive symptoms usually have irrational, internally contradictory justifications for their obsessive rituals.

Control

People can direct their thinking either towards specific topics or stop a train of thought. This is a fundamental capacity of human thinking ability. The person has the feeling of control. This control can be disturbed, both unnoticed by the person and noticed by the person. An example is obsessive rumination. A thought repeatedly imposes itself on the person, leading to a thought loop. The thinking must continue but brings no solution ("negative circular thoughts"). Here, emotional reasons are leading in most cases for the recurrence of thoughts. For instance, the grieving person repeatedly thinks about the loss when reminded of the lost partner in everyday life.

Attention disorders result in the inability to direct attention from one semantic area to another (Chap. 4 attention). A gatekeeper mechanism, discussed above, the "gating," apparently affects the thalamus. In thalamic nuclei, neurons of the frontal cortex can program a filter, as described above. This is apparently used for the organization of thought processes.

On the one hand, engagement with a topic is interrupted when attention is directed to another topic. This can normally be brought about voluntarily. Here, an attention shift occurs. In a syndrome of anxiety and grief, there is an inability to turn thoughts away from the specific thought content, or the thoughts return very soon as automatic thoughts.

On the other hand, thought control is also impaired in connection with the disturbance of interrupt processes of the brain. These interrupts can stop processes such as motor reactions (Gauggel et al. 2004).

The recurrence of a thought could be related to faulty neuronal activation, as in the epilepsy model (see aura). This can also persist for a longer time.

10.6.11 Role of Executive Functions in Thinking

Executive functions have already been discussed for the planning of a thinking task. They organize the entire sequence of thought processes. In school and professional training, there is exercising of executive functions. For example, people have trained sequences "what, who; where, when; why, for what purpose" when "considering" and discussing as well as presenting topics.

In trained individuals, multidimensional thought processes can be observed—as in medicine: first examination, findings, and diagnosis, then indications of therapy with consideration of contraindications (and interactions) before the indication of a drug or psychotherapeutic intervention.

Concluding Remark:

Some types of clinically diagnosed thought disorders are not presented in detail here. They are linked to the impairment of specific cognitive areas, such as the disorder of abstract thinking or concretism.

The change in the threshold of retrieving thoughts can lead to formal thought disorders, poverty of ideas on one side or pressure of thoughts on the other side. Specific aspects of thought disorders are also addressed at the end of the presentation of individual symptoms.

10.7 Psychopathological Symptomes of Thinking—Formal Thought Disorders

The symptoms of formal thought disorders have been differently described and defined; in addition to the definitions of the AMDP group (AMDP 11th ed. 2023), there exists a psychopathological scale of thought disorders specifically focussed on formal thought disorders in schizophrenic psychoses (Kircher et al. 2015).

Thinking Retarded
Definition. The flow of thoughts has become slower.

Example

A patient takes a very long time to answer simple questions, with no other psychopathological features or motivational problems providing an explanation (e.g., neither speech disorders nor amotivation or refusal), and even in his argumentation, the sequence of arguments is retarded. ◀

Position in Psychopathology.
AMDP 16.

Psychopathological Interactions.
General slowing, motivational problems (see above), the patient has given up contact in communication, is inhibited, regression.

Differential Diagnostic Distinctions.
Intended delay of answers, suspicion (checking the possibility that a statement could be used against oneself), refusal, thought inhibition see below.

Self-/other persons's judgment.
Other persons's judgment, history taken from other persons usually necessary.

Interview for Rating:
Observe the course of the interview in terms of time aspects.

Neuropsychology/objectification.
E.g., explaining proverbs; tests: fluency vs. finding similarities without time restriction.

Severity.
Degree of decelerationof the diagnostic interview.

Pathognomonic for:
Dementia, clouding of consciousness of the somnolence type, Huntington's disease.

Specifications:
1) limited to thinking: otherwise no general slowing, 2) general slowing, also motor slowing.

Personality influences.
Comfortable, cautious, "pedantic" personalities.

Neuroscientific/cognitive neuroscientific models:
Retrieval disorder 1) Shift of the activation threshold of neurons—difficult to activate, 2) difficult routine activation; a. change in form, (for example "catastrophic interference" e.g., after stroke, after epileptic seizure, in epileptic continuous activity), Cave: medical overdose, b) sticking—enechetic personality change, c) with general slowing in clouding of consciousness, 3) internal language processing of a thought too slow, so that the next association occurs retarded.

Thinking inhibited
Definition. Subjective characteristic of the perception of difficulty in thinking—subjectively inefficient thinking, because thoughts do not occur as usual. The patient experiences this as inhibition.

Introspective characteristic;
Discrepancy from the person's usual thought process.

Example

A patient cannot consider his situation; thinking "no longer succeeds, or it takes much more effort than before," important aspects do not occur to him, he remains in anxiety on catastrophic topics, etc. ◀

Position in psychopathology.
AMDP 15.

Psychopathological interactions:
- general inhibition, depressed mood, experience of insufficiency,
- rumination, inability to detach from affective-cognitive complexes (Chap. 11 emotion and affect) hinders thinking,
- blockage by delusion, affective-cognitive complexes.

Differential diagnostic distinctions:
Poverty of thought, without thinking drive, mental retardation,

1. Dementia syndrome: without associations,
2. general slowing,
3. interaction: the patient does not want to engage in the interview, wants to be left alone.

Further characterization:
To be understood as the subjective side of slowed thinking. Subjective impairment previously unknown to the person, being able to rely on promptly occurring thoughts for clear thinking; the person must now, unlike before, make an effort to retrieve and organize simple thoughts, which the person experiences as frustrating. Difference between thinking drive and efficiency.

Feeling of inhibition in the domain of thinking with sufficient thinking drive.

Self-/other person's judgment.
self-evaluation.

Interview for Rating.
"thinking subjectively against resistance?" "Too laborious?"

Severity.
From subjective thinking delay and planning disorder to transition into stupor, subjectively perceived as tormenting.

Pathognomonic for:
depression.

Specifications:
1. generally for all contents,
2. situational or content-related.

Neuroscientific/cognitive neuroscientific models
1. Retrieval disorder: for thinking, impaired in terms of impaired initiation (see below: drive)—e.g., impaired semantic recall (see e.g., verbal fluency),
2. Inefficiency of one's own drive in thinking (Chap. 7),
3. Feeling of effort as in mental "effort",
4. inhibition by "interfering drives", when an idea matures into motivation and action readiness, for example, an alarm thought with a feeling of anxiety disturbs.

Pressured thinking
Definition. Experiences of a multitude of ideas. The person give the impression of playing with the abundance of ideas; the abundance of thoughts imposes itself on the person. The focussing on a single target of thinking is therefore disturbed.

Example

A person is brimming with ideas that constantly come to him. As a result, he easily deviates from a structured conversation. When he is supposed to think about something, the influx of distracting ideas often proves problematic or annoying. ◄

Position in psychopathology.
AMDP 21.

Psychopathological interactions:
Concentration disorder, ambivalence and ambitendence due to the multitude of ideas, disturbance in the drive area e.g., starting and leaving off—in mania, confused mania: disinhibition, confabulation; in manic syndrome also: arrogance, only needing to think about something briefly.

Differential diagnostic distinctions.
Disturbance of thinking by a single emotional thought that repeats rapidly, as in brooding.

Further characterization.
In a way, the subjective side of racing thoughts with increased drive—the manifestation of increased drive in the area of thinking. Engagement for each new idea, rapid onset of interest.

Self-/other persons's judgment.
self-evaluation.

Interview:
Each time asking about the subjective side of a sequence of thoughts (how do you come to this argument now, how does this relate to the thought you just expressed?).

Neuropsychology/objectification.
Observation of the course of the conversation: number of little topic-related or unrelated ideas.

Severity.
In the interview, ranging from mild without impact to severe depending on the impairment of the interview or daily activities.

Specifications:
1) generally for all contents, 2) situational or content-related (see delusion induced disorganized thinking).

Conceptual problems of the feature:
Relationship to manic syndrome and distinction to thought control disorder, which is, however, also observed without increased drive.

Neuroscientific/cognitive neuroscientific models:
1) thinking drive is high, 2) control over thinking is reduced (overwhelmed by the abundance of ideas), 3) motivation fluctuation repeatedly leads to new intention that cannot be integrated into the flow of a thought, rapid engagement of interest leads to new ideas, 4) threshold of awareness of a content is lowered, so it becomes the subject of further conscious processing.

Flight of Ideas
Definition. The thinking of the person is interrupted by the abundance of ideas, through the multitude of thoughts.

Objective pressure of thoughts with increased drive (in contrast to thought control disorder, which also occurs without changes in drive). The person often do not suffer from it.

Example

A patient repeatedly jumps from one idea to the next in the course of his thoughts, with the arguments still showing a loose connection; he appears driven by the next idea that seems interesting to him. ◄

Position in Psychopathology.
AMDP 22.

Psychopathological Interactions.
In most cases, increased general drive; questionably selectively increased thinking drive.

Differential Diagnostic Distinctions.
a) Disturbance of thinking by a single thought that repeats, as in brooding, b) incoherence, c) associative loosening—reduction of the logical connection between the successive thoughts.

Further Characterization.
The occurrence of ideas is experienced by the examiner because the patient explains the ideas and can also comment on their chain of thoughts.

Self-/Other Person's Judgment.
Predominantly other person's judgment.

Neuropsychology/Objectification.
Observation of the conversation-flow characteristic: number of ideas—more or less topic-related or unrelated.

Severity.
Conversation unimpeded to: conversation not possible.

Pathognomonic for:
mania.

Neuroscientific/Cognitive Neuroscientific Models
See also above pressure of thoughts, Hoffman et al. 1986.

1. Specifications retrieved for a topic become the address for the next recall, but this is not controlled by a thinking goal—disinhibition,
2. Working memory impaired: retaining the thinking intention in sequences of thoughts is difficult but still possible.
3. Fluctuation of motivation (fluctuating interest—presumably therefore not noticed by the subject as a disorder),
4. Increased drive, possibly specifically in the thinking area.

Thought Control Disorder
Definition. The person experiences their thoughts as being beyond subjective control, i.e., the thoughts continue even though the person has no thinking intention for them, does not want to think them.

The person does not want to think, for example, because he wants to rest. Thoughts partly lead into a direction that the person does not intend. In contrast to pressure of thoughts, there does not have to be an increase in ideas.

Examples

- A person cannot rest because many different thoughts uncontrollably go through his head—for example, thoughts about daily events, which do not have to be days with particularly emotional experiences.
- A person with an incipient psychosis relapse reports that he can no longer think for himselve, he has no influence on his thoughts. "It is like always in my psychosis": the thoughts have become independent, and he passively watches as the ideas pass by in his head. ◄

Position in Psychopathology.
Not defined in AMDP.

Related Terms.
Executive disorder in the domain of thoughts.

Psychopathological Interactions.
Obsessive brooding, sleep disorder. Ego disturbances; foreign thoughts, thought insertion. No acoustic quality.

Differential Diagnostic Distinctions:
- Ego disturbance—the quality of being externally influenced in ego disturbance is not the case here,
- in obsessive rumination repetition of the same thoughts,
- individual automatic thoughts, usually well known to the person, for example catastrophic thoughts—generally with affective emphasis.

Further Characterization.
Usually perceived as unpleasant, depending on the content of the ongoing thoughts.

Self-/other persons's judgment.
self-evaluation.

Interview for Rating.
By themself non-controlled thoughts, patients complain about the passing by (»rattling through«) of thoughts without voluntary influence.

Severity.
Severe, when the person can no longer maintain sufficient space for their own thoughts, can no longer think in a planning manner.

Conceptual Problems of the Feature.
Apparently characteristic of the experience of thinking in schizophrenic disorders, relationship to ego disturbances, passivity of the thinking person.

Neuroscientific/Cognitive Neuroscientific Models
1. More generally defined by Benson (1994): »disorder in control of thought« for schizophrenia, disintegration of the voluntary thinking apparatus with loss of control over thought motivation, the direction of associative and executive attention,
2. Disturbance of the sensation of being the actor, i.e. executing a thought or an action (see ego disturbances). A disturbance of the sense of "being mine" has also been mentioned.
3. Inhibition system disturbed, resulting in the sequence of many unrelated thoughts, thereby also disturbing a single voluntary thought process,
4. Relationship to the passive listening to verbal auditory hallucinations, hearing voices; generation of thoughts in the CNS, which are then heard—without acoustic quality—experienced by the person as thought control disturbance.

Restricted thinking
Definition. The thinking remains fixed on one topic, the person can hardly/not be diverted from it, or will return to the one topic after a short time.

Example

A patient is completely absorbed by his sorrows, he only thinks about them and only talks about them in conversation. When trying to distract him to another topic, he says that this other topic has now become unimportant or he returns to his topic after 1 or 2 sentences. ◀

Position in Psychopathology.
AMDP 18.

Psychopathological Interactions.
Ruminating, delusion, obsessive rumination, poverty of thought,

Differential Diagnostic Distinctions:
- automatic thoughts, isolated, for example catastrophic thoughts—usually with affective emphasis
- intended persistence on a topic important to the person,
- perseveration,
- impoverished thinking, low IQ, slowing down,
- narrowed consciousness: additionally, inability to turn attention to something new—in acute stress reaction.

Self-/other persons's judgment.
Other persons's judgment.

Interview:
Course of Conversation Feature: when changing interview topics: hard/not to be diverted from the topic.

Severity:
- Degree of interview impairment,
- content: what is restricted thinking about? Thought, memory, worry, feeling.

Pathognomonic for:
Delusion, e.g., depressive delusion, but also in acute stress reaction, fanaticism.

Specifications.
Epileptic personality change, e.g. with the symptom of sticking.

Neuroscientific/cognitive neuroscientific models
1. attention management disturbed with deficit in disengaging attention (lack of flexibility in the control of focused attention).
2. affective-cognitive complex asserts itself against the shift of attention to new contents (topic/goal)

Perseveration
Definition. Immediate repetition of words (or short sentences); not for the purpose of special emphasis—the utterance initially fit the situation but becomes pathological through repetition.

Example

A patient with frontotemporal dementia (FTD) repeatedly says "You are a silly person," which could initially be interpreted as a curse in an agitation but, after many repetitions in many states of agitation, is characterized as perseveration. ◀

Position in psychopathology.
AMDP 19.

Related terms.
logoclonus.

Psychopathological interactions.
Word-finding disorder, poverty of thought, disinhibition.

Differential diagnostic distinctions:
- Thought narrowing,
- usual idiomatic repetitions "oh my God, oh my God",
- emphasis, as a rhetorical figure,
- palilalia—the utterance did not fit the situation, no increase in speed
- echolalia, rigid repetition of all words uttered by the interviewer,
- logoclonus—motor repetition of a word or part of a word, e.g., in extrapyramidal disorders.

Further characterization.
Repetition of language elements, words, or phrases.

Self-/other persons' judgment.
other persons' judgment.

Neuropsychology/objectification.
Observation of the conversation course, feature: immediate repetition, error counting.

Severity:
isolated, rare—to disruption of communication by perseverations.

Pathognomonic for:
aphasia forms, frontotemporal dementia.

Specifications:
a) words, b) phrases, sentences.

Neuroscientific/cognitive neuroscientific models:
Still unclear, apparently several influences come together

1. Facilitation of the last action, which is still pre-activated, leads to repeated triggering in the absence of alternative actions,
2. a language expression schema is predominantly activated.

Ruminating
Definition. Incessantly repetitive thinking of the same thought circles about a usually emotionally distressing/subjectively important topic that leads to no result—circular negative thoughts.

Example

A patient repeatedly thinks the same thought about his possible guilt in the failure of the marriage, he does not energetically resist it because he considers the topic always important to think about. He cannot escape the tormenting, circling thoughts—he experiences the thinking as an attempt at a solution, without a solution being achievable. ◀

Position in psychopathology. AMDP 20.

Related Terms. Ruminating.

Psychopathological interaction:
Delusion, complexes, ruminating can be perceived as tormenting, i.e., the patient cannot fully control it, i.e., "turn it off," overlap with "restricted thinking" on a target of thinking.

Differential diagnostic distinctions:
- Obsessive thoughts, compulsive ruminating—the inability to stop ruminating despite efforts.
- Pressing thoughts with mostly positively toned content in manic syndrome.

Further characterization.
Being attached to an affectively significant circle of thoughts.

Self-/other persons' judgment.
Self- and other persons' judgment.

Interview for rating.
Subjective—question about the amount of free time spent ruminating.

Severity.
Extent of subjective interruptibility of the circles of thoughts, impairment in daily activities due to ruminating.

Pathognomonic for:
Depression.

Specifications:
Spectrum of:

a) Believing to have to think about something to
b) Knowing that it is pointless to continue ruminating about something, but still doing it.
c) Tendency for self-punishment, being stuck in distressing thoughts repeatedly.

Neuroscientific/cognitive neuroscientific models
1. Complex of emotional and cognitive stressor—affective-cognitive complex (see below),
2. attraction effect of the worrying topic regarding attention—thereby failure of attention control in the thinking area,
3. Person experiences relief when considering the topic, like penance rituals (defence mechanism of undoing),
4. Repetition as an attempt to cope with the matter (to habituate, to learn to endure something).

Circumstantial thinking
Definition. Deviation of the thought process from the goal-oriented path, without this being intended by the person for any reason and without the person forgetting the goal.

If no question with a thinking-target is given, then the deviation to trivialities in relation to the currently prevailing conversation topic is to be assessed.

Example

A person is asked to describe how he came to the examination. He begins to describe initially occurring behavioral problems, but then deviate to explanations of biographical and sociological developmental stages of his youth, later to the problems neighbors have with each other, etc. ◀

Position in psychopathology.
AMDP 17.

Psychopathological interactions.
Disorder of working memory (goal representations and monitoring of intermediate goals), executive disorder (organizing the sequence of thinking and thus the report).

Differential Diagnostic Distinctions:
- manic flight of ideas (the deviation is always intended, the manic person wants to definitely mention this and that as well),
- amnesic—forgetting the thinking goal not only from working memory—but also, when asked what the question was, the person cannot remember.

- comprehension disorder, not understanding what the goal or topic is,
- premorbid existing intellectual performance reduction resulting in difficulty distinguishing important from unimportant,
- premorbid sthenic or easygoing attitude, also telling trivialities (in full detail)—also in obsessive patients,
- habitual: autobiographical, overtrained sequencing of reports in older patients.

Further Characterization.
Person is tempted in the thought process to activate contents that do not belong to goal-directed thinking, or represent trivialities. "Detours in the thought process" without the person having forgotten the goal.

self-/other person's judgment.
Other person's judgment.

Interview for Rating.
Inquiry whether the person still remembers the question. History taken from other persons regarding the premorbid conversational behavior.

Neuropsychology/objectification.
No formal tests, conversational assessment: Characteristic of deviation from the topic of the question .

Severity.
Extent of delay in the course of conversation, especially in biographical interviews, ranging from not disturbing to severe impairment of conversation management.

Pathognomonic for:
Psychiatric brain damage syndromes, frontal lobe symptoms.

Neuroscientific/cognitive neuroscientific models
1. Working Memory impaired
   - the target of thinking is deleted in working memory, or cannot organize the thought process (see below executive disorder).
   - from episodic memory the interviewer's question is retrievable (but in the current thinking, other, "far-fetched" thought contents are central),
   - with errors in monitoring the sections that need to be processed sequentially in thinking and updating what should be considered or presented as the next step.
2. Executive disorder: knowledge of the goal does not lead to the selection of thoughts essential for the goal.
3. attention not focused on the topic.

Thought blocking
Definition. A person suddenly loses the thread in thinking. He feels unable to continue what he was thinking or saying.

A person says his flow of thoughts has broken off. His head suddenly feels empty. It is not caused by a disturbance from the environment.

Example

- A patient thinks of a wish he wants to express and realize, but he needs to coordinate with his environment. Suddenly, he experiences that everything has disappeared from head, he has forgotten the matter, he only knows that he had intended to discuss something important.
- A patient reads a book and immerses herselve in the narrated situation. Suddenly, after reading a few pages, she no longer knows what the book is about and put it aside. ◄

Position in Psychopathology.
AMDP 24.

Psychopathological Interactions.
Thought withdrawal—experience that thoughts are withdrawn from the outside. This can be an interpretation by the person, a projection of the loss of thought onto the (hostile) environment; distracting hallucination, delusional idea, thought control disorder, inhibition.

In severe attention disorder, the arc of suspense cannot be maintained, for example in a conversation.

Differential DiagnosticDistinctions.
Thoughts are forgotten after a distraction in an amnesic disorder. Epileptic event.

Further Characterization.
Repeatedly inexplicable loss of the thread for the patient, which was not triggered by any mental event.

People with schizophrenic psychosis may not be able to retain the development of the situations when reading a novel.

Self-/other persons's judgment.
Self-evaluation, even if interruption of thoughts is observed, can only be judged as blocked if the patient expresses introspection about it.

Interview for Rating.
Inquire about inattention, whether something like this has occurred.

Severity.
Occasional to interview impairment,

Specifications.
Examination for focal neurological signs, signs of epileptic phenomena in the medical history.

Neuroscientific/Cognitive Neuroscientific Models

1. Function of the frontal sustained-activity neurons as carriers of working memory is disrupted in schizophrenia—"mental set" cannot be maintained,
2. Susceptibility of working memory: at the slightest distraction or too long a duration of a segment, the trace of the prevailing thought extinguishes.

Incoherent
Definition. The train of thought shows jumps that are inexplicable by the examiner. The internal coherence of thoughts is reduced. This hinders communication.

Example

The thinking of a patient jumps from one sentence about a subject abruptly to a completely different topic, then after another half-sentence, the thinking jumps again to a remote third area, or the patient does not explain why, in his opinion, the topics are related. ◄

Position in Psychopathology.
AMDP 25.

Related Terms.
Associative loosening, contamination as the mixing of one presented fact with aspects of another, eccentric thinking—as the expression of idiosyncratic, often delusional thought connections that are not explained to the conversation partner. Tangential thinking as a slower drifting away from the target of thinking, derailmentSee also Fig. 10.1.

Psychopathological Interactions.
Disinhibition, pressure of thoughts, clang associations as the cause of a thought jump, autistic lack of consideration for communicative inefficiency as well as disturbance of theory of mind, ego disturbance: thought reading; the patient believes the counterpart knows what he is thinking (he does not have to explain). Thought control disorder.

Differential Diagnostic Distinctions:

- jargonaphasia (semantic jargon), semantic paraphasias,
- uncooperativeness,
- manic thought disorder with acceleration: In this case, the jumps are intended by the person (becomes clear when asked why the topic was changed), for the distinction from manic or schizoaffective symptoms, it is typical for incoherence in schizophrenia: The train of thought jumps without increased drive of thoughts through the abundance of intentions.

- disruption of thought
- logical errors.

Further Characterization:
The jumps can, in individual cases, be related to unusual word usage with understandable association or with incomprehensible association.

The problem that some of the jumps become more understandable for biographical reasons with good knowledge of the patient occurs rarely.

Self-/other persons's judgment.
Other persons's judgment.

Interview for Rating:
Consider the comprensibility of the sequence of verbal expressions—assessment of the flow of thoughts, possibly inquire about wide thought jumps, how the person meant it—characteristic: illogical or unexplained transition from one thought to the next.

Severity.
Occasional unusual jumps to the incomprehensibility of verbal expressions.

Pathognomonic for:
Schizophrenic and schizoaffective psychoses.

Specifications:

- associative loosening: thoughts that do not fit into the train of thought are expressed, which are still comprehensible, distinction from circumstantiality,
- manic associative loosening: communicative, fewer interruptions,
- schizophrenic associative loosening: less communication intention,
- clang associations: The words of the train of thought show clang associations, the patient seems to be guided by clang associations in the continuation of the train of thought. Neuroscientific model concepts: intact phonematic processing with increased drive to think, intact repetition, but disturbed content processing. This can lead to clang associations or to form and express alliterations.
- tangential meaning: Words are used in unusual meanings.

Neuroscientific/cognitive neuroscientific model concepts

a) Incorrect, semantically unrelated or only slightly related association:
   1. Disturbance of the semantic network (Sect. 10.6.6),
   2. associative loosening—disinhibition is expressed in the activation of more distant associations,
      – less contextual effect on the precision of addressing a retrieval,
      – even clang associations become effective in the further development of thoughts (see above),
   3. Theory of mind disturbed, patient cannot imagine that the counterpart does not understand the verbal expression.
b) Disturbance of working memory: a target of thinking is forgotten and therefore other thoughts and communication motives come to the fore.

Incoherent answering
Definition. Deviating from the topic—despite understanding a question, deviating facts/thoughts are given as an answer.

Example

When asked about the reason for the disputes in the family, the patient responds with explanations on a religious topic, without addressing the question. When asked, he says he knows he should explain the reason for the disputes in the family; he insists, that he has answered the question. ◄

Position in psychopathology.
AMDP 23.

Psychopathological interactions.
Pressure of thoughts, incoherence, thought control disorder, not allowing oneself to be thematically restricted in mania.

Differential diagnostic distinctions:
- For the person, there is a connection, but they stubbornly continue their thoughts while the examiner tries to get his questions answered.
- As resistance, in defense and contempt regarding the situation or the examiners.

Further characterization.
Lack of consideration that the patient has not efficiently communicated the chains of associations occurring between question and answer—or assumes that these are known to the conversation partner, e.g. through thought broadcasting.

Self-/other person's judgment.
Other person's judgment.

Interview for rating:
Clarify whether something deviating was intentionally expressed, without regard to the interviewer's question. Clarify whether the person can still state the question; whether he assumes he has answered the question with his statement.

When noticing a question obviously not answered in the course of the conversation, ask and clarify to what extent the examiner's question or the interview situation was understood.

Severity.
Occasionally to the point of making an orderly exploration impossible.

Specifications:
- intended rejecting behavior by not addressing the examiner's questions—relationship to incompliance,
- inability or disinterest in addressing the interviewer's questions—violation of communicative rules,
  a) considering it as a consequence of autism,
  b) consequence of arrogance in megalomania.

Personality influences.
Schizotypal, schizoid, narcissistic, etc.

Conceptual problems of the feature.
Problem of insight towards one's illness and incompliance of schizophrenic patients, resulting in unwillingness and refusal to cooperate in the diagnostic interview. This often leads to the idiosyncratic and non-responsive addressing of topics that do not answer a question. Diagnostically, it is not always clearly distinguishable in some cases. Both variants can also coexist in a patient.

Neuroscientific/cognitive neuroscientific models
After understanding the question, the incoherence in the thought process causes the person to reach a distant association by the time of the response. The target of thinking set by the question cannot be utilized by the person. The person loses the mental context, the conversation goal (or sub-goal)—working memory deficit, relationship to disruption of thought.

Violation of communicative laws—"rule breaking behavior",

Neologisms

Definition. Coinage of new words.

Example

A patient speaks and writes a word "calmlove" (Fig. 10.1), ponders over the word and states that this word and the word "ecstasy" describe his life principles. ◀

Position in psychopathology.
AMDP 26.

Psychopathological interactions:
- disinhibition,
- autism or communicative disinterest,

Differential diagnostic distinctions:
- Aphasiological term, phonematic paraphasias make the word unrecognizable.
- Schizophasia with glossolalia, seemingly playful linguistic creations

Further characterization.
Often as a compound (e.g., Fig. 10.1 Ruhliebe).

Interview for rating.
history taken from other persons, letters, etc.

Specifications:
a) in the context of an aphasic language disorder, b) no aphasia.

Neuroscientific/cognitive neuroscientific models
Combination of effects:

1. attempt to express an unusual experience, but proceeding communicatively inconsiderately, i.e., the patient accepts not being understood,
2. disturbance of theory of mind: person does not know what the counterpart would understand,
3. autistic: inconsiderateness regarding comprehensibility by a social partner.

Rare Features
- Tangentiality: An answer only addresses the topic "tangentially," see incoherent answering.
- Illogicality: Loss of a logical sequence of expressed thoughts, see incoherence. Paralogy
- Overgeneralization: A characteristic of learning in disturbed neuronal networks; applying a rule from one context to another where the rule does not fit.
- Pompous language: see mannerism.
- Poverty of speech: see drive disorder.
- Empty speech: Chap. 9 Language—or in connection with severe incoherence
- Echolalia: Repeating the words of the conversation partner.

References

AMDP-System (2023) Manual zur Dokumentation des psychischen Befundes in Psychiatrie Psychotherapie und Psychosomatik, 11. edn. Hogrefe, Göttingen. Engl. translation: W Guy, TA Ban 2012, Springer Berlin

Benson FD (1994) The Neurology of thinking. Oxford Univ Press, New York

Brown RG, Marsden CD (1988) Internal versus external cues and the control of attention in Parkinson's disease. Brain 111:323–345

Carlsson A (2001) A paradigm shift in brain research. Science 294:1021–1024

Deco G, Rolls ET (2005) Attention, short-term memory, and action selection: a unifying theory. Prog Neurobiol 76:236–256

Fodor JA (1975) The language of thought. Crowell, New York

Fodor JA (1983) The modularity of mind. MIT Press, Cambridge

Fuster J (1990) Inferotemporal units in selective visual attention and short-term memory. J Neurophysiol 64:681–697

Gao WJ, Goldman-Rakic PS (2003) Selective modulation of excitatory and inhibitory microcircuits by dopamine. Proc Natl Acad Sci U S A 100:2836–2841

Gao WJ, Krimer LS, Goldman-Rakic PS (2001) Presynaptic regulation of recurrent excitation by D1 receptors in prefrontal circuits. Proc Natl Acad Sci U S A 98:295–300

Gauggel S, Rieger M, Feghoff TA (2004) Inhibition of ongoing responses in patients with Parkinson's disease. J Neurol Neurosur Psychiatry 75:539–544

Gottlieb J (2002) Parietal mechanisms of target representation. Curr Opin Neurobiol 12:134–140

Hoffman RE (1987) Computer simulations of neural information processing and the schizophrenia-mania dichotomy. Arch Gen Psychiatry 44:178–188

Houk J (2001) Neurophysiology of frontal-subcortical loops. In: Lichter DG, Cummings JL (Eds) Frontal-subcortical circuits in psychiatric and neurological disorders. Guilford Press, New York, pp 92–113

Kircher T, Krug A, Stratmann M, Ghazi S, Schales C, Frauenheim M, Turner L, Fährmann P, Hornig T, Katzev M, Grosvald M, Müller-Isberner P, Nagels A (2014) A rating scale for the assessment of objective and subjective formal Thought and Language Disorder (TALD). Schizophr Res 160:216–221

Kraepelin (1903) Die Erscheinungen des Irreseins. In: Psychiatrie, 7. edn. Barth, Leipzig
Lott PR, Guggenbühl S, Schneeberger A (2002) Linguistic analysis of the speech output of schizophrenic, bipolar, and depressive patients. Psychopathology 35:220–227
LeCun Y, Bengio Y, Hinton G (2015) Deep Learning. Nature 521:436–444
McClelland JL, Rogers TT (2003) The parallel distributed processing approach to semantic cognition. Nat Rev Neurosci 4(4):310–322
McClelland JL, Patterson K (2002) Rules or connections in past-tense inflections: what does the evidence rule out? Trends Cogn Sci 6:465–472
Oberauer K (2005) Control of the contents of working memory—a comparison of two paradigms and two age groups. J Exp Psychol Learn Mem Cogn 31:714–728
Pick A (1931) Aphasie. In: Handbuch der normalen und pathologischen Physiologie, Vol 15. Springer, Berlin, pp 1416–1524
Reischies FM, Mentzel A (2001) Neuropsychological deficits in acute schizophrenic psychosis without neuroleptic medication. Z Neuropsychologie 12:42–48
Reischies FM, Neu P (2000) Comorbidity of mild cognitive disorder and depression—a neuropsychological analysis. Eur Arch Psychiatry Clin Neurosci 250:186–193
Rummelhart DE, McClelland JL (1986) Parallel distributed processing. MIT Press, Cambridge
Sims A (2003) Symptoms in the mind, 3. edn. Saunders—Elsevier, Amsterdam
Singer JL (1993) Experimental studies of ongoing conscious experience. Ciba Found Symp 174:100–116
Spitzer M (1996) Der Geist im Netz. Spektrum, Heidelberg
Subiaul F, Cantlon JF, Holloway RL, Terrace HS (2004) Cognitive imitation in Rhesus macaques. Sience 305:407–410
Ungerleider LG, Mishkin M (1982) Two cortical visual systems. In: Ingle DJ, Goodale MA, Mansfield RJW (Eds) Analysis of visual behaviour. MIT Press, Cambridge
Wernicke C (1906) Grundriss der Psychiatrie in klinischen Vorlesungen, 2. edn. Thieme, Leipzig

Emotion and Affect

11

Contents

11.1 Introduction

Emotions affect a large proportion of psychiatric disorders and are involved in practically all psychopathological symptoms and syndromes. Unfortunately, many of the questions about emotions cannot be answered or are hotly debated; this concerns the various research directions: Research is being conducted in Affective Neuroscience, Psychiatry, Psychology, and also in the Humanities, where the positions represented there seem to be incompatible or far apart.

F. M. Reischies, *Psychopathology*, https://doi.org/10.1007/978-3-662-70293-2_11

This can be clearly demonstrated with anxiety, because some researchers believe that anxiety is always pathological, while others believe that anxiety is part of human existence and therefore normal. One basis for the difference in these positions is that different types of anxiety are assumed. Are there any emotional phenomena that are primarily pathological, i.e., whenever they occur, a psychopathological situation must be assumed? Is it always the quantity, too much or too little of the emotions, that constitutes the disorder, or the situational appropriateness? In other words, is a mild anxiety normal, but a panic attack is not? In addition, there is a fundamental dilemma: We could not be sure whether someone is experiencing a primarily pathological type of emotional sensation. For there is no direct comparison, no alignment with the type of sensation of other people.

Another question that should be posed at the beginning, for example, is: Is the conscious experience of emotions the decisive factor about them, i.e., the experience of emotional mood, or the unconscious effects of emotionality, or could it also be the physical and mental changes associated with them?

What can we reliably assume when we try to explain the disorder of emotions? Emotion psychology has yielded a wealth of insights, and many neurophysiological and psychopharmacological studies have been conducted. Due to the multitude of research approaches and studies, the knowledge, models, and theories about the field of emotions or affects are almost unimaginable.

Within this framework, only the aspects of emotional/affective disorder in mental illnesses are described. Some distinctions, general aspects of the psychopathology of emotion, and classifications of the field of affective disorders are important for the psychopathology of emotions, so they are presented at the beginning:

1. Emotion, mood, and affect,
2. Which sensations are regarded as emotions?
3. Subjective and objective aspects of emotions,
4. Psychopathological factors as opposed to normal emotionality,
5. Triggering, experience, and expression,
6. Affect control,
7. Primary, secondary, and instrumental emotions or affects,
8. Position in psychopathology,
9. Incompleteness of evidence.

11.1.1 Emotion, Mood, Affect, and Valence

Emotions we consider as a distinct class of sensations that we apparently share with higher developed animals. Emotional phenomena described in psychopathology can be distinguished into 1) an emotion as a single sensation, 2) a mood, an emotional state that lasts longer, and 3) an affect, which is characterized as a usually shorter and more intense emotional expression. Another phenomenon 4), which has recently come to the forefront again, is the sense of valence. It seems to be a basic sensation in the dimension of positive versus negative, which is generally widespread in the animal kingdom. The effort of the Research Domain Criteria (RDoC) initiative, for example, has defined positive and negative valence as one of the fundamental domains. This has stimulated neuroscientific research (Morris et al. 2022).

Affects are usually recognizable to observers; they are shown in behavior or in vegetative signs, such as blushing, etc. A person gets into a rage and is informed of this by other people, for example: "don't get so worked up!"—while the person had not consciously registered this circumstance. Emotions, moods, and affects can thus occur consciously and unconsciously. A person can describe an emotion and mood, but these will not necessarily be noticed by other people—except perhaps by very close and familiar persons and partners, who can more reliably infer a slight change in mood from the reaction. The mood can, for example, also be masked: The person wants to present a certain affective state outwardly, regardless of the actual mood.

Quantitative Aspects

The intensity of experiencing an emotion can constitute the disorder: In a disorder in quantitative terms, the strength of the emotion or affect exceeds the normal/healthy range—examples are extreme aggression or grief. It is important that the emotion initially represents a physiological phenomenon, not a pathological one. Only the intensity is too high compared to the norm. But what is the norm of emotional experience (Reischies 1990)? This is a question that cannot be answered precisely in principle.

In addition to abnormally strong emotions, there are also abnormally strong affects, which lead to wrong actions. This belongs to the area of affect control or the regulation of emotions. In this area, there are some disorders such as the too easy triggering of emotions in affect lability.

Furthermore, it should be emphasized that psychopathology usually deals with strongly pronounced psychological phenomena—not with minor, but possibly subjectively important emotional disorders.

Qualitative Aspects

Furthermore, the emotion could lie outside the spectrum of "normal" emotional diversity in qualitative terms. But a qualitative disorder of the sensation of emotions is again not easy to determine. How could one, for example, prove that one person feels anxiety differently than another person? Patients suffering from psychoses sometimes describe incomprehensible affects or moods. An abnormality in affect expression can be observed by the examiner in the example of parathymia (see below), where the patient expresses a mood that does not match his situation and what he verbally expresses. However, it cannot be said with certainty how abnormal the patient's emotional experience is.

11.1.2 Which Sensations Are Counted Among Emotions

A long and unproductive debate about the canon of emotions is ongoing, specifically about the question of which emotional phenomena should be considered as 1.) a basic emotion or as 2.) a complex emotional phenomenon subsumed under another or 3.) not as an emotion, but as a vegetative sensation. For example, how should disgust be evaluated, how should positive self-awareness be classified? Is positive self-awareness a fundamental emotion? Or should it simply be counted as part of positive emotionality, belonging to positive valence? Does it manifest in variants of pride? Positive self-awareness is related to narcissism as a personality trait. This debate is not addressed here. The presentation is oriented towards psychopathological disorders in the area of important or basic emotions, on which most researchers can agree (see below).

In principle, we do not include primary sensory sensations, such as those of brightness, in the spectrum of feelings, nor those of color, although there are already close relationships to emotions here, or smells, where even closer emotional relations are known. Furthermore, vegetative sensations such as appetite are excluded. We also do not count physical sensations such as freezing, shortness of breath, or pain as emotions. Pain often is at the center of somatization disorders and thus must be considered psychiatrically. It determines an important part of the sensations that belong to the negative area of valence.

The canon of central, psychopathologically relevant emotions includes anxiety, aggression, joy and sadness/depressed feeling. Surprise and disgust are added; they are certainly characterized as unmistakable emotions both facially and subjectively, but many consider them too short-lived and simple to be counted among the most important emotions. Psychopathologically, these two emotions also play a subordinate role. The feeling of attachment is considered by many researchers to be a fundamental emotion. The list also includes the feeling of interest, the desire for approaching someone or curiosity, which have been discussed in connection with drive and motivation.

Three of the four above-mentioned psychopathologically fundamental emotions are further subdivided and differentiated, e.g., 1.) anxiety into concrete fear and diffuse anxiety, 2.) aggression into rivaling aggression and predatory behavior, 3.) joy into pride, pleasure, gratification, etc.

According to some authors, more sensations are to be counted among the basic emotions: happiness, anger, contempt, satisfaction, embarrassment, excitement, fear, guilt, pride, relief, sadness, gratification, sensory pleasure and shame (Ekman 1999). Another aspect must be considered here. Some emotions are referred to as complex emotional sensations. Some researchers count guilt and shame among them. In addition to the basic or fundamental emotions, there are more complex emotional phenomena, such as romantic feelings, being in love, complacency, etc.

The basic or fundamental emotions are consistently identified on various levels:

1. through comparative studies in the animal world, phylogenetically,
2. through behavioral research studies in animals,
3. through psychological and introspective studies, and
4. based on linguistic analyses.

In his foundation of experimental psychology (Wundt 1874), Wundt proposed a basic, more elementary classification: that of positive and negative feelings. Accordingly, some researchers summarize happiness/joy, satisfaction, pride, relief, and gratification as positive emotionality. This classification is based on valence, an accompanying positive or negative sensation. Wundt suggested that we must assume a valence sensation occurring parallel to perceptions and emotions.

However, the valence classification seems too simple, as physiological systems for aggression, anxiety, and sadness can be delineated, thus justifying a sub-differentiation of negative emotionality.

The delineation of sexual emotionality is difficult and unsatisfactory. Here, sexual sensations are to be excluded as vegetative sensations, although psychopathological symptoms can be observed in this area.

11.1.3 Subjective and Objective Aspects of Emotions

Moods are predominantly subjective, affects are more objective, i.e., they usually have effects on behavior. The subjective side of emotions, the emotional experience, is contrasted with the objective side, the expression of emotions and the communicated emotion. Language has the dual aspect of 1. the prosody of speech melody, which expresses emotion, and 2. the content, in which emotional experience is conveyed. Additionally, language is also the vehicle through which speech acts are expressed in a behaviorally relevant manner.

How can we, apart from our own experience, know that the subjective quality of emotions exists?

The construct of emotion is recognized due to 1.) subjective evidence, 2.) evolutionary data, 3.) objective behaviors (e.g., facial expressions), 4.) action relevance (emotion as action readiness, prediction of actions facilitated by emotion), 5.) cognitive, 6.) intersubjective evidence, etc.

Neurophysiologically, very different mechanisms are involved that together constitute an emotion (Sect. 11.4 Neuroscience).

1. Let's start with the basic mechanisms: On the one hand, the Emotional-Motor-system (Holstege et al. 1996) has been characterized, which in the brainstem contributes motor schemas for the expression of emotion in behavior, especially in facial expressions, gestures, and prosody.
2. The physiological mechanisms of emotion also consist of more or less specific subcortical functional centers (Affective Neuroscience, Panksepp 1998). They are triggered when the conditons for that emotion are met. They activate the Emotional-Motor-system and vegetative accompaniments of emotion.

3 Finally, cortical mechanisms must be discussed: They serve various functions; the question is to what extent they are involved in emotional processes. Certainly, there are cortical emotional functions in the control of affect expression and in conscious experience (especially in the linguistic expression of emotion). Cognitive processing is essential for the triggering of emotions in everyday life—for example, emotions that arise in conversations or when reading poems. There are semantic triggers of emotions that are certainly processed cortically.

The 3 levels together determine the emotional symptoms of mental illnesses. However, many details are still unknown, i.e., which influences become effective in which symptoms (Fig. 11.1).

11.1.4 Psychopathological Factors in Contrast to Normal Emotionality

The psychopathology of emotional phenomena must be distinguished from the emotion psychology of so-called "normal" functional variance. The knowledge about the normal triggering and control of emotions is indeed important, but not sufficient to explain pathological phenomena. Even in mentally ill individuals, healthy physiological influences can manifest, which are then attributed to the "healthy parts" of the mentally ill person. However, in the case of emotional psychopathological features, qualitatively different factors must also be considered compared to the explanation of everyday emotional phenomena. The research task is to identify the neuronal mechanisms for this—in

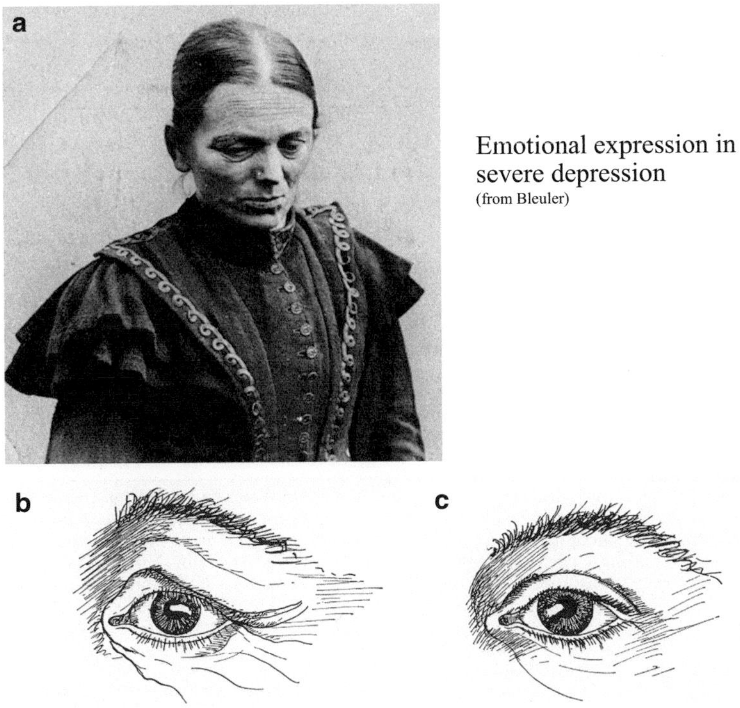

Fig. 11.1 Examples of psychomotor symptoms in depression (Bleuler 1979). **a** The head and gaze are continuously lowered, the shoulders and extremities hang with low tone; the handshake is limp, **b** Veraguth's fold of the upper eyelid in depression, **c** normal upper eyelid fold

the hope of better therapy. The neurophysiology of emotion is still in its early stages, but it has already been able to describe brain function systems on electrophysiological, imaging, and biochemical levels that are essential for certain emotions.

The psychopathologically central emotions mentioned above represent characteristic complexes from the areas of:

1. experience,
2. vegetative effects,
3. emotional expressions,
4. specific action readiness, and
5. cognition/thought content/language.

The psychopathologically central emotions can also be assessed in terms of their consistency (see below. "Mini-Syndromes"). This has far-reaching consequences: If a person says he is suffering from grief, then in psychopathological diagnostics, we expect consistent signs of this emotion on all these levels and then assess whether and to what extent the person is suffering from grief.

11.1.5 Triggering, Experience, and Expression

In an emotion, a distinction can initially be made between 1.) the triggering with triggering conditions and mechanisms, 2.) the experience, and 3.) the expression in motor skills, cognition as well as 4.) vegetative somatic phenomena.

Triggering of Emotions

Regarding the triggering of emotions, there are significant differences in the fundamental theoretical positions: The arousal-cognition explanation of emotion and the nativist position (see below).

In cognitivist emotion psychology, two aspects are emphasized:

a) agitation-arousal and
b) cognitive determination of which emotion is experienced.

Excitation-arousal

The excitation provokes an emotional reaction: A sequence is described: 1. Situational trigger—2. excitation—3. cognitive analysis—4. quality of the emotion.

Even though models of the arousal-cognition explanation of emotions can claim some experimental evidence, the evolutionarily developed diversity of specific emotions and many other aspects of emotions cannot be explained by it. Another objection relates to the sequence of events in emotion triggering: Naturally, during the development of emotions, there is usually an excitation and unfocused increase in attention in the sense of arousal. But it is not necessarily required. Everyone knows emotional mood states that are not initiated by arousal.

A milder form of alexithymia, the inability to consciously experience emotions, applies to many emotional phenomena—that is, people notice the arousal but cannot express the emotional quality at least linguistically.

Cognitive Information Processing for Emotion Triggering

A cognitive emotion model was presented that includes a cascade of cognitive decisions relevant to the triggering of emotions, such as novelty, danger, etc. (Scherer 2003, 2004). The following sequence is considered: trigger—cognitive analysis—triggering condition for a specific emotion—arousal and specific components of affect are triggered simultaneously. These models can be guidelines for researching emotion triggering. But for emotion triggering, as shown for anxiety (LeDoux 1996), there could be two pathways, a phylogenetically primitive pathway and a pathway of more complex cognitive processing in the cortex.

Nativist position

The nativist position stands in contrast to cognitive and arousal theories: It assumes fundamental emotions that have evolved evolutionarily and are therefore innate. We apparently share most emotions with higher developed animals. These archaic fundamental emotions correspond to various physiological mechanisms, each with specific triggering conditions. These can be differently controlled for each emotion.

As an example of the elaboration of triggering conditions, aggression should be used ("Disengaging in moral agency", Bandura 1999). In individuals who carried out aggressive actions, a sequence of development was described as characteristic:

1. A purpose of action is rationalized, religiously or otherwise motivated.
2. The consequences of the action are trivialized.
3. The victims of the action are dehumanized, declared as worthless people or animals.
4. Responsibility is seemingly taken away from the individual in a diffuse decision structure, the decision is anonymized.
5. Decision and immoral action are separated spatially/temporally.

These factors play a role in the political and criminal variant of aggressive actions. They describe the neutralization of aggression control. Psychopathologically, we are interested in the disruptibility of aggression control. In frontotemporal dementias, this aggression control is weakened, which can lead to uninhibited aggressive behaviors (see below). Even in Alzheimer dementia, impulsive aggressive actions can occur. These apparently proceed without the above-mentioned sequences of neutralizing aggression control.

Experience and Expression—Emotional Mini-Syndrome

Emotions and affects become apparent in several dimensions: One can speak of mini-syndromes (where the term "syndrome" is transferred from disorder-specific symptom complexes to emotion or affect): Affect as

a) emotional sensation, both conscious and unconscious (but accessible to attention)
b) cognitive processes (thought contents, ways of thinking, automatic thoughts, possibly also dysfunctional "cognitions"),
c) emotional-motor action readiness, i.e., a state of pre-activation of certain behaviors (Frijda 1986),
d) vegetative somatic characteristics.

According to Frijda, affects are related to specific action readiness. They could thus be evolutionarily justifiable in the sense that they are primitive switches for groups of action schemes already observed in animals. Emotions thus trigger an affect and secondly a cognitive attitude that leads to certain ways of thinking and above all to action readiness.

Some of the emotions frequently occur in the anticipation of events (Fig. 11.2), anxiety before an imminent harmful event, or anticipation of an imminent reward. Other emotions are more to be understood as emotional reactions to events that have occurred. It is clear that cognitive information processing must be different for these types of emotions.

The concept of an emotion mini-syndrome helps in psychopathological diagnosis. Because the question of what constitutes the primary feature of the emotion, the cognition, the subjective

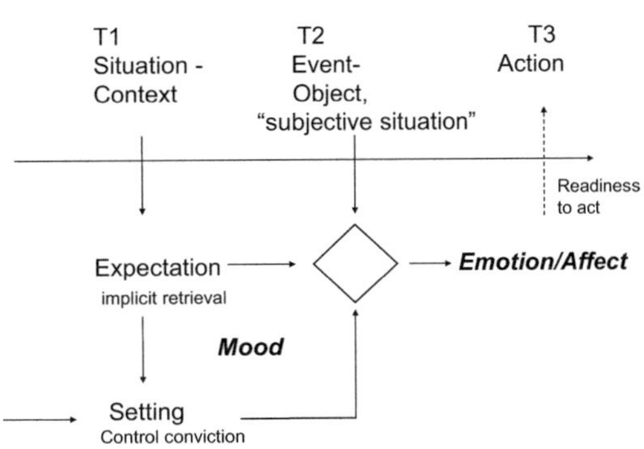

Fig. 11.2 Triggering of emotions/affects and moods: An initial situation (T1) includes an expectation of the future situation (T2), for example, an expectation of reward, which positively affects the basic mood—in terms of positive valence. The person contrasts the next expected event with attitudes, prejudices, memories, and control beliefs. An emotional reaction can arise after the occurrence of the next event as a result of emotional evaluation—for example, anxious tension or disappointment. Emotions can also occur before the event, for example, as anticipatory anxiety. The emotional reaction is closely linked to a corresponding action expectation (e.g., T3, joyful behavior, flight, or attack)

experience, the action readiness, or the arousal, may be irrelevant when considering the mini-syndrome of the emotion: Only the totality of these features constitutes the fundamental emotion.

Affect control

How passive is the person who gets into an emotion? Are people passive experiencing emotions and affects? There are a number of studies that describe the active role of cognitive attitude, the type of cognitive processing. In addition, there is the question of to what extent the emotion-triggering experience was actually sought out, the experience of an affect was even provoked. These levels of emotionality are a field of forensic assessment and psychotherapeutic treatment of emotional disorders.

Especially in the area of aggression, affect control is to be illustrated (see above). The control of aggressiveness usually does not stand out in the everyday life of a healthy person, seems to play a subordinate role. However, it is important in personality development, which cannot be described here. In the case of a disorder of control functions—e.g. after brain injuries—its absence becomes apparent. Then, for example, aggressive impulsivity occurs.

Affects can increase in intensity, so that the learned affect control fails. This can be observed in mania. The control of affects gains importance in psychopathology when the triggering conditions of emotions change, for example, when emotions are triggered more easily. Especially then, it is critical to what extent the person can control the affects.

In a situation where an emotion is triggered, it is decided whether the expression of an affect is given free rein or whether it is suppressed (like yawning at an evening party). Affect control is learned during childhood and adolescence and is part of a person's upbringing. The mechanisms of this development can be disturbed or lost in brain diseases. An overview of the model can be found in Fig. 11.3.

Primary, secondary, and instrumental emotions or affects

Another clinically helpful subdivision of emotional phenomena should be briefly mentioned here:

a) Primary affects are immediately triggered, e.g. anxiety in front of a fighting dog or joy over a win. They are triggered by an event or the information about an imminent event.
b) Secondary affects are emotional attitudes towards changes or reactions of the person, for example, the "fear of the fear", i.e. a person knows he will develop anxiety, which he is afraid of.
c) Instrumental emotions are used to achieve a purpose. They can be used manipulatively. For example, a person indulges in depression, tenderness, or aggression to achieve something from a partner. Affect control plays an outstanding role in this.

The psychopathology of emotions considers not only primary emotions but also secondary and especially instrumental emotions and affects. Indications of instrumental emotions can arise in the course of treatment, whereby, for example, the examiner or therapist becomes the target. Therefore, the analysis of emotion in each case should also be aimed at distinguishing primary from secondary and instrumental emotions.

11.1.6 Position in Psychopathology

Emotional disorders are central in psychiatry. Some researchers believe that psychiatric illnesses in general arise when emotionality is disturbed, i.e., emotions are diminished or become too strong (Panksepp 1998). Although this is not true for dementia, even in the purely cognitive domain of psychopathology, for example in the area of delusions and obsessive thoughts, emotional factors are often decisive. Delusion is not an emotional symptom but is classified as a

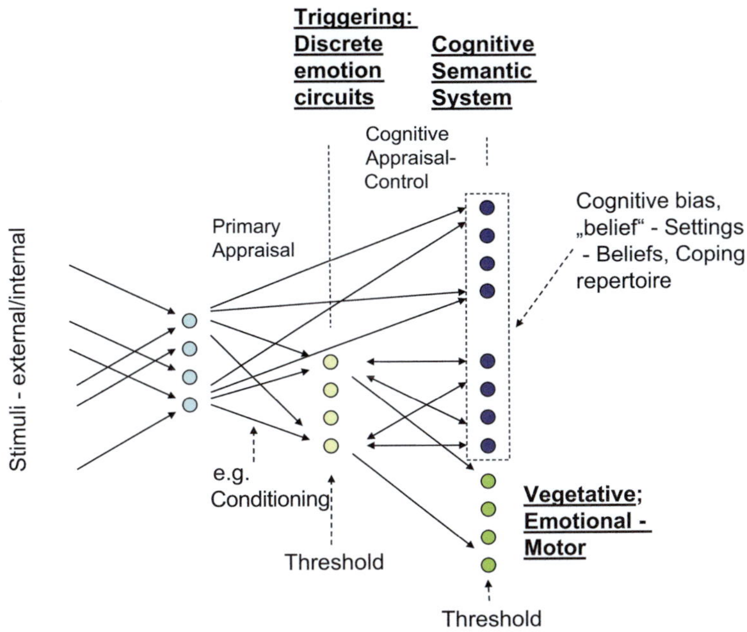

Fig. 11.3 Emotional information processing in the brain. External or internal stimuli are 1. primarily evaluated, for example, as an object of fear (primary appraisal). This leads to involuntary activation of the emotional systems for anxiety, aggression, joy, etc. ("discrete emotional circuits"). These can be conditioned. 2. Furthermore, a complex cognitive-emotional information processing occurs as "cognitive appraisal", which includes attitudes, control beliefs, etc. This neuronal network processing can also activate the "discrete emotional circuits", for example, when a condition for a specific emotional evaluation, such as an insult, is met. On the other hand, "cognitive appraisal" can also contribute to the control of the emotional reaction. 3. The expression of emotional activation is largely automated, controlled by the emotional motor system of the brainstem. Metabolic processes can change the synaptic connections between groups of neurons and especially the thresholds of activation of emotional reactions.

content-related thought disorder. Nevertheless, characteristic emotions usually accompany the various delusional contents, such as grandiosity, persecution, or guilt delusions. Another example is drive disorders. Interest is central as an emotional characteristic for drive disorders. In many areas of psychopathology, emotional symptoms play a role, whether as a main feature of a syndrome, as an individual symptom, or as an accompanying characteristic of psychopathological symptoms.

Even though it is undoubtedly true that emotions are neurally controlled, it is not argued that a disturbance of emotionality is a neurological disorder, but rather that certain functional systems in the brain are assigned to mental disorders—the "psychiatric brain".

11.1.7 Emotional Experience—An Epiphenomenon?

Against the significance of emotions, some theorists argue that moods represent epiphenomena, archaic functional systems that evolved early and have lost their significance. The subjective quality of emotions is not significant; only the behavior, which the subjective quality of emotions rarely affects, is decisive. Only the behavior of a person in the environment is important for mental illnesses. Is emotion an epiphenomenon of a person's behaviors? Pathological laughter or crying can clearly illustrate the separation of emotional behavior and emotional experience. A patient suddenly cries and reports after the state subsides that the crying came automatically, and he was not sad at all. The question, therefore, is whether the emotional quality of experience of emotions or only the physiological and behavioral reactions constitute the pathological characteristic of psychiatric disorders.

In contrast, examples of the crucial importance of emotional experience for psychopathological symptoms can be cited: An anxiety patient subjectively experiences a situation completely differently than another person. This is significant not only when he avoids similar anxiety-inducing situations in the future. Another example is addiction. Because of the pleasant feeling, the substance is taken again, even though the person knows that the addictive behavior will have negative consequences. Additionally, the experience of suffering in severe depression can lead to suicidal actions (Reischies 2021).

11.1.8 Incompleteness of Clinical Evidence

Problems arise in the diagnosis of emotional disorders. An adequate assessment of a person's emotionality is time-consuming. It requires an overall assessment of the person, the personality, and the social situation of the person. Emotional experience in pain and the ambivalence phase of the suicidal person are examples of the complexity of this field.

Emotional symptoms of mental disorders are clinically often not sufficiently examined. This does not apply to affects; they include behaviors that are observable by the environment. They are usually adequately described. However, milder emotional sensations and moods can remain entirely within the patient's experience, purely subjective. They do not have to be expressed, not even admitted when someone asks about them. Additionally, there are emotional states that the affected person is not even aware of.

We must acknowledge that the psychopathological findings cannot be fully and objectively examined; parts are fundamentally inaccessible to the examiner. On the one hand, psychoanalytic models of the unconscious should be mentioned. In clinical everyday life, this problem becomes evident, for example, in the signs of depression and anxiety in retirement requests. Furthermore, many patients cannot communicate the emotional experience—due to psychopathological reasons such as stupor, mutism, uncooperativeness towards one's illness, or due to general resistance phenomena in the area of interpersonal interaction with the examiners; they do not express the moods they suffer from, or do not express them adequately, more or less consciously.

Thus, the dilemma remains that the differentiated psychopathological examination of emotion is a core piece of psychopathology but often remains inaccessible to complete and objective examination. Among other reasons, this has led to the hope that finer methods to investigate the brain might possibly find objective correlates for moods and emotional sensations.

11.2 Clinic

11.2.1 Disorder of Emotions, Affects

In psychopathology, disturbances in the experience of emotions, the manner of triggering emotions, the expression of emotions and affects, and affect control are primarily considered:

a) Disturbance in the experience of emotions:
   - too few emotions are experienced: e.g., deficits in the triggering mechanisms—the perception of triggers or cognitive evaluation processes. It is also necessary to distinguish whether an emotion in the appropriate situations is not perceived, not allowed, not expressed, or can only not be verbally described.
   - too strong, e.g., emotional reaction exaggerated in experience, etc.—this is considered in terms of situational triggers and can naturally also manifest at the level of expression and action consequences,

- altered or not belonging to the normal kind of experience.

b) Triggering:
- too rapid triggering of affects,
- abnormally low response, in relation to the triggering situation; examples are on the one hand abnormally low emotional response or on the other hand absence of emotional reaction in situations that regularly bring other people into certain emotions (e.g., disturbed triggering mechanisms).

c) Expression:
- too little,
- too strong affect expression in terms of firstly intensity, secondly duration,
- specific pathological form of expression is socially unacceptable.

d) Cognitive aspects:
- excessively fixed content coupling to types of situations, semantic contents, etc. In this sense, affective-cognitive complexes should be considered (see below), for example, in phobias coupling to specific situations,
- dysfunctional cognitions, beliefs, and action-relevant thoughts. These dysfunctional cognitions, which are particularly considered in behavioral therapy, lie on the border between emotional phenomena and thought disorders.

e) Affect control:
- reduced affect control, affects that can normally be suppressed are expressed, such as anger. This involves on the one hand pathological impulsivity or inhibition mechanisms in the affective domain, on the other hand, for example, "letting oneself go,"
- suppression of emotions. The suppression of, for example, excessive emotions and affects may bind psychic energy with negative consequences for personality development.

f) Disturbances of the vegetative components of affects:
- exaggerated vegetative reactions, such as blushing, fainting, etc. These disturbances are particularly considered in psychosomatics .

These dimensions of disturbance can each apply globally, i.e., for all emotions, or be limited to one emotion, e.g., these dimensions may be disturbed only in terms of aggression, but not in a sad mood.

Emotional Exceptional States

In addition to psychopathological mood states, which can also be very mild, some emotional-affective exceptional states are described, which are usually accompanied by intense affect expression:

a) anxiety:
- Anxiety attack, panic.

b) Aggression:
- Rage, state of excitement with aggressive emotional tone—in contrast to agitation, where arousal is in the foreground and anxious emotional tone can also predominate.

c) negative affectivity, "desperate", self-insecure, depressive:
- acute withdrawal, emotional stupor
- Suicidal escalation with self-devaluation, leading to self-injurious actions (presuicidal syndrome).

Aggressive Misconduct

In the psychiatric clinic, misconduct with the danger of bodily harm to fellow patients and nursing staff unfortunately represents a continuous problem. This is especially true when a sudden attack occurs from a previously calm delusional or demented person. This happens suddenly, for example, due to hallucinations or delusional ideas, or it cannot be clarified in detail. The question is important whether the misconduct occurs with the experience of aggression, in an aggressive mood. If a patient carries out an mission within the framework of his delusional system, at least an aggressive mood or even anger might have been absent. This can also apply to a demented person with an impulse to hit.

Attempts have been made to use the term aggressive action as an umbrella term for these behaviors and to separate the emotional experiences that can underlie or accompany the outbreak of aggression from it. The distinction between on the one hand predatory behavior and on the other hand aggressive experience in rivalry has already been addressed. According to all findings of behavioral research, the lion will not feel aggression when killing a prey animal, a lamb (see e.g. Panksepp 1998).

Frustration arises in situations where a goal is not achieved. Then aggressive actions can occur. But the aggressive enforcement of goals itself does not necessarily happen with anger. Manic patients are partly irritable. They argue about everything and threaten. Here, a clear distinction must be made between rather playful striving and enforcement behavior on the one hand and on the other hand disinhibited anger.

Anger and frustration are rather emotions that are commonly referred to as "aggressive". A person can react angrily aggressive to a deprivation of liberty, for example, when being restrained. Loss of autonomy triggers anger, rage, and reflexive liberation actions. Anger over an insult can lead to aggressive revenge actions, to "revenge campaigns". Rejection, without a defeat in a rival combat having occurred, is accompanied by anger and rage.

Anger and rage manifest themselves in the daily routine of the psychiatric clinic often in a much more subtle way. Thus, splitting attempts between patients and the team, slander, intrigues, open insults, and rejections must be noted.

Hatred, in turn, as a long-term attitude and disposition assigned to someone, holds a special position. It is an affective-cognitive coupling, comparable to the coupling of anxiety to an object in phobia. Psychopathologically, hatred becomes important especially in delusion with its cognitive distortions. In many cases of fanaticism, at least overvalued ideas can be found (Chap. 13 Delusion—content-related thought disorders). However, fanaticism as a phenomenon does not yet seem to be sufficiently investigated.

Conclusion
Psychopathologically, it must be differentiated in the area of aggressive behaviors what can be attributed to behavioral patterns and what can be referred to as anger and rage among the accompanying emotional experience.

11.3 Diagnostics

The investigation and assessment of disturbances in the emotional, affective domain place the highest demands on the examiner. Reasons for this are:

a) that there is no possibility of comparison, no "gold standard," i.e., it is usually impossible to compare with what is "normal."
b) The situational context, which must be taken into account, requires extensive anamnesis efforts—it must be clarified: Is a mood disturbance, for example, a reaction to familial or professional conflicts, to the current psychiatric imagination itself, or to a pathological level of emotional reactivity?
c) The current emotional interaction with the examiner, for example, in the admission situation, is important in observing the mood: What role does the establishment of a therapeutic relationship with the examiner play, does it succeed, or are there resistances?

Problems with the Communication of Individual Normal and Pathological Emotions
Diagnostic problems persist due to the incomparability of emotions between people. Doubts about the adequate communicability of emotions through language are justified, as the words for experienced emotions may be idiosyncratic, i.e.,

a patient may understand "anxiety" differently than the examiner.

The reason for this is that words for emotional experience cannot be matched by pointing to something as with objects, e.g., "I understand by 'xyz' this…". In this language-game, terms can be clarified by referring to something concrete. However, this does not succeed for the quality of emotional experience.

If it is already difficult to communicate, for example, what a person feels with a specific color, it is impossible to comprehend the experienced quality for colorblind individuals. Therefore, it is never certain which qualities known to the examiner are meant by a person or even something foreign to him, which he could never experience (like the color perception of a colorblind person). In this context, not all problems of everyday psychological description of psychopathological facts and the critical discussions in the philosophy of mind can be presented.

Even if there are fundamental problems with language communication about emotional experience, the clarifiable communication barriers should be removed.

▶ The question in psychopathological examinations is always: Has the examiner adequately understood the patient's emotional situation? What did the patient mean? What is the appropriate description of the patient's subjective and objective emotional status?

Several factors play a role in this:

- emotional experience of the examiner,
- empathic quality.
- The interview on emotionality should exhibit some special qualities:
- The interview should work with open questions,
- if a suggestion for description is made, such as "is it something like anxiety?", then it must be asked later in summary whether it was meant as the examiner understands it. Otherwise, there is a danger that the examiner asks suggestively.

Problem of Assessing the Appropriateness of an Emotional Reaction

Emotional reactions can not always be empatheticly understood; there are limits to empathy. For instance, mothers and, to some extent, fathers will confirm that the intense emotions triggered by their own baby were surprising. They could not have predicted these feelings. Similarly, it can be expected that a person who does not know such emotions cannot diagnostically assess their appropriateness. In a certain sense, this also applies to being in love, which is unimaginable for prepubescent young people. How is it with aggression: Even in antiquity, an aggressive state was described as a state of "temporary madness."

Are depressive patients more realistic in their pessimistic assessments of future developments? This has been investigated in psychological studies (Haaga and Beck 1995; Hancock 1996). In psychopathology, the question must be of interest whether there is a systematic misjudgment in normal cases, a positive emotional tone that ensures situations are not seen as frightening, the future is seen as rosy, etc.

The question of how the positive emotional tone arises is unresolved. Undoubtedly, the effect is evolutionarily advantageous. One could think of an innate mechanism. Alternatively or complementarily, a developmental mechanism must be considered. The child particularly experiences full positive feedback from the parents when it beams, laughs, and tries everything without hesitation.

In addition to the systematic slight predominance of positive emotionality, which includes the satisfaction with one's own situation expressed in all surveys, there are some non-emotional components: The neglect of information, experiences, and knowledge that could cloud the picture. Emotions have an important property in directing attention to an object, be it the beloved person, the discovery of a feared animal, or, for example, a feared symptom of the body. This circumstance of influencing attention, cognitive processing, and rational judgment by emotions is further addressed in the section on content-related thought disorders.

The positive emotional bias, i.e., a positive "bias" that produces a positive memory, a positive self-image, a positive outlook on the future, etc., is particularly important in psychopathology because the underlying mechanism can also be disturbed. In depression, this seems to be the case.

Review of Emotional Symptoms in the Interview or Examination Situation
If emotional psychopathological features might be present, each feature should be checked:

a) how it is described verbally, especially the subjectively conscious side of the feature,
b) how the expressive behavior is (observation in the interview, on the ward, or also from reports of relatives),
   - how intense the disorder is described: unusual, strongly pronounced, normal variant,
   - duration unusually long-lasting,
   - reduced affective/emotional action readiness,
   - affective overall situation: mutual inhibition of affects.

Are individual affects disturbed, or is it a far-reaching change in emotionality? For this, the consistency with the emotion concept as an "emotional mini-syndrome" is examined:

- cognitive: what the person thinks during the emotion,
- action preparation: what they are preparing for, what they are set on,
- vegetative somatic features,
- motor signs: e.g., trembling, restless pacing, etc.

In the expectation of events: In what mood is the person 1) e.g., anxious, depressed, joyful, 2) to what extent situation-related 3) triggering of emotion: situational condition of triggering inappropriate, 4) threshold too low/high.

The consistency of the communicated and expressed emotion with the behavioral observation must be present (consistency of the findings). This is important for possible doubts regarding statements about emotions, for example, when there is suspicion of aggravation, if a retirement request becomes apparent; in case of suspicion of simulation or manipulative behavior.

Further Objectification.
Behavioral observation and observation of the thought process in dealing with, for example, triggers, threatening situations, or matters to which an emotional reaction was shown. It should be clarified with the patient by offering alternative perspectives to what extent the symptom is meant by the patient as initially expressed.

Aspects of establishing a relationship in the examination/therapy situation
An important aspect is the examination situation itself. For psychopathological diagnostics in general, but especially for the diagnostics of emotional symptoms, securing the relationship between the examining and the affected person is of utmost importance.

If the affected person transfers emotions to the examining person

- Expectations, feelings of attraction
- histrionic contact initiation, unauthentic, seeming fake
- Shyness, emotional reluctance to show emotions in front of strangers (cultural, religious attitudes),
- help seeking behaviour,
- Manipulation (even unconsciously), emotional behavior with "emotional act" character, e.g., tears are provoked, an outburst of aggression is staged,
- Consistency

Here, the specific psychodynamic positions cannot be addressed, for example, that an emotion could already indicate a defense formation in a conflict or the projective identification with the unconscious attempt to achieve a certain emotion and reaction from the examining person.

Affect control
In the case of affect disorders, there is often, especially in mental illnesses, an inadequacy of behavior, in which an affect-control disorder can become apparent. The extent can be assessed, for example, by the degree of inadequacy of behavior.

How pronounced are affective-cognitive complexes (e.g., coupling of phobic anxiety to a specific situation, such as riding in an elevator), with what intensity is there an emotional reaction.

The affect control is often only adequately assessed in the history taken from other persons, for example, from relatives: Previous affect control, learning history (e.g., compensation efforts), changes, critical situations, triggers, extreme situations, etc.

Situational Control:

- Is the affective reaction in the triggering situation still controllable
- Is the control of future triggering situations successful—avoidance
- Reaction of the person to the affect outburst:
- Shame, etc.,
- Attempt at reparation, undoing.
- Disturbance of emotionality at the level of consciousness:
- Reduction or increase of attention to emotions or triggers (e.g., control of attention in spider phobia)

Due to social competence and early childhood learning of emotional matters, psychiatric examiners usually implicitly consider the above-mentioned diagnostic features during the interview process. An explicit appreciation of the above diagnostic features is necessary for problematic cases and difficult differential diagnoses.

Here, a delicate circumstance must be addressed. There is a dependency of clinical psychopathology on the characteristics of the examiner. If the examiner has emotional or personality-related impairments, the emotional psychopathological assessment can be distorted. It is the task of every examining person to know their personal psychological peculiarities. This must be taken seriously in training.

11.3.1 Reaction of the Person to the Experience of the Emotion

Psychopathologically important is the reaction of the person to a panic attack, to an outburst of anger. This is not the place to describe reaction forms, especially defense, avoidance, or personality traits as well as the genesis of personality in the experience of emotions (see textbooks of psychotherapy). Inhibition of aggression and avoidance of anxiety as well as the cognitive maneuvers of the person for the defense of anxiety and hurt underlie many psychopathological features and clinical pictures. In particular, the effort of control, correction, and compensation or overcompensation of the self-experienced emotional problems again leads to psychic symptoms.

In the diagnosis of the coping repertoire, the defense mechanisms, and more generally the personality traits, the handling of emotionality takes a central place. Psychiatric diagnostics address the experience of a person with their anxiety, their pride, a strong fear of shame and grief, frustration and anger, rage, and attempts are made with the patient to trace their adaptation to individual emotionality. How much avoidance of anxiety and hurt plays a role in the person's behavior? How are self-confidence and satisfaction with oneself maintained? What beliefs and cognitive constructs emerge in the process? How does the person try to cope with losses anticipatorily? How does the person avoid openly aggressive behaviors and how do they defend against overwhelming anger and daily annoyance?

11.4 Neuroscience

11.4.1 Introduction

Emotions cannot yet be sufficiently explained neuroscientifically in all facets of their appearance, this applies especially to the conscious experience of emotion. There are a number of fiercely contested positions. Many researchers consider their approach as the only valid one. The neuroscientific explanations depend on the emotion model: Are emotions physiological processes and their more or less conscious experience; or are emotions ways of perception, adaptive dispositions towards situations; are they types of evaluative judgments or evolutionary interaction modes of our social brain?

How the individual patient feels anxiety, for example, in the specific moment is not accessible to reductionist science. The legitimate approach of neuroscience is at least to explain the information processing for the way of experiencing basal, fundamental emotions (overview e.g. Borod 2000; Dolan 2002; Dalgleish 2004). Panksepp (1998) has summarized a number of features of emotion physiology in 6 points (see the following overview).

Characteristics of Emotions according to Panksepp

1. The neural processing of emotions is genetically determined, innately prepared for the access of unconditioned stimuli—for example, the emotional system responds immediately to dangers such as shortness of breath, the death of a loved one, etc.
2. Emotions include adaptive reactions to dangers or other significant situations of the living being. Emotional reaction modes include
   a) behavior, i.e., influences on the activation and inhibition of motor systems.
   b) Changes in the autonomic nervous system and
   c) hormonal effects
3. Effects on sensory systems—e.g., emotionality determines the selection of stimuli
4. Stimulus duration—after the triggering stimulus, emotions have different durations
5. Conditionable, i.e., emotional reactions can come under the control of conditioned stimuli. There is an emotional memory system
6. Reciprocal interactions with the physiological systems for cognitive decisions and awareness

Physiological Emotion Specificity

Do specific neural systems exist for all fundamental emotions, or are they only present for some of the phylogenetically important emotions such as anxiety and reward, i.e., for negative and positive emotionality? The neuroscience of emotion currently essentially follows a nativist approach: It assumes a group of physiological, evolutionarily developed, basic emotions.

Much evidence supports physiological emotion specificity. Neuroscientists are searching for specific systems of the emotional brain; or have identified groups of neurons that are at least associated with aspects of emotion (functional brain imaging diagnostics, see overview: Dolan 2002).

For no area of psychopathology are more hormonal and pharmacological influences known than for the emotional area. Humanity has learned through a long history of experience which herbs and substances can alter the emotionality of individuals. However, the abundance of emotionally effective hormones and pharmaceuticals does not prove that there are diffuse biochemical-neuronal mechanisms for emotionality. On the contrary, it indicates that specific systems for the various emotions are established in the CNS, which work with different transmitters or receptors. Furthermore, the finding suggests that the physiology of emotions is specifically hormonally controlled. These systems are more or less pharmacologically influenceable.

The triggering of some emotions has been investigated, such as the triggering of aggression in the hypothalamus or anxiety in the amygdala and the basal forebrain. In animal experiments, stimulation in these areas causes the expression behavior characteristic of the emotion; whether the subjective emotional quality is also achieved remains unresolved. However, how the neuronal triggering functions in these core areas is still largely unknown. Imaging findings suggest that during imagined unrestrained aggression, the medial orbitofrontal cortex is inhibited (Pietrini et al. 2000). This is consistent with the model that the medial prefrontal cortex normally exerts an inhibitory control and that specific deactivation of neurons in this cortical area enables emotional behaviors or emotional experiences.

Much is now known about emotional motor functions and expressions and the consequences of emotions. In recent years, mechanisms of affect control have become known, such as influences of the medial prefrontal cortex on the hypothalamus and the periaqueductal gray.

11.4.2 Different Levels of Emotions

Certainly, emotions are not solely equated with the information processing of the cognitive criteria that trigger them, the "appraisal." For example, the discovery that a colleague's remark was an impertinence triggers the emotion anger— the emotion is not exhausted in the cognitive processes of criterion processing. For the psychotherapy of emotional disorders, addressing the cognitive criteria of emotions is very valuable. Emotion encompasses more than cognitive triggering. The fulfilled criteria of emotion lead to the activation of subcortical centers of the specific emotion. An action readiness is triggered. Think of an evolutionarily old, archaic switch. More or less specific ways of thinking ("cognitions") accompany a motor action readiness. Finally, the emotion-expressing motor functions are activated in the brainstem centers, whether it be gestures, facial expressions, or even just tension. Additionally, vegetative symptoms of affect may occur. For each level of emotionality, there are neuroscientific mechanisms, which, however, are still unknown in many details. Ekman (1999) proposed the concept of emotions as affect programs. According to this, emotion refers to a complex "program" that runs after the triggering and for the duration of the emotion. In an emotion, the specific elements of the different levels become active together, creating the multifaceted picture of emotional experiences and behaviors. Differences between the emotional and the cognitive system, both of which are understood as adaptive systems, are described, for example, by Gainotti (2000). Interindividual differences are found at the various levels, including different learning and memory systems. For emotions, more than for the cognitive system, the conditioning processes described below are important (Buechel and Dolan 2000).

Specificity of Emotional Information Processing at Different Levels

Table 11.1 provides an overview of the different levels using the example of 4 emotions

Using examples, we will subsequently consider the specificity of the centers for emotional information processing in the brain.

Emotional Motor System (Holstege et al. 1996)

Emotional motor functions are specifically controlled in the Emotional Motor System. For example, in the case of a central paralysis of the facial muscles on one side, involuntary, spontaneous smiling remains intact, while the voluntary movement to distort the mouth as in smiling is paralyzed. This example already proves the different activation of emotional and voluntary movements. The phenomenon is also known from the difference between voluntary smiling at a photo session and natural smiling. The emotional expressive movements are controlled in a brainstem system called the Emotional Motor System (Holstege et al. 1996; see Fig. 11.4). It is a core area found in a section of the reticular formation that extends over many levels of the brainstem.

Pathological laughter or crying can illustrate the separation of emotional behavior and emotional experience. As described above, emotional expressive behavior is observed without emotional experience; it occurs in brain disorders that a patient cries but, when asked, states that he has not felt a sad emotion. A patient can, for example, report, "it laughs me," i.e., he does not feel humor or joy while laughing, which can accordingly seem displaced to others (Wild et al. 2003).

Table 11.1 Different Levels of Four Emotions

	Anxiety	Sadness Depression	Aggression	Joy
Trigger: Information Processing "Appraisal"	Danger	e.g., Loss	e.g., Rival	Surprising Reward
Subcortical:	Amygdala	e.g., anterior cingulum, hypothalamus, inhibition of the reward center, neural structures for processing negative valence	Hypothalamus	Ventral Tegmental Area, Nucleus Accumbens
Action readiness	Flight	e.g., Withdrawal, retardation	Attack	e.g., Sociability, Play
Effector: Emotional Motor System	Brainstem	Brainstem	Brainstem	Brainstem, Cortex

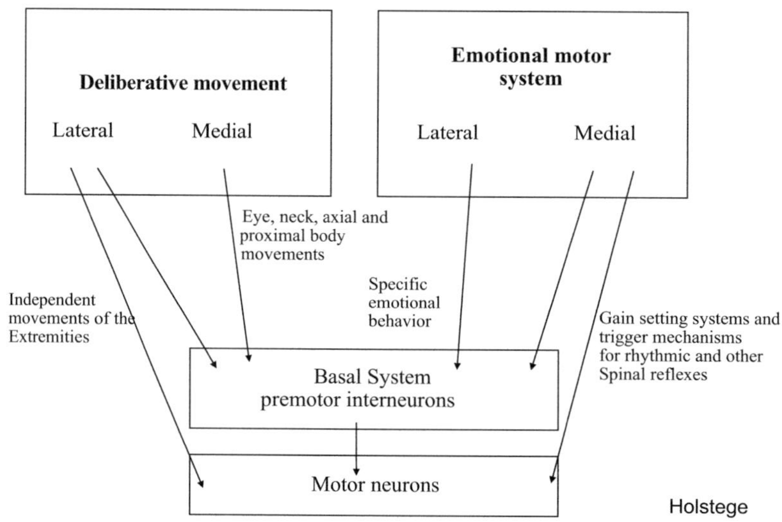

Fig. 11.4 An Emotional Motor System controls the motor functions of emotional behaviors (Holstege et al. 1996). It is responsible, for example, for natural smiling, which is inaccessible to the voluntary control of most people. Thus, emotional expressive movements are motorically controlled separately from voluntary movements

Core Areas of Emotions in the Brainstem

Besides the motor areas for emotional expression, there are core areas that are activated when cognitive processing triggers an emotion. Many are located in the hypothalamus, and those for anxiety are presumably in the amygdala (see below). A rapid access pathway to the amygdala has even been described, which reaches this core area directly from the thalamus. This allows a living being to prepare flight movements early in case of danger, independently of the slow, precise cognitive processing in the cortex (LeDoux 1996).

It is further assumed that there are brain regions responsible for central emotional processing. These will be presented in the following. Panksepp (1998) assumes different levels and subcortical centers of emotional information processing. However, he presents a model of a neural network that has areas of input neurons, several levels of central information processing, and an area of output neurons responsible for motor effects (see below, Fig. 11.3). It is not only assumed that information processing is unidirectional, i.e., from input to output, but also that there is an interaction between the levels. In other words, central neurons in the brainstem can influence experience and cognition—thus, there appears to be an interdependence of functional levels: Cognitive processes were crucially involved in triggering the emotion and are in turn self influenced by the "emotion program" triggered by it.

The phenomena of alexithymia and dissociation of emotions also show that emotional expressive behavior and vegetative somatic emotional manifestations can occur without emotional experience, although the mechanisms of these clinical phenomena are not yet fully understood (Taylor and Bagby 2004). This is evident in affective prosody, which often gives interlocutors more clues about the speaker's emotional processing than the speaker self consciously experiences, can express, or wants to express. The function of the different levels of emotional information processing can be dissociated . The conscious ways of experiencing emotions and affects are to be separated from central and motor affect processing.

Conscious Experience of Emotions

Where in the brain does the emotional quality that constitutes the experience of emotion arise? EEG studies in various states have shown differences that could indicate cortico-thalamic specializations, and brain imaging studies have suggested the involvement of different brain regions in various emotions (Phan et al. 2002). However, due to the phylogenetically early occurrence of emotions in evolution and in child development, it is also assumed that the cortex in its entirety is not necessary for emotional experience in humans. In contrast, the early-developed, so-called limbic areas might have a function in emotional experience, or the experience itself might be related in an as-yet-unknown way to the function of brainstem nuclei. The conscious emotional way of experiencing and the level of language processing of emotional experience are again to be separated. The possibility of musically emotional experience shows this dissociation. For many people, the diverse emotional nuances of music are not expressible in language.

An indication of limbic information processing related to emotional experience can be sought in imaging findings on pain experience. Findings on the activation of specific regions of the anterior cingulum in pain perception provide a clue to a role of this region in the experience of pain (Price 2000). Although there are justified doubts about the nature of the role of the activated region in the information processing in imaging findings, an "involvement" in the examined function seems to be demonstrable. However, whether other regions might contribute much more specifically cannot be definitively excluded with these findings. An area of the anterior cingulum located anterior to the described region has been associated with the emotional system in lesion studies in humans (Bush et al. 2000; Hornak et al. 2003), and even further anterior, below the "knee" of the anterior cingulum, is the region found to be critical for depression in imaging studies (Drevets 2003; see also overview Phan et al. 2002).

Using the example of pain experience, a possible role of the reticular formation in the brainstem for an early form of experience can likely be demonstrated. It could form a bridge to the experience of pain (and more generally of negative valence and suffering, Reischies 2021) assumed to be present in less highly developed animals.

The Process of Triggering Emotion—Unconscious and Conscious Emotion

Triggering an emotion is a complex process. How can this be investigated? One must assume that an emotion is triggered in a person or an animal when the behavioral characteristics and vegetative somatic signs of the emotional syndrome are present. If a patient cannot or does not want to provide information about the emotional experience, can we assume with some certainty that he is feeling the emotion?

In everyday life, we assume that the person is likely to feel the emotion if we can recognize their "emotion mini-syndromes" (i.e., the specific signs in facial expressions, gestures, behavior, cognition, and the vegetative system). The situation is reminiscent of a little boy who has a wound and says, "an Indian knows no pain," but the fellows know better based on their observations.

However, in this conclusion about a person's experience, we can be mistaken: In patients with a disorder of self-perception, who cannot recognize that he is, for example, reacting angrily, one must speak of an objective triggering of anger if the surroundings register clear signs of anger. The emotion anger is triggered without the person experiencing it himmselve (see alexithymia).

This has been shown particularly impressively for anxiety, where, as indicated above, a special processing pathway of faster information processing from the thalamus to the amygdala could be demonstrated (LeDoux 1996). The process of emotion triggering has been described in more detail in further studies on humans. Already when a person sees the wide-open eye of another person (which can be a sign of anxiety), this triggers an activation of the amygdala neurons (Whalen et al. 1998, 2004). However, the activity remains essentially confined to the amygdala. The vegetative signs of the emotion cannot be detected, and the person does not show the characteristics of an empathically triggered negative emotional reaction. In the further process of emotion triggering, apparently, other brain areas must be activated. In the case of bilateral damage to the amygdala, the perception of anxiety in the facial expression of others is impaired (Adolphs et al. 2005).

Triggering Emotion through Cognitive Information Processing

Many researchers have dedicated their investigations to the cognitive mechanisms that become effective in triggering emotions. When a person realizes that a certain critical situation is the case, the specific emotion is triggered (Scherer 2004). Usually, this is the main mechanism for triggering emotions. The evaluation of situations however, does not only consist of checking objective cognitive criteria. The appreciation of statements from others involves various experiences and memories, e.g., old scores to settle. Additionally, the basic mood state of the person evaluating a statement from another person plays a role. Everyone knows the situation where a cheeky remark is countered with a "sharp" retort or humorously neutralized in a high-spirited mood; however, in a depressed basic mood, this can be dysfunctionally processed as a sign of contempt from others.

How are basic moods triggered? This is an unresolved question. On the one hand, it could be 1) longer persistent but only partial activation of the emotion centers that cause a corresponding mood: irritability, an anxious or joyful basic mood. On the other hand, one can assume 2) a form of integration of the positive and negative events of recent times—resulting in a persistently positive or negatively pronounced valence. This affects the positive or negative basic state. 3) Psychiatric pathology knows a multitude of "endogenous" fluctuations in the basic mood state, which are partly genetically determined (see, for example, cyclothymia). These "endogenous factors" can indeed interact with the environment but can also trigger an emotional basic mood state without an external event or cognitive evaluation.

Summary

After the triggering of emotions through cognitive information processing, both subcortical and cortical effectors are activated, as well as the neuronal structures involved in the emotional experience, which we do not yet know. Additionally, psychopathologically, the control functions of affective expression still need to be clarified further. The following will present neuropsychiatric research findings on these questions.

11.4.3 Neuropsychiatric Findings

Neuropsychiatry has long been dedicated to the disruptibility of emotional behavior or experience by brain lesions or degenerative brain diseases. In this process, some syndromes have been characterized, which, however, cannot be presented in detail here. Only the reference to neurophysiological mechanisms, which could be demonstrated by the syndromes, is of interest for psychopathology.

Frontal Brain Symptoms in the Emotional Domain (Benson 1994; Hornak et al. 2003)

- pseudodepression(drive disorder, abulia)
  - Aprosody (Ross 1981)
- Pseudopsychopathic syndrome
  - disinhibition: wit
  - Euphoria (Reischies et al. 1988)

Temporal Brain Lesions with Emotional Symptoms

- Klüver-Bucy syndrome (among others: fearless, hypersexual syndrome)

Diencephalic Lesions Laughter and rage states can be triggered.

Brainstem lesions; Emotional-Motor system (Holstege et al. 1996)

- pseudobulbar affect
- pathological laughter (Wild et al. 2003)
- emotional facial expression preserved in paresis of voluntary motor function, "laughing apraxia" see above.
- Depression psychomotor: eyes, posture, etc.

11.4.4 Neuroscientific Models of Specific Emotions

Neuroscience of Negative Emotionality: Startle Reaction

The sudden fright in the face of something unexpected leads to a typical reaction, the startle reaction, which has emotional components.

In the case of an unexpected announcement of a negative event, there are, with some specificity, motor reactions such as eye closure or eye widening, straightening up, and muscle tension (preparation for flight). Vegetative features are increased heart rate and blood pressure. The part of the reaction that relates to attention and arousal has already been mentioned. The emotional component is related to anxiety, the anticipation of negative events. Something surprising can also happen that is related to joy (joyful surprise).

The startle reaction is an evolutionarily successful process that prepares a living being nonspecifically for impending actions, triggering a general arousal. The specific action readiness is determined by the type of emotion. Information processing must quickly make the decision about attack or flight. The switch "flight" is associated with anxiety, the switch "fight" with aggression. In fractions of a second, the decision is made about gain or loss and thus joy or sorrow.

The scare corresponds to the schema that initially activation is ramped up and only then does the quality of the emotion appear. The resulting emotion can only be specified through the information processing of the situational perception.

The scare provides an initial nonspecific preparation for action for fight or flight. It appears to be a phylogenetically early developed reaction mode. It is well-researched due to the clarity of the triggering conditions and reaction findings (Koch 1999). The information about a loud noise that triggers the scare is transmitted in rats from the cochlear nuclei to the giant neurons in the caudal pontine reticulum, a part of the reticular formation. From there, the motor, autonomic, and cognitive reactions are triggered. The physiology of the startle reaction in humans has particularities; however, the basic structure of the physiological system that mediates the reaction is apparently very similar to that in animals (Koch 1999). In patients with anxiety disorders, the level of the startle reaction is increased (Grillon 2002). The activation of the startle reaction in an anxiety situation is linked to an activation of the amygdala and the anterior cingulate (Pissiota et al. 2003).

The modulation of the startle reaction is known from many studies. The startle reaction habituates quickly. The level of the startle reaction that sets in after habituation is dependent on many influences. In addition to habituation and reduction of the startle reaction through positive emotions, there is a sensitization and increase in the reaction level through, on the one hand, pain stimuli and, on the other hand, conditioned fear reactions (Koch 1999). For this reason, the startle reaction has become a vehicle for anxiety research.

Anxiety

As we have seen, scare can be the entry point into anxiety, which is triggered by an event. However, anxiety has many other aspects. The works of LeDoux (1996) and (Davis et al. 1997) have contributed to a better understanding of the physiology of anxiety. The fear reaction to an event that has occurred or is expected consists, for example, of freezing with muscle tension and trembling or motor restlessness and vegetatively in increased blood pressure and pulse rate. In the case of prolonged anxiety, bladder and bowel symptoms can also occur. The arousal level is increased. These effects are apparently mediated by the central nucleus of the amygdala. From this center, all the crucial brainstem nuclei are activated (Davis et al. 1997; Fig. 11.5).

How is the information processed that leads to the fear reaction? It is assumed that some immediately fear-inducing stimuli, e.g., a very loud bang or snake-like movements on the forest floor, are already processed in the brainstem nuclei or in the thalamus and are directly forwarded to the amygdala. There, a rapid reaction can be activated (LeDoux 1996). The detour with object recognition in the "What-Pathway" takes longer but is the more important path for fear generation in humans. Only when object identification is performed inferotemporally is the information forwarded to the amygdala and the hippocampus. From the hippocampus, episodic information, i.e., memory of a dangerous situation, can be retrieved and then conveyed to the amygdala (Paton et al. 2006). In the amygdala, the information is processed in the basolateral nucleus and forwarded to the central nucleus (LeDoux 1996).

The bed nucleus of the stria terminalis, which also has connections to the brainstem nuclei, has been discussed as one center for anxiety. It is assumed that it can react to the neuroendocrine substance CRH (corticotropin releasing hormone) without direct stimulus influence and mediates anxiety (Davis et al. 1997). In connection with these two core areas, a differentiation between stimulus-dependent fear and non-stimulus-bound, diffuse anxiety has been speculated. Certainly, the psychological disorders of phobia with stimulus-dependent fear and panic attacks without triggering stimuli show differences. However, whether these can be sufficiently explained by the involvement of the closely interconnected core areas of the amygdala and the bed nucleus of the stria terminalis remains to be clarified.

With the activation of the central nucleus of the amygdala and neuroendocrine effects, it can be explained how fear objects or fear situations can be answered with specific action preparation (flight) and emotion. Because both the central nucleus of the amygdala and the bed nucleus of the stria terminalis can activate the brainstem nuclei that cause the fear equivalents, such as sweating and increased heart rate, etc. (LeDoux 1996; Davis et al. 1997).

Learning Phenomena

The fear system usually learns quickly. Fear conditioning occurs when an unconditioned fear stimulus is paired with a neutral stimulus. The system responds to the initially neutral stimulus after the conditioning as a stimulus belonging to the situational context of the fear stimulus with a fear reaction. In the future, the anxiety will be triggered already at the appearance of the formerly neutral and now conditioned stimulus.

An important finding is the persistence of the learned stimulus-response association. When animals are brought to a fear reaction with tones of certain frequencies, neurons are found in the amygdala that persistently respond to this specific frequency (LeDoux 1996). These neurons

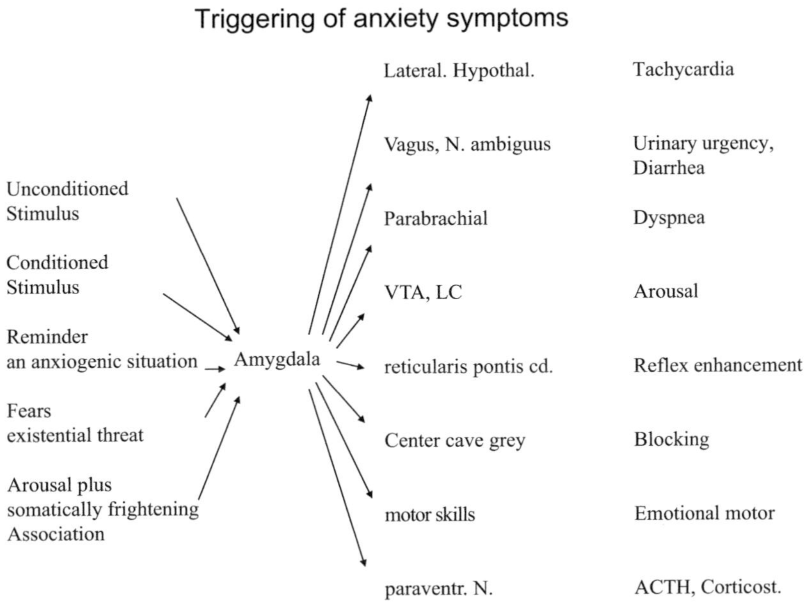

Fig. 11.5 Neurobiological research attempts to find and characterize the CNS centers of the "discrete emotional circuits." The amygdala has been identified for the central circuitry in connection with the emotion anxiety. The neurons of the amygdala are activated by various stimuli, on the one hand immediately after the sight of a fear object, on the other hand mediated by cognitive processing (for example, the housewife realizes during the billing that money for an outstanding bill is not available). From the amygdala, a series of subcortical or brainstem regions are activated, which mediate the vegetative and motor forms of the fear reaction (so-called fear equivalents)

remain active even when the anxiety no longer occurs because the animal has learned that the formerly neutral stimulus poses no danger. A decrease in the fear reaction, when in the extinction phase the specific tone no longer occurs with a threatening situation, is apparently not achieved by a decrease in the activity of the amygdala neurons but by an external control of the amygdala activity.

In recent years, it has been shown how neurons of the frontal brain control amygdala activity. Milad and Quirk (2002) have demonstrated an inhibition of the amygdala output after an unlearned fear stimulus. In this information processing, frontal neurons received the information about the fear stimulus. These neurons sent activity back to the amygdala in a specific manner, which suppressed the output of the amygdala. Specifically, neurons are inhibited that relay the information to the brainstem nuclei after the triggering of anxiety. This has succeeded in showing a mechanism of cortical control over emotional information processing (Deng et al. 2017). Investigations using functional magnetic resonance imaging also point in this direction, showing a decrease in amygdala activation and a parallel increase in frontal activation when anxiety subsides (Hariri et al. 2003). This would be consistent with the idea that certain frontal brain areas play an important role in the suppression of anxiety reactions.

The data can explain why anxiety symptoms from traumatic life events so often re-emerge uncontrollably in old age and in degenerative brain diseases with damage to the frontal brain, whereas they were under control in younger adulthood. It may be possible to find more of these mechanisms for emotional information processing in other emotional core areas.

Negative Emotionality

Negative feelings include, among others, sadness and pain. Imaging studies found medial prefrontal activation in the grief phase when viewing photos of the deceased person, an area that is also involved in the pathophysiology of depression (Gündel et al. 2003). The involvement of the anterior cingulate, the dorsomedial thalamus, the periaqueductal gray, and the insula in human grief or depression has been discussed—particularly regarding the activation of comparable regions in an animal experiencing stress from a separation situation (Panksepp 2003).

The pain system has been well studied. Although pain, as a primarily somatic sensation, belongs more to internal medicine and neurology, abnormal pain occurs psychopathologically—for example, as head pressure in depression, where the pain threshold is generally lowered. Also, as coenesthesia in schizophrenia, pain is reported, such as excruciating pain in the genitals, which patients experience as being caused by other people (see ego disturbances).

The sensation of mental effort, the pronounced exertion, can be felt when tasks requiring maximum concentration are performed. This is increased in depression and decreased in mania. Many studies have reported activity in the anterior cingulate during strenuous tasks such as the Stroop test (Chap. 4 attention). Lesions in this region lead to a disturbance of emotionality with a reduction in attention (Bush et al. 2000). The anterior cingulate apparently has many other functions, with mediating effort being one of them.

Negative Valence

In neuroscience, aversive reactions of animals after stimulation of brain areas have been studied. There is still uncertainty about how negative valence is processed in the brain, on the one hand at a basal level in less developed organisms and on the other hand in humans. Various sensory stimuli, such as pain stimuli, hunger stimuli, sensory reactions to shortness of breath, but also the feeling of illness with nausea and fatigue should be integrated into the sensation "negative valence" in a still unknown way. In addition, there are negative cognitive assessments of the subject's situation in humans, etc. A model of a basal integration of negative stimuli into negative valence and suffering, which can be conceptualized as extremely negative valence, sees negative valence as an evolutionarily early signal for behavioral adaptation (see Reischies (2021).

Neuroscience of Positive Emotionality

In psychopathology, the loss of joy, or the loss of positive basic mood, is diagnosed as a symptom of the depressive syndrome. The young neuroscience of emotions has been able to clarify at least one thing: The information processing for positive emotions is organized differently than that of negative emotionality. This may be related to the fact that it interacts with other physiological systems. While negative emotions are more about rapid reaction, about fight or flight, positive emotions are more about motivation and selection of promising activities. In feedback with the orbitofrontal cortex, the expectation of reward for each activity is estimated. For this reason, a central nucleus for positive emotion, the Nucleus Accumbens, is found in the basal forebrain.

Classical and instrumental conditioning

Classical conditioning has been intensively studied in neuroscience (see above). An event triggers an emotion and the organism learns to predict the emotion. Vegetative reactions and cognitive events can also be associated with conditioning processes. However, one of the main domains of conditioning is learning in the affective sphere.

This physiological reaction in conditioned fear response plays a significant role in the regulation of emotions; thus, fears occur in events that the person has experienced in association with negative events—this triggering process can occur unconsciously, especially uncontrollably by the person.

In contrast, instrumental conditioning involves an action by the organism that leads to feedback from the environment. This feedback is associated with positive emotions in the case of a reward and with negative emotions in the case of punishment. Through this, the organism learns to adapt its actions to the conditions of the environment. Positive and negative valence is closely coupled with this feedback (positive or negative). The reward system is closely linked to instrumental conditioning and plays a role in the neuroscience of addiction, depression, and schizophrenia.

The amygdala apparently not only plays a role in fear processing. The early processing of emotional stimuli occurs in the amygdala, both for negative and positive valence (LaBar et al. 1998; Büchel and Dolan 2000; Paton et al. 2006). The amygdala is also an important station for conditioning, both for positive and negative stimulus associations (see Rolls 1999). Only for the flexible processing of feedback stimuli, whether rewards or punishments, i.e., motivating and demotivating stimuli, is the orbitofrontal cortex apparently necessary.

Orbitofrontal cortex

Neurons in the orbitofrontal cortex are activated by objects that represent a value for the organism—mostly a positive value, but to a lesser extent also a negative value. It is assumed that these orbitofrontal neurons represent a CNS representation of a value system (Rolls 1999).

The information about an object is first processed in the lateral orbitofrontal cortex. The visual object information comes via the fasciculus uncinatus from the inferotemporal cortex (the "What" system). If necessary, additional inputs from the amygdala, which has already coded the valence of a stimulus, namely to what extent it is an anxiety-laden object, are passed on about a specific object.

What is the peculiarity of the orbitofrontal neurons? From various sources of neuroscientific analysis such as lesion studies, from the electrophysiological characterization of information processing by individual neurons, and imaging techniques, it has been clarified that the rapid re-evaluation in a value hierarchy apparently takes place in the orbitofrontal cortex, in collaboration with the subcortical nuclei (see above).

An example of the everyday importance of flexible value assignment is food selection, such as at a buffet. If a salad does not taste good on the first round, which otherwise belongs to the person's favorite dishes, the person will not choose it again on the second plate. Rolls found out (1999) that monkeys have many different food sources during the day. They must evaluate these according to the current quality, for example, the ripeness of fruits. Certain aspects of negative feedback after the individual's actions are apparently also processed in the orbitofrontal cortex. In this context, the negative aspects are not those of punishment, but for example, devaluation, which is needed for the flexible changing of preference decisions (Reischies 1999a, b).

- The orbitofrontal cortex is not specifically necessary for the fear reaction, but for unlearning an action when—unexpectedly—negative consequences have occurred. This explains the disturbance of feedback-dependent flexibility in decision-making behavior in orbitofrontal lesions (Rolls 1999).

The relative reward value of several objects also seems to be differentially represented in the orbitofrontal cortex (Tremblay and Schultz 1999). Therefore, it has been suggested that information processing for motivational regulation takes place there.

The orbitofrontal neurons are activated by objects that contain valences in both directions, positive as well as negative, but the positive evaluation predominates. For a long time, it was unclear how the brain divides the processing of negative and positive information. It is assumed that the special processing of negative evaluation towards anxiety runs via the amygdala. The amygdala also receives information about objects that are positively evaluated (Paton et al. 2006). An animal can also learn reactions to positive stimuli if the orbitofrontal cortex is damaged (see Rolls 1999). Only the flexibility of assigning values to objects is performed in the orbitofrontal cortex.

The orbitofrontal cortex is subdivided into a lateral part, which is more closely related to the incoming information about stimuli of various modalities, and a medial part, which has close relationships with subcortical brain areas and seems to be particularly important for emotionality and vegetative regulation. The described information processing includes a complex representation and updating of the representations of the values of objects in the cortex.

Where is the behavior of joy generated? Is the orbitofrontal cortex the critical location and does the described information processing have to do with the experience of joy?

Orbitofrontal cortical-subcortical projection loops (Frontal Loops)

The subcortical brain areas with which the orbitofrontal cortex closely collaborates are the Ncl. accumbens, the ventral part of the caudate, and the ventral tegmental area. From the ventral tegmental area, a significant group of dopaminergic neurons innervates the Ncl. accumbens.

The orbitofrontal cortical-subcortical projection loops (orbitofrontal loops) have the following stations: From the orbitofrontal cortex 1. to the ventral striatum, the Ncl. accumbens, and to the ventral part of the caudate. From there, 2. the ventral pallidum is reached. The neurons of the pallidum have high spontaneous activity and tonically inhibit the 3. station, the mediodorsal thalamus, which projects back to the prefrontal cortex (Middleton and Strick 2000; West and Grace 2000).

The mediodorsal thalamus and also parts of the anterior thalamus are involved in the orbitofrontal cortical-subcortical projection loops. The general physiology of the projection loops includes a specific disinhibition of the thalamic activation of the cortex, as the striatum inhibits the spontaneously active neurons of the pallidum via GABAergic neurons. These, in turn, inhibit, again GABAergically, the thalamic neurons. Through this double inhibition, only specific thalamic activity, which the cortex controls, is left activated, i.e., is not filtered out. The cortex thus controls its own activation (Carlsson 2001). Besides filtering information that the thalamus should let through, the frontal loops apparently have another function. The frontal loops, which are organized in countless parallel channels from the cortex back to the cortex, represent recurrent information for the cortex, which may be necessary for maintaining sustained, enduring activity—necessary in terms of working memory (see Gao et al. 2001; Gao and Goldman-Rakic 2003; Houk 2001), in addition to a possible role in the selection of further cortico-cortical neuronal networks (Chap. 10 thinking).

The mesolimbic dopaminergic system

In the reward system of the CNS, dopamine plays an important role (Wise and Rompe 1989). The dopaminergic neuron of the mesolimbic system, found in the ventral tegmental area, is known in many aspects of its anatomy and physiological properties. It modulates the information processing in the frontal loops in a complex manner.

A dopaminergic neuron of the ventral tegmental area is active when a reward is given or expected (Schultz 1998). It apparently integrates a wealth of information for this purpose. The activity is passed on to the N. accumbens. There, activity has also been measured in humans in situations of expected reward (Marschner et al. 2005).

In addition to a phasic activity of the dopaminergic neurons, a tonic extracellular increase in dopamine concentration in the Ncl. accumbens is also observed, presumably due to dopamine that is not released synaptically (West and Grace 2000).

The effect of the activity of this dopaminergic neuron has a central position in psychopharmacology. On the one hand, drugs and illegal substances that increase dopamine concentration cause an increase in positive emotionality, as well as drive and cognitive functions. On the other hand, neuroleptics that inhibit the effect of dopamine and the activity of dopaminergic neurons, for example, through a depolarization block (West and Grace 2000), cause negative mood.

There is a wealth of information about the effect of neuroleptics, which negatively affect the signal processing of dopamine. The activity of the dopaminergic neuron of the ventral tegmental area is altered, as well as the effect at the receptor and synaptic efficiency. In the

Ncl. accumbens, this is achieved through D2, D3, or D1 receptors; in the frontal cortex, predominantly other receptors are involved, e.g., D4 or D1 receptors (Bronstein and Cummings 2001). The pharmacology of this neuron, which is important for psychiatry, is described in more detail in textbooks on psychopharmacology. The disinhibition of the indirect loop of the dorsal striatum through D2 blockade explains the Parkinson-like undesirable effects of neuroleptics.

Here, the focus should primarily be on anhedonia, the inability to experience joy, as a side effect of neuroleptics with a primary effect on the D2 receptor. This is partly responsible for the fact that patients who benefit from neuroleptics, such as patients with schizophrenia, prefer to discontinue their medication. After discontinuing neuroleptics, they report a resurgence of their positive emotionality. The Ncl. accumbens receives afferents not only from the cortex, especially from the medial orbitofrontal cortex (Middleton et al. 2001), but also from the amygdala and the hippocampus. The axons of the dopaminergic neurons partly inhibit presynaptically afferents from other regions. They can change the connectivity in the frontal loops. A so-called indirect pathway of the frontal loops, as in the motor system, is not known for the medial orbitofrontal loop.

Where the information processing for positive emotionality, joy, happiness, etc., takes place cannot yet be determined from previous neuroscientific studies. So far, we only know that positive emotionality is associated with the activity of dopaminergic neurons. The coupling of positive emotionality and initiation of motor activity in the striatum confirms the concept that emotions are coupled with action settings or action tendencies (Frijda 1986).

The described system of the orbitofrontal loops, Fig. 11.6, is also central to motivation and drive and is described there in terms of the evaluation of action initiatives. For thinking and other cognitive functions, the physiology of the frontal loops is also important (Houk 2001), and the crucial aspects for this are discussed there (Chap. 10 thinking).

Opioid system

Another system is linked to the experience of positive emotion, the opioid system (Panksepp 1998). It includes neurons that release endorphins and receptors that, for example, respond to morphine. Opioid receptors μ, delta, and kappa have different functions and are distributed differently in the brain. The opiate drugs are μ-agonists. How does the binding of opioids to the corresponding receptors affect positive emotionality? Insights into the mechanism have emerged from addiction research. It is believed that the opioid system ultimately also activates the dopaminergic reward system. The opiate drugs apparently utilize the enkephalin activation of the VTA neurons (ventral tegmental area) of the reward system. This occurs through the inhibition of the GABAergic, inhibitory interneurons of the VTA. Thus, the neurons that, for example, release dopamine in the Ncl. accumbens are disinhibited.

The activation of the endogenous opioid system would thus be something like the information processing of a primary reinforcer, such as food for a hungry laboratory animal. The opioid system also seems to be initially responsible for the expectation of positive feedback from the mother and later from social partners in the development of a child (Panksepp 1998; Moles et al. 2004). It is therefore about the feelings associated with emotional interindividual bonding.

Expression of Positive Emotionality

Pathological laughter has already been reported. Here, the disinhibition of emotional motor functions is the cause of the behavior. Laughing fits are known in epileptology. In this context, it is presumably the epileptic activity in the hypothalamus that triggers laughing behavior. In the lateral hypothalamus, there are neurons that are associated with the orbitofrontal system of value representation—predominantly of positive values (Rolls 1999). Additionally, other brain areas seem to be involved, with a distinction being made between emotionally and voluntarily initiated laughter, and different brain regions being found responsible for the two behaviors (see Wild et al. 2003).

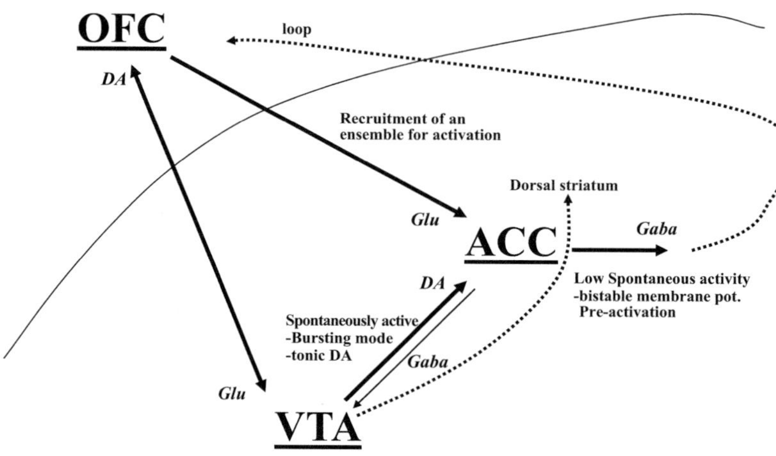

Fig. 11.6 The neurons of the ventral tegmental area (VTA) have axons that innervate the Ncl. accumbens (ACC, in the ventral striatum) and also the overlying striatum, the Ncl. caudatus, and the globus pallidum. Another portion of axons extends to the prefrontal cortex. Specifically, the orbitofrontal cortex (OFC), in turn, activates the Ncl. accumbens. It is the beginning of the cortico-subcortical projection loop of the orbitofrontal cortex, which continues to the ventral pallidum and mediodorsal thalamus. The orbitofrontal cortex presumably organizes the information processing for motivation. It contains neurons that encode the preference for certain stimuli and also neurons that signal the flexible relation of the current "value" of feedback or rewards for the individual. The dopaminergic innervation (DA) has an activating effect on both mental and motor activity and supports motor learning as well as the flexibility of cortical value representation. Additionally, it plays a role in the reward system, which is associated with addictive behavior.

Conclusion

From the presented information, an initial outline of a system of positive valence, or emotions associated with positive valence, emerges. It initially includes the recognition and relational processing of objects concerning their value to the person. The subcortical nuclei and brain regions such as the Ncl. accumbens, the ventral tegmental area, and presumably the ventral hypothalamus, hold a central position in the triggering of behavior. Currently, it can only be speculated that these regions also evoke the experience of positive valence or joyful events. The neurons of the emotional-motor system (see above) in turn control the motor functions of specific joy behaviors, such as laughing, smiling, etc.

Aggression

Aggression holds a special position among affects. It cannot be simply classified into positive and negative emotionality. At this point, the advantage of an additional independent instance of valence becomes evident, which variably represents the positive or negative direction of the evaluation for the subject in both sensation and emotion (this also applies, for example, to other emotions and pain, which can also sometimes receive a positive value).

Furthermore, there are many different ways of expressing or showing aggressiveness in behavior. The intense affect of aggression disrupts cognitive processing, and one rightly speaks of blind anger. Thus, it is the prototype of emotions that exhibit an interaction with the cognitive system.

- Severity: mild (aggressive conversation)—severe (e.g., manslaughter).
- Directness: direct (physical attack)—indirect (trap, intrigue).
- Use of physical force: with (e.g., kick)—without (insult).
- Targeted at the body: yes (stab)—no (flailing).

- Accomplices: no (alone)—yes (in group, manipulation of teams, intrigues).
- Preparation: impulsive (defense, affect)—planned (intrigue against rivals, gang fights).
- Trigger: situational (gang finds a victim)—non-situational (old enemy deliberately eliminated).
- Reactivity: reactive (defense, provoked)—proactive, spontaneous (rival combat).

There are significant differences between the various forms of aggressive behavior—on the one hand, indirect verbal aggression, such as slander or insult, poisoning, and on the other hand, an impulsive punch to the face. Nevertheless, in most cases, the emotion of aggression is present.

To explain the variance in aggressive behaviors, one must distinguish between prolonged hatred and a short-term exceptional state like rage or aggressive impulses. Hatred is not only related to emotional moods but also to cognitive beliefs and dispositions, "if he comes with that again and says it, then I will strike back".

A distinction should be made between spontaneously aggressive actions and reactions or defense. For in psychopathological assessments, spontaneous aggressiveness is more informative than reactive aggressiveness, where a person was provoked.

The most important aspect of aggression, however, is that practically none of the typically aggressive actions can be unequivocally and in every case classified as aggression. It is known that patients with personality disorders, especially those with narcissistic antisocial characteristics, often do not feel aggression during aggressive acts—they exhibit a kind of equivalent to predatory behavior. In other words, when they attack a person, it is not out of anger, but almost always out of calculation, with the attitude, "I am entitled to this"—somewhat like the lion is "entitled" to kill the lamb as food. Some patients with an irritable mania can also be classified in their behavior in this way. This has significant consequences for psychopathology. The diagnosis of aggressiveness as a psychopathological feature of emotions can only be evaluated in the overall context of a diagnosis. This is also valid for many other emotions, but to a limited extent.

Neuroscientific Studies on Aggression

The neuroscience of aggression is only partially understood. According to behavioral research findings, the different types of aggression are organized differently. Predatory behavior is apparently triggered in the lateral hypothalamus (Siegel et al. 1999; Fig. 11.7). As mentioned above, many researchers do not consider predatory behavior to be a form of aggression that corresponds to what is referred to as human aggression in everyday life.

Defensive aggression is triggered in the medial hypothalamus (Gregg et al. 2003). It has closer relations to the affect of fear. At this point, the Fight-Flight Dimension comes into play (Chap. 7 Drive). Activity of neuron groups involved in defensive aggression leads to the activation of neurons in the periaqueductal gray. They are closely related to the flight reaction. There is apparently a mutual inhibition of these neurons and the neurons of the lateral hypothalamus, which mediate predatory aggression, with this inhibition being exerted via GABA receptors. The behavior of predation is associated with the attack pole on the Fight-Flight Dimension. Other researchers have studied aggression in rival fights. In this case, a rodent is placed in another's cage, and the resulting aggressive combat actions are examined. However, stress reactions and post-fight differences between winners and losers are rather confounding variables when it comes to a more precise determination of the neurobiology of aggression.

The hypothalamic regions for aggression should be considered subcortical centers for the aggression program. The information is relayed by the mentioned neurons to other brainstem centers responsible for pupil dilation, increased heart rate and blood pressure, piloerection, and the generation of affective accompanying sounds. Facial expressions, gestures, and body posture of the affect aggression are presumably also organized via neurons of the emotional-motor system (see above).

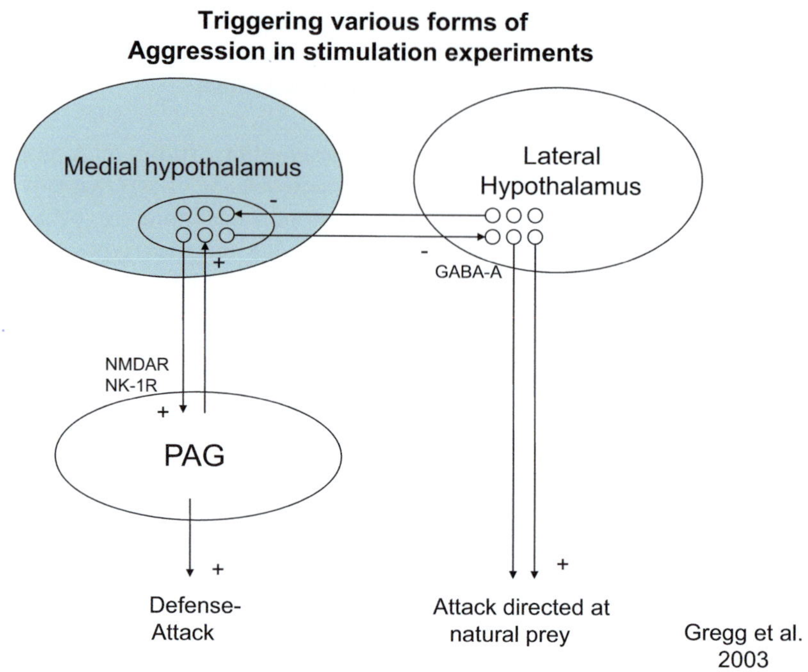

Fig. 11.7 Cell groups in the hypothalamus control aggressive behaviors in animal experiments. Cells in the medial hypothalamus are responsible for the attack for defense, which trigger aggression motor skills via the periaqueductal gray (PAG). Cell groups in the lateral hypothalamus, which are found to be responsible for aggression directed at natural prey, are in mutual inhibition with those mentioned in the medial hypothalamus (Mod. after Gregg et al. 2003)

To what extent the findings of aggression research can be transferred to human psychopathology is, of course, questionable. However, the regulatory processes that can be studied in animals are likely also present in humans, although additional control mechanisms, such as the cortical control of aggression triggering, are likely to have been added in humans (see above Pietrini et al. 2000).

11.4.5 Neuroscience of Affect Control

A person can not only control their motor actions and have more or less perfect control over impulses, but they also have a certain control over their emotions and affects. Two areas of control are to be distinguished:

1. The cognitive influence on emotion triggering. This can be found in textbooks of psychotherapy, such as cognitive behavioral therapy.
2. A person has control over the expression of affects. They can suppress laughter, secretly experience joy, stop aggressive behavior, etc.

This second emotional control works more or less well. Although it is not always possible to suppress inappropriate laughter, crying, and aggressiveness, most people manage to control it at least in the most important situations. On the one hand, the expression of affect is prevented or at least reduced or shortened. The attempt to prevent innate motor skills sometimes leads to strange results, such as when suppressing yawning.

The very unfortunate old term “affect incontinence” primarily describes a deficit in the area of affect expression: a disorder of the control of affect expression—patients cannot suppress a strong affect or limit the extent of affect expression. As mentioned above, the disorder of pathological laughing and crying indicates the vulnerability of the ability to control affect expression. Pseudobulbar palsy with significant damage to the connections from the cortex to all subcortical emotion centers is well known, especially from vascular damage to the brain. In this clinical syndrome, there is affect lability with unusually quickly triggered affects, and affect control disorder.

While the control of the expression of emotions undeniably exists, on the other hand, control over the experience of emotion is more problematic. Frontal cortical mechanisms of anxiety control have already been presented (see above). Clinically, it is noticeable that PTSD (post-traumatic stress disorder) can be reactivated in old age, which had receded into the background, i.e., was controlled, in adulthood. A mechanism was already mentioned in the presentation of the control of acquired anxiety reactions (see above). This involves an inhibitory control of the amygdala in relearned anxiety reactions through feedback from frontal neurons that receive information about the arrival of the anxiety stimulus from the amygdala (Milad and Quirk 2002; Fig. 11.8).

The discussed mechanism of suppression of anxiety reactions assumes an interaction of frontal control mechanisms with the amygdala. In general, there seems to be an "interface" in the medial frontal cortex between cortical information processing and brainstem areas or the hypothalamus (Price 1999). The influence can involve different mechanisms. An influence of these neurons on emotional, instinctive, and vegetative mechanisms is to be assumed. The loss of control of affect expression, of vegetative reactions in emotional responses, or possibly also in the experience of emotions is likely to be associated with damage to this brain region. In cases of damage to this region critical for emotions, which is bilaterally organized, i.e., affects the corresponding brain areas of both hemispheres, emotional changes are observed (Bush et al. 2000; Hornak et al. 2003). In frontotemporal dementias, which specifically affect the frontal brain, and in Pick's disease, which also affects the frontal lobe, disinhibitions of affect expression, but also of affect experience, are observed (Reischies 2005). Specifically, the mediofrontal brain areas appear to be damaged in frontotemporal dementia. To what extent frontal information processing in general or specifically frontal control mechanisms of emotionality are related to serotonergic innervation (New et al. 2002) is still unclear. Certain therapeutic improvements after serotonin reuptake inhibitors in frontotemporal dementia do not yet allow further conclusions. Valproic acid, which not only achieves general sedation but particularly enables better control of aggressive impulses, is also partially effective. This is used in mania therapy and in the treatment of frontotemporal dementia.

Control of Self-Administration of Pleasant Stimuli

When affect control or emotional regulation is mentioned, it is usually in the areas described above. But there is another field of influence on emotions in the area of positive valence. People can promote their positive emotions. The term self-indulgence seems more appropriate than self-reward. For it is not a reward in the strict sense, what would a person be rewarding himself for when he treats himself to ice cream, a praline, or a cigar? It is usually something that in colloquial language is more likely to be described as lack of discipline or "letting oneself go."

When a person indulges in something pleasant to eat or drink, such as their favorite food, a glass of wine, a warm bath, or a moment of joy in a game, he can initially enhance his own feeling of happiness (Chap. 7; textbooks of behavioral therapy). He applies direct, primary reinforcers, such as sugar, but also indirect reinforcers like money, recognition, and applause. Generally, it is considered that the positive feeling increases with the "dose" of what is applied. However, the joy is dampened by the expectation of negative consequences, such as waking up with an empty wallet after a shopping spree. One can assume a maximum of the positive effect of self-administered reinforcers. This occurs due to the reduction by negative

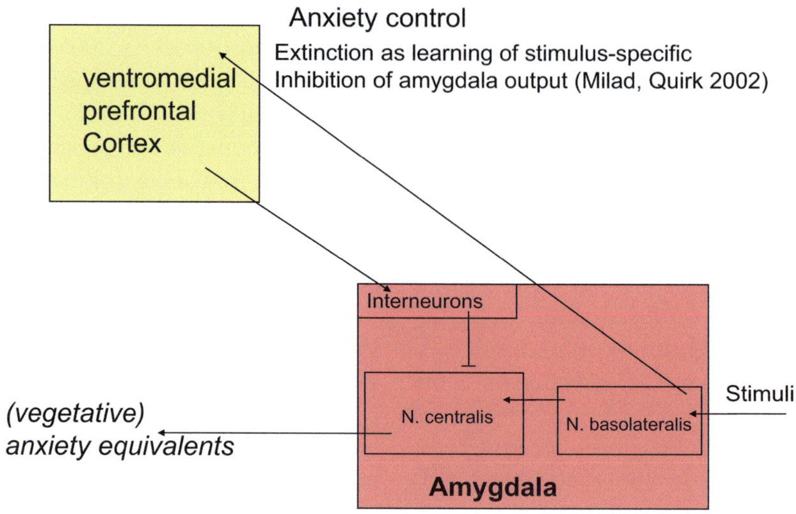

Fig. 11.8 Inhibition of amygdala activity (Mod. after Milad and Quirk 2002). The neurons of the amygdala initially respond immediately to an anxiety object after the anxiety reaction has been conditioned; however, the prefrontal cortex can inhibit amygdala activity. This has been shown especially for the medial prefrontal cortex. When an extinction of the conditioned anxiety object has been accomplished, neurons respond to the activity of the basolateral "input nucleus" of the amygdala and can in turn inhibit the central nucleus of the amygdala via interneurons—and thus the output of the nucleus. This blocks the activation of the outputs shown in Fig. 11.5 to the nuclei that mediate the anxiety reactions. Conditioned anxiety thus seems to be able to be unlearned through active inhibition.

consequences in the upper "dose range." Thus, it results from the balance of the expectation of positive emotions and negative consequences.

Addiction usually also involves tolerance development and withdrawal symptoms. This refers to the somatic factor, i.e., the factor of adaptation of physiological processes to the drug effect. One effect of the drug is that, in the course of addiction development, it must be self-administered to avoid withdrawal symptoms. However, this is not sufficient to explain the development of addiction in most cases.

Additionally, there is a tendency for "dose escalation" in response to a reduction in the positive effect on the reward system (which particularly reacts to unexpectedly high rewards). A model of shifting the sufficient dose to ever higher doses that need to be administered has been established. This includes an increase in the dose of the drug or the amount of winnings in gambling, relative to what is necessary to trigger a feeling of happiness in healthy people. In the example of the addicted gambler compared to the non-addicted gambler, low winnings lead to a lesser positive emotion, and the joy increases with higher stakes and winnings. For the non-addicted gambler, there is a maximum stake and thus the expectation of winnings, after which, with too high stakes, the expectation of negative consequences prevails, and considering the overall situation, the game for these high stakes is avoided. Functional imaging procedures in card games with addicted and non-addicted gamblers have shown that "normal," smaller winnings could only trigger lower activity in the ventral striatum of addicted gamblers compared to non-addicted gamblers, who showed more pronounced activation. This finding is also observed in drug addicts.

Thus, the value system seems to be reshaped in the development of addiction, with the maximum expected joy being shifted in such a way that joy can only be felt when relatively high risks must be taken. This is only possible if the person evaluates the expectation of negative consequences lower than a healthy person. When thinking about cigarette smoking, it becomes clear how specific the reshaping of the value system can be. Although the smoker structures their day around this addiction need and bears severe consequences, they can function normally in all other areas. This is also the case for the majority of heroin addicts in methadone substitution programs.

An explanation for the shift in the maximum of self-indulgent stimulation could be that through the experience of excessively strong pleasant stimulation, such as from ecstatic exaggerations or great feelings of happiness, the reward system is adjusted, with two explanations being discussed: On the one hand, a change in the reward system through learning of relative reward stimuli, and on the other hand, a metabolic adjustment of the trigger point in the reward system, specifically in the Ncl. accumbens or in the afferent neurons of the ventral tegmentum. Is there a special drug effect of heroin in the adjustment of the reward system? This occurs

a) due to supernaturally high reward values that were experienced, or
b) due to the specific drug effect that directly adjusts the reward system and fixes it in the adjusted situation.

The term "self-indulgence" is unfortunate because in the pathological case of addiction, self-indulgence turns into self-neglect; perhaps the term "autohedonia" would be more appropriate. The introduction of autohedonic stimuli is also subject to control: How is it prevented that all people are constantly occupied with organizing and consuming opium, sugar, winnings, etc.? Normally, a person can control the self-administration of pleasant stimuli. This happens partly through executive planning, where pleasant things are reconciled with necessary daily duties. This avoids the bad consequences of enjoying the pleasant things, drugs, etc. Planning is also successful through the anticipation of negative stimuli, the consequences of overindulgence by self-administration of positive stimuli.

11.4.6 Summary of the Neuroscientific Aspects of Emotion

Initial research results indicate a subcortical processing of the respective emotion program. Specific centers mediate the triggering of the emotion of specific vegetative somatic reactions, motor readiness, innate movement programs, and motor expressive behavior. In part, we know where neuron groups can be found that perform this function. The specific psychopharmacological influenceability suggests the involvement of various neurononal systems.

For the neurologist Damasio (1994), emotions involve the brain's ability to assess bodily reactions to past and future expected reactions, both in the autonomic nervous system and in the voluntarily controlled system. He speaks of somatic markers.

The emotional system is further explained as an archaic system, which 1) is at first differentiated according to the valence systems and 2) can adapt behavior from the feedback of body states to the preceding experiences (negative or positive valence) and expectations—especially after one's own actions (Reischies 2021). This explanatory approach is initially very abstract. For the evolution of the emotional system, such a self-control system is assumed. However, it became significantly more differentiated in the development to humans, both in the triggering of emotions and in aspects of affect control. In humans, cognitive and intentional aspects play a major role in the triggering of affect, and cortical effects of emotion regulation and affect control gain a certain influence on affect expression. These mechanisms are particularly susceptible to disturbances.

11.5 Psychopathological Symptoms of Emotion and Affect

Preliminary Remark
The classification of emotion features follows the valence polarity— negative and positive

valence—i.e., initially, features associated with the depressive syndrome are described, then those associated with the manic syndrome. Negative valence is not presented as an independent emotional feature; it to some extent merges into the feature of depressed mood. The symptom of depressed mood has no specific quality for the experiencing subject, compared to anger or sadness. It is uncharacteristically negative, ranging from mild negative mood, which is often not recognized by the person himself, to excruciating suffering—the extreme negative valence.

As already indicated, valence is conceived as an independent emotional dimension that runs parallel to emotions, perceptions, or activities and conveys a positive or negative sensation to them. This makes it possible to explain that an attack with an aggressive feeling can be perceived as negative or positive, and pain can be perceived as devastatingly negative or—in the context of pleasure—positive.

a) Negative Valence
   anhedonia , depressed mood, feelings of guilt, feelings of shame, complaintiveness, feelings of insufficiency, inner restlessness, anxious, phobic anxiety, hypochondria, somatization, disturbance of vital feelings, suspicion
b) Positive Valence
   euphoric, ecstasy/rapture, increased self-esteem
c) Other features related to emotion:
   dysphoric, irritable, aggressive behavior, increased agitation, increased feeling of disgust,
d) Then follow features of emotional responsiveness and affect control and finally
e) Obsessive compulsive symptoms

11.5.1 Negative Valence—Depressive Syndrome

Anhedonia

Definition.
Reduction of positive emotion in the number of joyful reactions as well as in the subjective and objectively observable quality of the joyful reaction (extent and duration—each compared to earlier), reduction of joy-related action readiness.

Example

- A person can no longer feel joy when they receive a call from their children or when visitors come and bring something, although they state that they would have been very happy in the same situation earlier.
- A person in a severe grief reaction cannot feel joy,
- A person who is distanced from a paranoia appears unmotivated and shows no initiative and only gets up to eat and go to the toilet. When asked, they say that nothing brings them joy anymore, they cannot be motivated by anything. ◀

Position in Psychopathology. Not in the AMDP, but in the definitions of negative symptoms in schizophrenia and the depression of many syndrome descriptions or classification systems,

- Disturbance in one of the fundamental emotions.

Related terms. Joylessness, see also loss of interest.

Psychopathological interactions:
- Feeling of numbness often meant as joylessness, while anxiety can still be felt (see below).
- anhedonia occurs, for example, as part of the depressive syndrome, with a feeling of numbness, no longer feeling love, no longer feeling appetite, reduced appetitive behavior,
- anxiety.

Differential diagnostic distinctions. Feeling of numbness also for negative emotions, such as grief in the feeling of numbness.

Self-/other persons's judgment. In mild expression predominantly self-evaluation, but in longer observation validatable other persons's judgment (through history taken from other persons—supported by behavioral observation).

Interview for rating. Question about joyful experiences, behavioral observation, history taken from other persons.

Neuropsychology/objectification:

- Behavioral observation of the emotional "mini-syndrome",
- Attempt to elicit reactive joy, to induce cheerfulness.

Severity. Assessment of the degree and inadequacy of behavior, reduced ability to feel joy up to the complete inability to feel joy even in usually very positively rated situations.

Personality influences. People who do not show emotions, or affect-poor personality.

Conceptual problems of the feature. The phenomenon is characteristic of the depressive syndrome and at the same time more unspecific—it can help to better describe schizophrenic patients and those with neuropsychiatric syndromes. Anhedonia refers to the extreme, the complete loss of joy.

Neuroscientific/cognitive-neuroscientific models

1. Disturbance of the reward system—reduction of reward-related brain activity in the basal forebrain, orbital frontal brain, and partly also the amygdala,
2. unclear to what extent anxiety and affective-cognitive complexes can inhibit positive emotionality,
3. neuronal bifurcated connection from the amygdala a) to neurons of the orbitofrontal cortex and b) of the Ncl. Accumbens—blocking of the reward center by neurons in the habenula of the thalamus (Matsumoto and Hikosaka 2007; Hikosaka 2010).

Depressed Mood

Definition.
Mood with predominant sensation of negative valence, downcast, gloomy, depressed—with an increase in negative emotions and the feeling of reduced action readiness.

Example

- A person feels bad in terms of mood, says everything is a torment, feels physically exhausted and not ready for the demands he sees coming. He sits slumped with reduced muscle tone and stares silently ahead—his eyes fixed unwaveringly on a point in front of him on the floor. When spoken to, he responds with a dull, pressed voice (see Fig. 11.1).
- A patient is downcast, in contrast to her otherwise predominantly cheerful mood. She is socially withdrawn. She displays a serious facial expression, her eyes are often lowered, and eye contact is fleeting. The speech melody is more monotonous than usual. ◀

Position in Psychopathology. AMDP 63.

Related Terms. Depressed, downcast, feeling unwell, uncomfortable, psychic suffering.

Psychopathological Interactions. Common occurrence with many features of the depressive syndrome with possible interactions: grief, despair over an event and sorrows, anhedonia and loss of interest, anxiety and feelings of hopelessness and helplessness.

Differential Diagnostic Distinctions. The feature "depressed mood" is often part of the depressive syndrome and therefore not easily distinguishable from other simultaneously occurring dimensions of the depressive syndrome:

- anhedonia, drive disorder, pseudodepression in frontal lobe disorder,

- anxiety with action readiness for flight/social withdrawal.

Further Characterization. Negative valence, the depressed mood has no own emotional quality (compared to grief or disgust), it is therefore usually described with the associated, persistently negative feelings, without anxiety being predominant (only e.g. anxiety dimension of future worries—for example due to lack of action readiness, delusional or dysfunctional future worries).

Self-/other persons's judgment. More weight on the self-evaluation (if it appears reliable—otherwise main weight on other persons's judgment of the emotional "mini-syndrome").

Interview for Rating. Subjectively introspectively downcast, depressed, consistency.

Neuropsychology/objectification:
Consistency of the subjective side with behavioral observation: objective signs in posture, tone, reflexive mobility, gestures, facial expressions, prosodyand sound of a voice, sorrow lines, partly crying,

- reaction to content-related provocation of negative emotion (grief, guilt etc.).

Severity Assessment of the severity and inadequacy of behavior, purely subjective to obviously objective—people report being in a state of suffering, of unbearable torment.

Specifications. self-reported or only upon questioning.

Conceptual Problems of the Feature. Should be supported by behavioral observation.

Neuroscientific/cognitive-neuroscientific models
1. Predominance of negative valence
2. anxiety-induced: amygdalar fear-related activity, a) primary or b) disorder of the frontal inhibition of the amygdala,
2. cerebral inhibition system overactive (relationship to fight-flight system),
3. Emotional-motor system shows a predominance of grief-related affective motor activity,
4. affective-cognitive complexes have developed, resulting in the inhibition of positive associations.

Hopeless/Pessimistic

Definition.
Thoughts about the immediate, near future and the more distant future are determined by increased sorrows, with the probability of negative outcomes of current developments coming to the forefront. The expectations are affectively negatively tinged.

Example

A patient with a depression doubts whether he can recover, whether his family can continue to live in good circumstances, and above all, whether the hospital treatment can be paid for, even though he knows that he is insured and financially secure. ◀

Position in psychopathology. AMDP 64.

Related terms. Pessimism, fear of the future.

Psychopathological interactions. Interactions in the depressive syndrome with anhedonia, low mood, depressive delusions, helplessness, suicidality (conversely, hopelessness is also a prerequisite for suicidality), brooding.

Differential diagnostic distinctions:
- appropriate reaction to real acute resource loss with realistic future concerns,
- help seeking behaviour,

Further characterization: A more cognitive feature of the depression syndrome,

- cognitive selection and focus on the future negative; dysfunctional cognition.

Interview for rating. Questions about the future with follow-up questions on whether sorrows could be justified, history taken from other persons.

Neuropsychology/objectification. Observation of dealing with hopeful future prospects.

Severity. Assessment of the extent and inadequacy of behavior, from normal variance of realistic pessimistic assessment to devaluation of all personal preferences due to merely possible, but assumed certain, losses and failures.

Pathognomonic for: depressive syndrome, pessimistic basic attitude in personality trait.

Specifications. Spontaneously expressed or only upon inquiry.

Personality influences. "Pessimist" as a personality variant.

Conceptual problems of the feature. Purely subjective feature, which is expressed through speech acts. This may possibly express help seeking behaviour.

Neuroscientific/ Cognitive Neuroscientific Models

1. affective-cognitive complex in the field of expectations with mutual reinforcement of a) selection of negative associations and prospects and b) affective evaluation of negative developments.
2. Anticipatory anxiety with action readiness; the person sees himself in the expectation of negative development of events (e.g., depressed view of his own resources for managing and coping with future developments).
3. Blocking and devaluation of positive development potentials a) through anxiety and b) brooding with pressing negative thoughts that inhibit consideration of positive developments.
4. Assessment bias—dysfunctional thinking with acceptance of negative assessment and rejection of positive development evaluation,
5. The apparently physiologically present (and anthropologically functional) more positive attitude relative to the objective facts regarding one's own chances is disturbed.

Guilt Feelings

Definition.
Negative assessment of one's own action—the perspective is retrospective with recalling one's own mistakes or moral failures—as well as negative reinterpretation of positive achievements,

- predominantly cognitive feature of the depressive syndrome.

Example

A woman reproaches herself for agreeing to build a house, because during the construction of the house, her husband died of a heart attack. She has strong guilt feelings for having "driven her husband to death." ◄

Position in Psychopathology. AMDP 73.

Related Terms. Self-reproaches, self-devaluation.

Psychopathological Interaction. Brooding, overvalued idea, other dysfunctional cognitions, delusion.

Differential Diagnostic Distinctions. Public Shaming, Feelings of Shame, depressive delusion. Habitually socially humble demeanor.

Further Characterization. Mostly dysfunctional cognitions, negative selection of memories, reinterpretation of memories towards one's own guilt. Relatively higher weighting of the supposed mistake (or one's own failure) in relation to the person's expectations or standards.

Interview for Rating. Question whether the person has something to reproach themselves for, e.g., brooding over it, history taken from other persons.

Neuropsychology/Objectification. Observation of dealing with alternative assessments of situations that have led to guilt feelings.

Severity Assessment of the extent and inadequacy of behavior, selection of negative events up to delusion-like reinterpretation of clearly positive achievements as failures and guilt.

Specifications. Spontaneously or only expressed upon inquiry.

Personality Influences. Conscientiousness.

Conceptual Problems of the Feature. Purely subjective feature, which is expressed through speech act. Questionable independence from the spectrum: delusion—dysfunctional thinking.

Neuroscientific/Cognitive Neuroscientific Models

1. Affective-Cognitive Complex with mutual reinforcement of negative memory selection and affective evaluation of negative past developments.
2. Memory—Selective recall from episodic and autobiographical memory,
3. Assessment bias with acceptance of negative assessment and rejection of positive evaluation of past developments.

Feelings of Shame

Definition.
Feeling of exposure to others of (supposed) mistakes and deficiencies. In doing so, the person sees moral expectations or performance expectations of the environment as disappointed. The expectation of physical appearance can also seem violated, for example, regarding subjectively unacceptable physical characteristics (of the body or appearance) that suddenly become visible.

Examples

- A patient remains silent in the examination situation, which is extremely uncomfortable for him, as topics are addressed that he believes expose him.
- A patient believes he can no longer be seen in the circle of colleagues and friends after a behavioral disorder has occurred.
- A person fears showing himself to friends after his high-flying career plans have been thwarted. ◀

Position in Psychopathology. New AMDP as additional item ZP9.

Related Terms. Modesty.

Psychopathological Interactions. Conscientiousness, social anxiety.

Differential Diagnostic Distinctions. 1) Feelings of guilt—more in retrospect regarding external norms versus 2) Shame more in the present or immediately impending disclosure of discrepancies to expectation, exposure; dysmorphophobia; social anxiety.

Further Characterization. 1.) High expectations of oneself are 2.) supposedly not met.

Interview for Rating. Questions about experiences of shame and fear of shame, history taken from other persons.

Neuropsychology/objectification: Vegetative signs (blushing in embarrassing situations)

- Observing the confrontation with a shame-inducing situation.

Severity. Assessment of the extent and inadequacy of behavior, a) intensity and frequency, which justify the dysfunctionality, b) the extent of reactions to embarrassment should be described. Effects of fear of shame, efforts to avoid shame.

Specifications:

- concrete shame in the situation,
- expectation of an embarrassing disclosure, fear of shame
- Processing of embarrassing situations—reactions to embarrassment, development of avoidance and change of attitudes.

Personality Influences. More common in certain individuals and in youth (or potentially a kind of behavior in establishing relationships).

Conceptual Problems of the Feature. Often not sufficiently separated from feelings of guilt. Neuroscientific/cognitive neuroscientific models

1. learning history with model learning of adopting expectations, identifications, partly religious, moral development - development of demands on one's own actions and appearance and acceptance of internal but also external evaluation instances,
2. regarding performance and moral claims as well as aesthetic standards,
3. Reactions and conscious measures of the person after an embarrassment, avoidance, compensation efforts
4. Anticipatory anxiety before an embarrassing disclosure.

Complaintive – moaning

Definition.
A person expresses suffering culturally inappropriately strongly, with pronounced help seeking behaviour. In doing so, they accept the harassment of others (even if this proves to be dysfunctional); the complaint behavior is repetitive.

Complaints can be presented morosely/dysphorically (sullenly) or full of reproaches.

Example

A patient walks up and down the corridor groaning and seeking attention, repeatedly knocks on the door of the clinic staff, and is clingy in direct contact. He repeatedly calls his children, asking them to organize more help for him, etc. ◄

Position in psychopathology. AMDP 70.

Psychopathological interactions. anxiety, inner restlessness, pronounced dissatisfaction with oneself and one's situation.

Differential diagnostic distinctions:
- Manipulative behavior ,
- Increased drive, sometimes difficult to distinguish from manic-depressive mixed state (in mania increase in targeted drive).

Further characterization. Demonstrative help seeking behaviour by emphasizing one's own suffering.

self-/external rating. External rating.

Interview for rating. Interview with introspection, history taken from other persons.

Neuropsychology/objectification. Behavioral observation—spontaneous everyday behavior, communication behavior, expressive behavior (consider cultural peculiarities)—reaction to attention.

Severity. Assessment of the extent and inadequacy of behavior, conspicuously strong help seeking behaviour to stereotypically presented complaints that hinder communication.

Pathognomonic for: Mostly an element of the depressive syndrome (agitated depression, "whining depression"), but also in somatization or hypochondriacal complaints, etc.

Specifications. Predominant help seeking behaviour versus affect control disorder regarding the expression of one's own suffering.

Personality influences. Histrionic personality.

Conceptual problems of the feature:
- Speech acts that express features of the depressive syndrome,
- Behavioral variant of the depressive syndrome (social withdrawal is more common).

Neuroscientific/cognitive neuroscientific models
1. Depressed suffering leads to inner restlessness, which the patient acts out.
2. learning history: e.g., trained in nursing homes when caregivers only respond to loud lamentations—the person can particularly poorly endure negative states.

Feelings of Insufficiency

Definition.
The confidence in one's own strength and skill to master the future is diminished to extinguished. The concrete expectation of one's own performance in the current situation is inappropriately strongly reduced.

Example

A patient with excellent performance as a young doctor suddenly feels overwhelmed and inferior and thus presents himself as so incapable that the interlocutors get the impression that he has chosen the wrong profession. ◀

Position in Psychopathology. AMDP 71.

Related Terms. Loss of self-confidence, self-esteem.

Psychopathological Interactions. If the person is performance-oriented, assessments of worthlessness occur more easily; depressive dysfunctional cognition, e.g., the generalization of random failures, etc.

Differential Diagnostic Distinctions. The assessment of a weakening, clumsiness, or cognitive impairment must be inappropriate, exaggerated, or the subject of a depressive delusion.

Self-/other persons's judgment. Other persons's judgment.

Interview for Rating. Questions about the evaluation of performance, being up to the tasks, history taken from other persons.

Neuropsychology/objectification. In the interview, observation of the engagement with positive aspects of one's own resources or performance.

Severity. Self-confidence reduced to globally extinguished – with reinterpretation of previous high achievements and the boundary of inadequacy delusion—inadequacy of behavior

Specifications:
- excessive unrealistic performance expectations,
- with or without premorbid performance orientation
- domain-specific or generalized.

Personality Influences. Premorbid high performance orientation.

Conceptual Problems of the Symptom. Assessment of appropriateness can be difficult in cases of mild feelings of inadequacy.

Neuroscientific/Cognitive Neuroscientific Models Affective-cognitive complex with mutual reinforcement. Selection of topics about current incapacity or powerlessness and drive inhibition and recollection of mistakes and failure experiences. Affective evaluation of negative performances—present and past.

Inner Restlessness

Definition.
Sensation of an unexplainable restlessness, which is perceived in the body or psyche and experienced as negative or tormenting

- often reported as rising from the chest

Example

- A patient with severe depression states that due to a feeling in the chest, which is unbearably tormenting and can be described as restlessness, he cannot continue living like this. ◀

Position in Psychopathology. AMDP 69.

Psychopathological Interactions. Negative valence, depressive syndrome, feeling of insufficiency, feeling of guilt, anxiety, depressive delusion

Differential Diagnostic Distinctions:
- Unlike motor restlessness, there is no urge to move
- Pressing thoughts,
- Restless legs,
- Akathisia—restlessness predominantly in the legs, motoric.

Further Characterization. Unjustified arousal that leads to nothing, but causes restlessness .

Self-/Other Person's Judgment. The statement of the person is necessary and other person's judgment.

Interview for Rating. When asked if restlessness is felt, follow-up questions based on observations, history taken from other persons.

Neuropsychology/Objectification. Observation in relaxation situations.

Severity. Assessment of the severity (interference with the interview) and inadequacy of behavior: Slight reduction of possible calmness to unbearable restlessness.

Specifications:
- Inability to relax—with/without physical tension,
- Experienced restlessness—psychological, somatic.

Conceptual problems of the feature. Sometimes the feature is described by the person as anxiety.

Neuroscientific/Cognitive-Neuroscientific Models
1. Strong negative valence perceived in the body as tormenting
2. arousal, anxiety equivalent, agitation in the somatosensory system,

Anxious

Definition.
The person perceives the emotional state as strongly negative and usually accompanied by a vegetative reaction and tension. This refers anticipatorily to a threatening situation or the expectation of an imminent danger or impairment.

- The person identifies the feeling as "anxiety" or negative condition.
- Panic, anticipatory anxiety, or anxious avoidance behavior

Example

A patient suddenly starts sweating and trembling. He says he doesn't know what's wrong with him, but he has anxiety, about to die or somehow go crazy, become insane. He grabs his chest and checks his pulse, which is increasingly tachycardic. He hyperventilates. When asked, he states that he feels extremely uncomfortable. ◀

Position in Psychopathology. AMDP 65.

Related Terms. Fear referred to as anxiety in concrete threat situations, general anxiety, panic attack, being easily scared (often associated with lack of self-confidence, despondency). An acute state of anxiety is referred to as "state anxiety" and a persistent disposition to anxiety is referred to as "trait anxiety".

Psychopathological Interactions. Lack of self-confidence and underestimation of one's own strength—on the fight-flight dimension.

Differential Diagnostic Distinctions:
- phobic anxiety, situation-bound anxiety
- appropriate emotional reaction to dangerous situations or caution and avoidance behavior,
- aggravation, simulation, when the state of anxiety is only reported without any objective sign or reaction to the anxiety being found.

Further Characterization. Immediate experience of specific feelings of threat or their equivalents in concrete impairment or anticipatory of negative events or experiences, whether they are real or only imagined. Expectation of suffering; there is apparently no specific sensation for anxiety, but predominantly somatic characteristics of emotional experience.

Self-/Other Person's Judgment. Emotional mini-syndrome that exhibits subjective and objective characteristics.

Interview for Rating. In mild anxiety without external signs, prompt introspection about possible feelings of anxiety, history taken from other persons.

Neuropsychology/Objectification. The behavior and confrontation with the situation perceived as threatening are observed.

Severity. Expression and inadequacy of behavior are assessed,

a) which anxiety reactions, anxiety characteristics—the relation of negative events to the extent of anxiety,
b) extent of vegetative, motor reaction.

Specifications:
- psychotic anxiety (diffuse form of anxiety that is to be classified with a feeling of threat within the framework of paranoid schizophrenia)
- being easily scared,
- or remaining anxiety (all other forms of anxiety);
- in the anxiety syndrome—a predominance of the emotional, cognitive, vegetative, or motor symptom area.
- inadequacy of behavior, real vs. imagined threat situation, acute or future threat
- expected emotional state
- extent of efforts to overcome anxiety

Neuroscientific/cognitive neuroscientific models
Anxiety is explained as a symptom of the immediate expectation of a painful event.

1. Dysfunctional amygdala activity leading to unwarranted anxiety signals,
2. concrete psychomotor-vegetative anxiety reaction—activation of the fight-flight system with predominance of the flight component, i.e., predominance of the related perceptual activity,
   - in learning history possibly a consequence of imprinting through severe inferiority/victim situations,
3. anticipatory anxiety with evaluation of response options,
4. emotional-motor system, anxiety motor reactions activated,
5. lack of extinction or inhibition of amygdala neurons by the medial ventral prefrontal cortex (Milad and Quirk 2002)
5. anxiety reaction apparently belongs to the central information processing in the amygdala (LeDoux 1996), neuronal connection for the anxiety reaction: thalamus, lateral nucleus of the amygdala, central nucleus of the amygdala, brainstem.
   - stimulation of the amygdala: anxiety, generally negative emotions, rarely positive emotions (see Gloor 1997) functional activation by emotionally negative stimuli; loss of anxiety syndrome after bilateral lesions of the amygdala.

Phobic Anxiety

Definition.
Unjustified fear in a specific situation with an imagined threat—usually accompanied by avoidance behavior.

Example

A patient cannot walk over a bridge. When he approaches the bridge, anxious restless sensations begin with trembling, sweating, and tachycardia, accompanied by thoughts that the bridge is unsafe, especially regarding the railing, which could fail in a gust of wind (this is objectively not the case); or he might fall over the railing into the depths. He stops and looks for a way out of the situation, i.e., how he could reach his destination without crossing the bridge. ◀

Position in psychopathology. AMDP 29.

Psychopathological interactions. Learned, conditioned aversive reaction.

Differential diagnostic distinctions: Anxiety without a clear trigger.

Self-/other persons' judgment. Combined.

Interview for rating. Question about the feeling of anxiety and the situational coupling, behavioral observation, and history taken from other persons.

Neuropsychology/objectification. Behavior and confrontation with the situation perceived as threatening are observed—anxiety during the imagination of approaching the fear object?

Severity:
- Assessment of the extent and inadequacy of behavior ,
- Extent of the psychological, cognitive, and vegetative motor anxiety reaction.

Specifications:
- Many names for objects of fear—distinguished are the concrete fear of objects/animals or specific situations such as height or confinement and
- the social anxiety—for example, fear of being seen in public.
- Psychotic anxiety towards a person who is delusionally perceived as an enemy (let the initial situation be described),
- Extent of the efforts to overcome the phobic anxiety to achieve a normal social functioning level vs. giving in to avoidance behavior.

Personality influences. Lack of self-confidence, self-insecurity, problematic confrontation with death

Neuroscientific/cognitive neuroscientific models
1. Prototype of affective-cognitive complexes, a stimulus is conditioned to affect, anxiety reaction with flight tendency (in the fight-flight system) with subsequent increase in avoidance behavior,
2. Conditioning/tuning of amygdala neurons persistently to properties of the object of fear (if not inhibited by frontal neurons—i.e., failing control of the amygdala's anxiety triggering by medial ventral prefrontal activity),
3. Stabilization of avoidance behavior—due to the reward each time by avoiding negative emotionality (behavioral therapeutic approach),
4. Prevention of extinction through avoidance behavior (by means of labilization of the memory trace in the postulated reconsolidation process).

Suspiciousness

Definition.
Expectation of negative attitude or hostile actions against oneself—Watching for signs of hostile attitude or impending attacks/hostilities.

Example

An older man assumes that his relatives are only after his money, interpreting every visit and every kindness as an effort to ingratiate themselves or as inheritance fraud or attempts to steal or cheat.

- A woman is overly anxious during a taxi ride, watching whether the driver takes a detour or if he grabs her wallet or suitcase and drives away when paying. ◀

Position in Psychopathology. AMDP 29.

Related Terms. Assumption of hostility, aversive relationship assumption

Psychopathological Interactions. Hyperarousal, content-related thought disorders (paranoia), anxiety, aggressiveness.

Differential Diagnostic Distinctions. Anxiety symptoms, realistic hostility (e.g., in emigration, uprooting situations), delusion.

Interview for Rating. Question about trust towards strangers, history taken from other persons (e.g., clinic, practice staff).

Neuropsychology/objectification. Observation in confrontation with new people

Severity. Assessment of the degree and inadequacy of behavior up to the inability to trust another person and severe impairment (because everyone in the environment would have bad intentions).

Specifications:

1 with delusion,
without delusion,
- general insecurity and suspicious search for dangers,
- suspicion towards specific persons or institutions.

2 Area-specific: e.g., pathological jealousy

Neuroscientific/cognitive neuroscientific models. affective-cognitive complex—Danger is perceived in situations where others would consider this fear to be inappropriate.

1. anxiety, aggression—shift on the fight-flight axis,
2. Projection mechanism: one's own aggressiveness is not perceived, a) but aggressive reactions of the environment are anticipated and b) the atmosphere is changed by affective expression, thereby self-provoking signs of tension in others,
3. learning history of reducing internal tensions when attention is turned to an external danger

Perplexed

Definition.
The person feels exposed to a situation he does not understand. The person is perplexed, astonished, amazed—noticing the failure of his own resources to help himself or to obtain help.

Example

- A patient does not know immediately after an car-accident what has happened, what is "wrong" with him. He appears, waking up from unconsciousness, bewildered by what is happening to him.
- Prototype: perplexity upon awakening from a coma. ◀

Position in Psychopathology. AMDP 59.

Related Terms. Astonished, helpless.

Psychopathological Interactions. Disorientation, especially situational orientation with relationship to the disturbance of awareness of the environment, memory impairment, memory disorder, concentration disorder.

Differential Diagnostic Delimitations. Dissociative states

Further Characterization. Subjective side in brain damage syndromes with disorientation, feeling of "not knowing what to do next".

Interview for Rating. Question about how the person feels in the situation

Neuropsychology/objectification. Investigation of orientation and amnestic symptoms, behavioral observation, dealing with the mastery of the situation.

Neuroscientific/cognitive neuroscientific models
The person does not yet understand the situation, for example in reorientation after an event.

Somatic sensations and their disorders
The next symptoms relate to the body, the bodily sensation, or the attention to the possible bodily symptoms of diseases. The distinction between the person's body, which we fellow humans can perceive (like the skin), and the subjective body that the person experiences themselves, is helpful. The difference in perspective brings useful clarifications in the body-related symptoms.

Hypochondriac and somatization symptoms are presented. Central is the anxious attention related to the body. Problems arise with psychosomatic features, e.g., pain symptoms in mental illnesses, alexithymia, and a feeling of physical freshness or fatigue, as in the vital symptomatology of depression.

Table 11.2 provides an overview of various terms in this area.

Hypochondriacal Anxiety

Definition.
Anxious thoughts or belief that one is suffering from a dangerous disease for which there is no evidence, or the anxiety of dying soon from a diagnosed disease that is harmless according to medical diagnosis.

Example

- A patient has anxiety about having or contracting AIDS. He constantly thinks about ways of infection and doubts all reassuring medical findings.
- A patient repeatedly thinks he is seriously heart-diseased and will die of a heart attack. Examinations are conducted, but he does not trust the negative findings, believing that the next, more specific examination or a more capable specialist will show that he is right in assuming he has heart disease. ◀

Position in Psychopathology. AMDP 28.

Related Terms. Nosophobia.

Psychopathological Interactions.
- Depression
- Somatization (focus on symptoms, not on a disease, as in hypochondria. In somatization, the patient suffers from the symptom, for example, pain; in hypochondria, the anxiety concerns the disease behind a harmless symptom, including fantasies of death),
- Cardiophobia (both panic attacks with tachycardia and the anxiety of dying immediately from heart dysfunction occur, especially the anxiety of not surviving the current episode),

Differential Diagnostic Distinctions. Hypochondriacal delusion is to be distinguished (Chap. 13 Delusion—content-related thought disorders).

Further Characterization. The person is convinced of being misdiagnosed and reacts overexcitedly when reading reports about the supposed disease in the media. He neglects other aspects of life management.

Table 11.2. Differentiation of various terms in the somatic area—using the example of pain

Designation	Stimulus	Pain	Expression	Comment
somatization	none	yes	yes	attention to symptom
hypochondria	none or insufficient	yes	variable	concept of illness incorrect
body hallucination	none	yes	questionable	partly bizarre
simulation	none	none	yes	conscious symptom fake

Interview for Rating. Question about the concept of illness, whether a somatic disease is responsible for the person's suffering, history taken from other persons.

Neuropsychology/Objectification. Behavior and dealing with the perceived threatening physical danger are observed, dealing with negative findings.

Severity:
Assessment of the extent and inadequacy of behavior

a) Preoccupation in intensity and time consumption with the concern about illness,
b) Extent of actions resulting from the symptoms, such as doctor consultations, hospital admissions.

Neuroscientific/Cognitive Neuroscientific Models.
1. Specific anxiety theme, affective-cognitive complex with the content of disease,
2. Learning history—experience that internal tensions and ambivalences are alleviated when the person focuses on illness anxiety; modeling in the family
3. Regressive functional disorder, the patient gives up self-control and current goals, and the fantasy arises that his life is in danger

Somatization

Definition.
Fixation of attention on physical symptoms or suffering from diagnostically nonspecific symptoms such as pain; difficult to assess due to bodily misperceptions or misjudgments.

No pathophysiological correlate can be found for the reported symptoms, or none sufficient to explain the extent of the described complaints.

In many cases, the environment is to be made aware of the patient's suffering.

Example

- A man focusses attention only on the pain he feels in his back. No pathological finding was found during examinations. The patient spares himself, although he is told that he should start back training to strengthen the muscles.
- An elderly woman spends most of the day dealing with bowel movements, anxiously paying attention to every bowel movement. ◀

Position in psychopathology. Not listed in AMDP, but constitutive for, e.g., somatization disorder and to be distinguished from hypochondria.

Related terms. fixated on physical complaints

Differential diagnostic distinctions:
- without belief of suffering from a specific disease (hypochondria),
- Coenesthesia, body hallucinations,
- Simulation ("secondary gain from illness", theatrical presentation, tendency to response distortion, therefore history taken from other persons, longer observation periods—also clinically),
- depersonalization.

Interview for rating: Questions about complaints, subjective assessment on a scale, differentiation and variability of the description; valid history taken from other persons ,

- Exclusion of simulation, which is difficult to prove.

Neuropsychology/objectification:
- Behavior and dealing with the physical symptoms experienced as threatening are observed.

- Pain: Observing the dealing with pain; What do you call "pain" in the skin, for example with a needle and pinching/pressure?

Severity. Assessment of the severity and inadequacy of behavior, suffering from isolated somatization phenomena to complete preoccupation and lack of turning away from the symptoms.

Specifications:

- with vs. without anxiety ("belle indifference" type).
- Fixation of attention on a somatic symptom that is explained by somatic findings and is amplified by the fixation of attention (psychosomatic type),
- Anxiety equivalents: chest pain, dry mouth, nervous bladder, etc., which occur more frequently,
- Dissociative and conversion disorder:
- There are complaints about a perception disorder, e.g., visual disturbance, changes in consciousness, etc., dissociative type
- There are symptoms of striated muscle disorder, e.g., paralysis, conversion type

Personality influences. Histrionic personality.

Neuroscientific/cognitive neuroscientific models

- Turning towards symptom perceptions that cannot be medically explained, resulting in the amplification of dysfunctional bodily perceptions (with the limiting condition that this turning is not conscious, or a simulation is present), attention-dependent symptoms of the body (see e.g. Ramachandran 2004), learning history: milder somatic disorder features (heart palpitations, realistic pain, etc.) are anxiously picked up, attention is focussed on them, and the symptom is thereby provoked,
- Turning away of attention, for example, in the dysfunction of a limb: A patient is strangely uninvolved during the examination of a gait disorder that seems to be due to the weakness of a limb, for which no pathological finding can be demonstrated.
- Anxiety equivalents due to the connection of the amygdala with brainstem nuclei (Davis et al. 1997),
- learning history with model learning or internal tensions lead the person to turn his attention to the body—with the result of reducing the tensions—possibly symbolism of the symptoms regarding the problem situation of the specific person, whereby the individual problem situation has contributed to a selection of the symptoms.

Dysmorphophobic Anxieties

A person experiences a flaw in appearance, the body is perceived as misshapen, which is why they feel shame in contact with others.

It is usually a body schema disorder that manifests in the perception of one's own body. For example, in front of the mirror, the person looks worried about how others would perceive their body, the flaw. Influences of personal and socially communicated ideal images have an effect. Distinction from delusion.

Disturbance of Vital Feelings

Definition.
A disturbed bodily feeling with powerlessness, fatigue and loss of physical freshness. In contrast to the experience that the body otherwise functioned well, naturally. The feeling of somatic well-being is disturbed.

Example

- A patient experiences heavy limbs, making every movement feel like work, everything becomes arduous. He feels impaired by the loss of physical vitality.
- A patient experiences a powerlessness in the movements of the legs, which is also accompanied by a strange pain in the muscles and tendons. ◀

Position in Psychopathology. AMDP 62.

Psychopathological Interactions: In a morning low, the person pays attention to the bodily feeling with a certain concern and anxiety after waking up.

Differential Diagnostic Distinctions:

- Sickness behaviour, experienced in severe infection or heart failure, somatic pain, muscle diseases, etc., which can explain the perception of physical discomfort,
- Feelings of insufficiency,
- depressive inhibition with a feeling of being slowed down in movements
- Coenesthetic complaints, subjective body hallucinations

Self-/other persons's judgment. self-evaluation.

Interview for Rating. Question about physical freshness: Introspection.

Neuropsychology/objectification. Behavioral observation in everyday life, in coping with daily tasks.

Severity. Mild lack of physical freshness and vitality up to complete subjective failure of movements due to the torment they cause.

Pathognomonic for: depressive syndrome.

Specifications. If specific somatic disease signs occur, they should be documented as specifications.

Conceptual Problems of the Feature. Problematic use of the term "masked depression," where more somatizing complaints, which are at the forefront of this kind of depressive syndrome, are meant rather than the disturbance of vital feelings.

Neuroscientific/Cognitive Neuroscientific Models

No convincing models yet—possibly pathophysiological interaction with physical inhibition in depression

1. negative valence manifested in the body domain
2. somatic representation in the CNS disturbed,
3. effort-system disturbed, perception of effort thereby predominant,
4. negative somatic condition and latent pain, which are otherwise quickly forgotten in everyday life, become conscious.
5. in depressive illnesses possibly caused by muscles (model of mitochondrial disorder)

11.5.2 Positive Valence

Euphoric

> **Definition.**
> Inappropriately good mood or cheerful, with corresponding facial expressions and gestures; with action readiness for possibly inappropriate actions.

Usually with high self-esteem, the feeling of being physically and mentally highly capable,

Examples

- A young woman suddenly feels wonderful, contacts everyone and radiates joy; she believes she has good future prospects. She is in a joking mood and laughs a lot.
- She gives friends and acquaintances small gifts that clearly exceed her financial means, as she lives on social assistance.
- A patient with multiple sclerosis, who has become bedridden over the course of the illness, appears cheerful. When asked if he feels depressed at times, he states that this was once the case, but that time is now over, and he is in a good mood. ◀

Position in Psychopathology. AMDP 66.

Related Terms. Bliss, inappropriately increased joy.

Psychopathological Interactions. Increased self-esteem as a feature of the manic syndrome, judgment disorder, delusions of grandeur.

Differential Diagnostic Distinctions:
- silly mood, in a social group with good humor, joy as an appropriate affect, suddenly relieved by positive situational change,
- inappropriate jocularity (frontal lobe syndrome),
- increased drive, restlessness each without consistent positive emotions,
- simple judgment disorder without consistent positive misjudgment of one's own situation.

Further Characterization. Positive emotions that cannot be explained by a realistic assessment of the individual's situation.

Self-/Other Person's Judgment. Other person's judgment of the mood, the inappropriateness of positive emotions.

Interview for Rating. Question about possible reasons for the obviously good mood, about plans and history taken from other persons.

Neuropsychology/Objectification. Behavioral observation and observation of dealing with negative aspects of the current situation of the person.

Severity. Assessment of the extent and inadequacy of behavior, purely subjective to severe behavioral disorder with socially inappropriate actions.

Pathognomonic for: mania, personality change in brain damage syndromes.

Specifications: inadequacy of behavior
- cheerful mood without drivenness and drive disorder,
- strong urge to act.

Personality Influences. Cheerful, always overactive personality.

Conceptual Problems of the Feature. The emotional side should be described independently of interactions with other psychopathological features, i.e. euphoria should be described separately in cases of delusions of grandeur.

Neuroscientific/cognitive neuroscientific models 1.system of positive valence is overactivated, thus lowering the activation threshold of positive emotionality and affects,
Involved are neural systems that are associated with reward and positive emotions (see above),
2. Judgment disorder, anosognosia (e.g., MS patients, Reischies et al. 1988),
   - Expectation of positive reinforcement falsely high,
3. disinhibition,
4. Reduction of amygdala tone with anxiety-free state (after lesion: Klüver-Bucy syndrome).

Ecstasy, Rapture

Emotionally exceptional positive state usually with excessive joyful agitation, altered perception, and changes in consciousness.

Can be expressed, for example, in expressive gestures, sometimes appearing bizarre, and increased psychomotor activity.

The attention and thinking is restricted to the joyful experience

- relationship to alterated conscious experience.

Increased Self-esteem

Definition.
Inappropriately positive assessment of one's own performance or value, social rank or reputation, actions, thoughts, or moral quality.

Positive reinterpretation of neutral or even morally reprehensible behaviors or mistakes.

Example

A woman believes she will easily find a job because she appears highly capable to employers. She considers herself to be a genius and expects to become wealthy soon—also because she is creative and will make inventions. Already in the ward, she helps fellow patients as a co-therapist to get well. ◀

Position in Psychopathology. AMDP 72.

Related Terms. Grandiose ideas.

Psychopathological Interactions. Pressure of thoughts, euphoria, increased drive

Differential Diagnostic Distinctions:
- Grandiosity in the context of schizophrenia or mania,
- Narcissistic personality disorder

Self-/other persons's judgment. other persons's judgment.

Interview for Rating. Interview focused on self-image, plans for the future, history taken from other persons.

Neuropsychology/objectification. Behavioral observation and observation of dealing with negative aspects of the current situation of one's own person, limitation of resources, etc.

Severity. Assessment of the extent and inadequacy of behavior: Excessively positive self-assessment beyond a normal level of self-confidence up to a massive misperception of an appropriate self-image and reinterpretation of mistakes—borderline to grandiosity delusion.

Personality Influences. Narcissistic personality.

Conceptual Problems of the Feature. Prototype of a feature that depends on the self-concept of the social person—with implicit rank assessment—cognitive-emotional feature of the manic syndrome.

Neuroscientific/Cognitive-Neuroscientific Models
1. Increased positive emotionality (see above).
2. affective-cognitive complex with mutual reinforcement of selection of positive memories and positive affective evaluation of past and present developments,
   - selective recall of positive memories, memory retrieval bias,
   - judgment bias with acceptance of positive evaluation and rejection of negative evaluation of past and future personal developments,
   - relatively too positive assessment of the expectation of reward both in considering the future and the past,
   - possibly coupled with poor judgment.

11.5.3 Aggression

A quantitative gradation between dysphoric, irritable, and aggressive behaviors appears clinically necessary.

Dysphoric

Definition.
Aggressive discontent, sullen, or angry mood. The morose mood is expressed verbally (e.g., grumbling) and in emotional expressive behavior, e.g., facial/gestural, without becoming immediately threatening.

Example

A patient is noticeably in a bad mood, reproachful. His wife has a problem, not him. She should have been in treatment. He does not see that it is his changed mood that contributed to the admission. He takes every opportunity to complain. ◄

Position in psychopathology. AMDP 67.

Related terms. Sullen, in a bad mood, disgruntled, morose, grumbling, frustrated.

Psychopathological interactions. Agitation, tense, increased drive, negative valence, arrogance.

Differential diagnostic distinctions. Irritable (see below).

Further characterization. Covert aggressive attitude that does not immediately lead to overt verbal or physical aggressive behaviors.

Self-/other person's judgment. Other person's judgment.

Interview for rating. Questions about anger, aggressive feelings, intentions and impulses, course and situational context; history taken from other persons.

Neuropsychology/objectification. Behavioral observation in everyday situations and observation of dealing with specific issues that lead to angry reactions—confrontation the patient with the interviewers' impression.

Severity. Assessment of the extent and inadequacy of behavior, purely subjective to social consequences due to dysphoric behaviors.

Specifications. Querulous personality traits.

Neuroscientific/cognitive neuroscientific models

1. Aggression—increase and dysfunctional neuronal activity in the areas: diencephalic mechanisms, emotional-motor system, fight-flight dimension,
2. Situational triggering of aggression with active control.

Irritable

> **Definition.**
> Irritable-aggressive reaction pattern with a lowered threshold for openly aggressive behaviors. In this context, a noticeably tense affectivity prevails, with fluctuating affective outbursts. Aggressive behavior is exhibited after only slight provocation.

Example

For no significant reason, a patient who has previously behaved inconspicuously stands threateningly in front of a fellow patient. ◀

Position in psychopathology. AMDP 68.

Related terms. Aggressive, aggressive dynamics, excitability.

Psychopathological interactions. Increased drive, megalomania, in irritable mania the behavior can arise from impatience when the person feels held up in their grandiose ideas.

Differential diagnostic distinctions. dysphoric as the corresponding basic mood.

Further characterization. Affect with a readiness for physical aggression. The examining person involuntarily adopts a defensive posture.

Self-/other persons's judgment. other persons's judgment.

Interview for rating. Questions about anger, previous experiences with aggression outbursts; history taken from other persons particularly important.

Neuropsychology/objectification. Behavioral observation in everyday situations, expressive behavior, arousal, aggressive expressions.

Severity. Occasionally tense calm with the probability of eruptions up to persistent aggressive reactivity with threats or execution of physical aggression, making cohabitation impossible.

Personality influences. Impulsivity of the person, narcissism: patients believe that the behavior is their right; antisocial personality—reduced empathy

Neuroscientific/cognitive neuroscientific models: Disinhibition or surmounting of inhibitions through the extent of aggression.

Aggressive Behavior

> **Definition.**
> Manifest—or concretely threatened—aggressive, harmful behavior

Example

- A tense patient already lashes out during attempts to approach, without any contact being made or any provocation.

- A patient actively seeks out conflict and physical confrontation.
- A man is tense and highly agitated—he curses, screams, and threatens a person with severe violence. ◀

Position in Psychopathology. AMDP 94.

Psychopathological Interactions. Disinhibition, dysphoric mood and irritable aggressive reactivity, tension, increased drive, irritable mania. Megalomania

Differential Diagnostic Distinctions. Criminal harmful behavior in the context of antisocial acts, carried out in conscious decision against social and legal norms.

Further Characterization. Harm to others or immediate danger of harm to others.

Self-/other persons's judgment. Other persons's judgment.

Interview for Rating. Question about previous outbursts of aggression; history taken from other persons.

Neuropsychology/objectification:
- Behavioral observation in everyday situations regarding immediate threats of violence and execution of aggressive behavior towards others, or
- Extent of the necessity for self-protection of the examiners.

Severity. Assessment of the severity and inadequacy of behavior, from isolated threats to the necessity of social consequences due to aggressive behavior towards others (e.g., to restrain).

Specifications:
- Objects: violence against property—violence against people;
- Type: verbal—physical;
- Trigger: spontaneous—provoked, by conflict etc., delusional thoughts
- Reaction to the outburst of aggression: recognizable clear insight into misconduct—no insight .

Personality Influences. Antisocial personality.

Conceptual Problems of the Feature:
- The danger of harmful actions towards others (with physical harm to the victim or killing) is the psychopathologically and clinically relevant feature; the reactivity of an aggressive action, i.e., aggression as a reaction or as provocation etc., is difficult to objectify in some cases.
- Separation of aggressive behaviors from the affect of anger or rage.

Neuroscientific/Cognitive Neuroscientific Models See above; aggressive behavior controlled by neuron groups in the diencephalon:

- Predatory aggression in carnivores,
- Rage—bloodlust in martens etc.,
- Flight against resistance, self-defense aggression,
- Rivalry fight aggression.

Frustration Intolerance

Situations in which the person must remain are experienced as unbearable, with feelings that are very unpleasant for the person.

For example, a situation in which the person is unpleasantly confronted by negative feedback, their plans are thwarted, or they have to wait a long time for an expected reward.

The person wants to end the situation, to flee from the situation, but cannot.

The person reacts with tension, agitation, or motor restlessness, dysphoric to irritable.

Interview for rating. experience with postponing gratifications, history taken from other persons.

Neuropsychology/objectification. Behavioral observation over a longer period.

11.5.4 Other Emotions

Excitation-Tense

> **Definition.**
> A person is in a state of strong excitement and inner tension, without developing, for example, anxiety or aggression; with increased motor reactivity and spontaneous motor activity as well as increased vigilance.

From this state, aggression, panic, or more rarely, joy can develop.

> **Example**
> A patient in the emergency room of the hospital has increased tension, increased muscle tone, and is slight trembling. He looks around the room restlessly—reacts to everything promptly—like a shot; he shows rapid limb movements and changes in posture. A state of excitement, in which he threatens to "explodc" at any moment (regarding physical violence against others or himself). ◀

Position in psychopathology. Not present in AMDP. A feature from emergency psychiatry.

Related terms. High arousal, undirected attention.

Psychopathological interactions. Increased drive, state of heightened motivation, arousal, motor tension.

Differential diagnostic distinctions. irritability refers to an affective attitude that already possesses an aggressive emotional tone, inner restlessness.

Self-/other persons's judgment. self- and predominantly other persons's judgment.

Interview for rating. Question about reasons for the noticeable agitation, history taken from other persons (premorbid level, etc.).

Neuropsychology/objectification. Observation of the dynamics of behavior and assessment of muscle tone in body postures, examination of muscle tension (e.g., when shaking hands in a greeting situation).

Severity. Slightly increased arousal level to extreme tension.

Neuroscientific/cognitive neuroscientific models
1. situational hyperarousal, undirected attention greatly increased—due to affects, due to the chance of a great gain, or loss (or danger),
2. motor tension: co-activation of agonists and antagonists during motor pre-activation in readiness for movements.

Increase in the Feeling of Disgust

> **Definition.**
> Very easily triggered or more intense feeling of disgust—associated with aversion and rejection.

> **Example**
> A woman with schizophrenic psychosis feels "disgusted" by many things (as she says), especially on the street, sexually disgusted by women, possibly triggered by sexual body hallucinations. ◀

Related Terms. Aversion

Psychopathological Interactions. Discomfort, anorexia, delusion, coenesthetic hallucinations (especially sexual); vegetative: nausea.

Interview for Rating. Question about experiencing aversion, history taken from other persons.

Neuropsychology/Objectification. Behavioral observation in everyday situations.

Severity. Mildly pronounced, but subjectively unpleasant to subjectively unbearable, disturbing every contact.

Conceptual Problems of the Feature. Little-studied psychopathological item with disturbance of one of the fundamental emotions.

Neuroscientific/Cognitive Neuroscientific Models
1. Amplification of disgust through pre-activation, or lower triggering threshold of the specific neuronal system for it
2. the person experiences a tension reduction when he intensifies his feelings of disgust. (see Phillips et al. 1997).

11.5.5 Emotional Responsiveness and Affect Control

Decreased Number of Affects

Definition.
Reduction in the number of different affects in everyday life.

Example

- A patient is in the interview without affective facial expressions, gestures and prosody and spends the day on the ward without any recognizable or reported emotional reaction.
- A person reports outwardly without affective expression about the terrible future prospect, which results from his depressive delusion. ◄

Position in psychopathology. AMDP 61.

Differential diagnostic distinctions:
- Feeling of numbness emphasizes the subjective side, especially of positive emotions
- Affective rigidity includes the ability to oscillate and reactivity
- Alexithymia emphasizes the self-perception disorder and the disorder of verbal expression with potentially normal affect.

Further characterization:
- Reduction of spontaneous affective reaction in the dimensions of different affects,

Self-/other persons's judgment. other persons's judgment.

Interview for rating. Question about the experience of different emotions; attempt to elicit emotions.

Neuropsychology/objectification. Behavioral observation in everyday situations (e.g., how many affects are shown in the interview), affective expression in relation to possible triggering situations.

Severity. Individual affects shown – up to the complete absence of affective expression.

Personality influences. Inability to show affects as associated with sociopathy (term: affectionless psychopathy)—today rather associated with lack of empathy.

Neuroscientific/cognitive neuroscientific models
1. Emotional-motor system inactivated, blocked—no expressive behavior,
2. Questionable whether an overly rationalizing behavior style can lead to a poverty of affect.

Feeling of Numbness, Emotionless

Definition.
A person experiences a decrease or no emotional reaction to environmental events or mental processes, compared to the emotional responsiveness they previously knew; with a characteristic pattern of a more pronounced reduction in positive feelings and in sadness, while negative states, or anxiety, can only be felt if the symptom is strongly pronounced.

Example

A patient with severe unipolar depression says he feels nothing anymore, the food tastes like cardboard. He can no longer even be sad and cry, which he reproaches himself for because of a funeral in recent weeks. When he sees something on a walk, his feelings no longer react as they used to.

A patient reports that when praying, he no longer feels the rich emotional experience he used to have. ◀

Position in Psychopathology. AMDP 60.

Psychopathological Interactions. anxiety, depressive delusion, anhedonia

Differential Diagnostic Distinctions:

- In a state of anxiety, the patient reports feeling anxiety. The person with a feeling of numbness does not suffer directly from anxiety, but often the negative state is heightened.

Self-/other persons's judgment. self-evaluation.

Interview for Rating. For example, ask about the variety of emotional experiences when watching a movie

Severity. Reduction to the loss of emotional reactions.

Pathognomonic for: Depressive episode.

Conceptual Problems of the Feature. A pattern of losses of emotional sensations.

Neuroscientific/Cognitive Neuroscientific Models

1. Activation of neuronal activity in the reward-motivation system is disturbed as well as in other affective systems, especially the emotional-motor system,
2. Amygdala hyperactivity, neuronal connection to the ventral striatum and orbitofrontal cortex (possible functional impact: anxiety blocks the reward system),

Alexithymia

Definition.
Reduced ability or inability to have conscious access to emotional processes and to talk about them.

Example

A patient is unable to see that he reacts emotionally aversively. He assumes he is reacting rationally. ◀

Position in Psychopathology. Not in AMDP.

Related Terms. relationship to dissociation from emotions.

Psychopathological Interactions:
Anosognosia

- Upbringing to deny emotionality,
- Dissociation from emotional aspects and affects,
- Linguistic inability to describe differentiated emotional experiences.

Differential Diagnostic Distinctions:

- blunted affect and feeling of numbness,
- Consequence of rejecting psychological aspects of one's own situation, such as in somatization or so-called psychosomatic complaints.

Self-/other persons's judgment. other persons's judgment.

Interview for Rating. Question about the description of the subjective side of the person's suffering (e.g., psychosomatic illness)

Neuropsychology/objectification: Behavioral observation in everyday situations, during exploration, and in behavior during group sessions. In this context, emotional aspects of the person seem perceptible to outsiders but remain inaccessible to the person.

Severity : Difficulty up to complete inability to experience feelings.

Neuroscientific/cognitive neuroscientific models

1. At the level of conscious experience (with the possibility to communicate about it), an emotional reaction is not available to the patient,
2. Deficient self-perception
3. learning history with tension reduction by distracting from emotions that reached the level of consciousness, and distraction with rational occupation, e.g., in unlearning anxiety,
4. Rationalizing cognitive style,
5. Inaccessibility of emotional experiences due to the disturbance of critical brain regions (Hornak et al. 2003).

Feeling of Emptiness

The person feels unpleasantly devoid of feelings, intentions, ideas, and thoughts. The mood is negatively tinged.

Relationship to burnout, lack of drive, loss of interest, and boredom.

Reduced Affective Resonance

Definition. Reduction of emotional resonance capacity, emotional responsiveness, i.e., when an emotion is triggered, the intensity of the affect -swings is reduced.

Example

A patient with a severe depression shows hardly any emotional movement, even when talking about his condition with relatives—if he seems to have a feeling, it appears to be only very mild. He remains in his depressed basic mood state the entire time. ◀

Position in psychopathology. AMDP 79.

Psychopathological interactions: Affect poverty, anhedonia; "Apathetic," where the triggering of affect is difficult—a term often used unclearly.

Differential diagnostic distinctions. blunted affect emphasizes primarily the number of different emotions shown.

Further characterization. affective rigidity refers to the reduction of emotional dynamics in everyday contact.

Self-/other persons's judgment. other persons's judgment.

Interview for rating. Ask if there have been any intense emotions recently, history taken from other persons.

Neuropsychology/objectification:

- In the interview, various affective dimensions must be stimulated—behavioral observation (affective resonance in conversational interaction),
- both spontaneous and externally stimulated affective resonance must be assessed.

Severity. Mild reduction to complete abolition of any emotional/affective movement.

Pathognomonic for: Although common in a depression, remaining in a jokingly euphoric mood is also referred to as affective rigidity.

Neuroscientific/cognitive-neuroscientific models

1. still unclear; activation (a) of a mood possible, but (b) not of the variably pronounced emotions and affect expressions
2. Emotional-motor systems afference, efference, or "center" disturbed, with accompanying reduction in the experience of the emotion.

Affective Lability

Definition.
Affects are triggered more immediately than usual, both spontaneously and externally stimulated, and by minor occasions than usual; this can be observed both in the triggering of an affect and in the switching between affects.

Example

- A patient suddenly starts crying at inappropriate occasions—for example, at the mention of an event that does not necessarily have to be sad. When distracted by joyful things, he can laugh—still with tears in his eyes. ◀

Position in psychopathology. AMDP 77.

Related terms. Colloquially for the depressive syndrome: susceptible to tears; regarding aggressive emotionality: irritability (see below); irritable weakness.

Further characterization. The dynamics of emotionality in affective lability concern the rapid response, not the intensity of the affect.

Self-/other persons's judgment. other persons's judgment, lesser importance of self-evaluation.

Interview for rating. Question about changes in emotional response, history taken from other persons.

Neuropsychology/objectification. Attempt to address emotional topics with behavioral observation.

Severity. From slightly faster triggering to impairment of communication due to frequent triggering of affects.

Specifications: 1) Triggering of affects with negative or positive valence 2) Triggering of irritable-aggressive affect (see feature irritable)

Conceptual problems of the feature. The term "irritable" in the classification criteria means "to react quickly or to minor occasions with anxiety or aggression," which is subdivided here.

Neuroscientific/cognitive neuroscientific models

1. disinhibition with lowered threshold regarding the activation of the emotional-motor system; model of pathological laughing or crying, without feeling joy or sadness,
   - corresponding to affect rigidity, it is questionable whether a central function for multiple emotion systems exists, which is related to the general triggerability of emotions,
   - pseudobulbar palsy with extensive damage in the white matter of the brain hemispheres.
2. Pre-activation in an emotional brain system, with corresponding lowering of the threshold for emotion triggering.
3. Control education: control of certain emotions can vary between cultures.

Affective Flattening

Definition .
Affects are shown, but not to the extent of the person's involvement as before, are more fleeting, and have less impact than before.

Example

- A patient laughs foolishly after greeting his caregiver, as if he had made a joke about her, but does not show a lasting humorous mood.
- A patient seems to feel no emotional response, but occasionally reacts with a brief affect; relatives believe the emotional "depth" no longer seems to be as it was before. ◀

Position in psychopathology.
Not in AMDP

Psychopathological Interactions.
Parathymia, affect lability .

Differential diagnostic distinctions: Affect lability refers to the dynamics of affect response, while affective flattening targets the discrepancy between expressed and experienced emotionality,

- Cheerfulness as a learned defense,

Further characterization. Emotional access to the person seems less possible.

Self-/other persons' judgment. other persons' judgment—preferably also longitudinal observation.

Interview for rating. Inquire how intensely the shown emotion was experienced (example: if the patient suddenly and briefly cries, ask how intense the sad feeling was).

Neuropsychology/objectification: Several emotional stimuli should be provided in the interview (topics from various emotional areas, including humorous remarks).

Severity : Mild: Emotions are less intense and fleeting— to: no more emotional contact possible.

Pathognomonic for: Schizophrenic defect states—"hebephrenic laughter"

Neuroscientific/cognitive neuroscientific models
- see above model of pathological crying,
- possibly also a difficulty in accessing emotional experience.

Parathymia

Definition.
Emotions are expressed that do not match the emotions expected in the respective situations. The emotional expression occurs spontaneously, but also situationally as an emotional reaction.

Example

A person laughs during the discussion of serious future problems at sad events. ◀

Position in psychopathology. AMDP 76.

Related terms. Inadequacy of affects.

Psychopathological interactions. Paramimia, faulty facial expression, grimacing, misdirected affective gestures.

Differential diagnostic distinctions: Influence by cognitive phenomena, with emotional reaction to phonemes or focus on delusional reinterpretations of the situation,

- "Tears of laughter," a normal psychological phenomenon, easily breaking into tears briefly under affective tension.

Further characterization. Emotional misactivation; questionable correspondence in the emotional experience of the person.

Self-/other person's judgment. Other person's judgment.

Interview for rating. In each case, when there is inappropriate affect expression, inquire in an attempt to elucidate the emotional experience and clarify whether it might be a reaction to hallucinations.

Neuropsychology/objectification: Behavioral observation in the interview.

Severity. Occasional to emotional inaccessibility due to incessant parathymic expressive behavior.

Pathognomonic for: Schizophrenia.

Specifications. Grimacing as an extreme form of disturbed affective facial expression.

Conceptual problems of the feature. Conceptually important, whether the displayed affects might be appropriate to abnormal associations or hallucinatory experiences (this seems to be the case in many instances);

Neuroscientific/cognitive neuroscientific models 1.An affective expression is activated without the situational trigger having led to it.

2. Misactivation of the emotional-motor system—newborns show facial restlessness with many communicatively significant elements.

Affect Control Disorder

Definition.
Intensification of affect expression in extent and duration or rather the weakening of control; the affect expression is usually inappropriately strong.

Example

A patient is unable to control anger for an extended period of time, he rages, screams, threatens, without relatives or police, who try to influence him, being able to achieve a moderation of the aggression. ◀

Position in Psychopathology. AMDP 78.

Related Terms. Old term: Affect Incontinence, Excessive Affects.

Psychopathological Interactions. Disinhibition.

Differential Diagnostic Distinctions. Intended; feigned loss of control to achieve a goal.

Self-/Other Assessment. Other person's judgment.

Interview for Rating. Question about the experience of affect control (attempt at control), life history, history taken from other persons.

Neuropsychology/Objectification. Behavioral observation.

Severity. Mild overshooting to unrestrained "freaking out" in one of the affects.

Personality Influences: Narcissistic anger

Specifications:
a) all affects are affected, b) predominantly one affect is affected
a) emotion too intense for the person's affect control capabilities, b) involvement of a component of "letting oneself go"

Conceptual Problems of the Feature. The old term Affect Incontinence is very unfortunately chosen.

Neuroscientific/Cognitive Neuroscientific Models
1. Disinhibition of an affective brain system (in the emotional motor system), e.g., epileptic activity,
   - Pseudobulbar Palsy in extensive damage to the white matter of the brain hemispheres,
2. General disinhibition and behavioral control disorder in frontal lobe lesions and manic syndromes,
3. Learning history, education of control abilities of certain affects.

Self-Control Disorder with Addictive Substances

Definition.
Pleasant stimuli, such as illegal drugs, are sought, pursued, and consumed even at the risk of disproportionately high negative consequences.

Substance-bound through the administration of a drug or non-substance-bound, such as through pathological gambling.

Example

- A patient harms himself through the consumption of alcohol and drugs, even though he knows that this will harm his well-being and is life-threatening in the long run. ◀

Position in Psychopathology. Not in AMDP—central for still voluntarily changeable addictive behavior

Related Terms. Indiscipline in resisting addictive substances, self-indulgence, addictive behavior, weakness of will.

Psychopathological Interactions. Depressed mood and anxiety can lead to the consumption of substances that have calming primary effects (comfort eating).

Further Characterization: Disorder of control in self-relationship, i.e., the functions to limit oneself are weakened—in contrast to an overly strict self-relationship

Differential Diagnostic Distinctions: Socially adapted administration of reinforcers is to be distinguished, decompensating control of self-administered positive reinforcers can be assessed.

Interview. Questions about the description of the subjective side of the consumption of addictive substances. History taken from other persons

Neuropsychology/Objectification. If necessary, behavioral observation during an abstinence attempt.

Severity. Difficulty in limiting oneself to otherwise harmless pleasures, which, however, can lead to everyday relevant impairments, up to the complete inability to refrain from even highly risky administration of positive stimuli.

Pathognomonic for: Dependence .

Personality Influences. Antisocial Personality with lack of evaluation of negative repercussions, impulsivity.

Neuroscientific/Cognitive Neuroscientific Models.

1. Self-stimulation experiments in animals in regions with pleasant valence effects led to unrestrained self-stimulation and neglect of other activities
2. Reduction in the processing of information about negative consequences (for example, in the amygdala) or disturbed elaboration of the representation of negative consequences and their processing in executive planning.

Self-Harming Behavior

Definition.
Actions are directed against one's own person, the physical or social person; however, they do not aim at dying.

Example

- A person pulls out his hair,
- A person bangs his head against the wall,
- Skin cuts in states of arousal in borderline personality disorder, in dissociative states
- Giving notice to quit the apartment and workplace in depressed despair. ◀

Position in psychopathology. AMDP 96.

Related terms. Self-injury.

Psychopathological interactions. Desperate agitation, aggressiveness, learned help-seeking behavior

Differential diagnostic distinctions. Suicidality with a death-oriented intention to act.

Further characterization. Classification of behaviors that are carried out from various psychopathological causal contexts, with the intention of causing harm to oneself—as opposed to addictive behavior.

Self-/other person's judgment. other person's judgment.

Interview for rating. Questions about the development of the intention to act, intentions, somatic examination, observation, scars.

Neuropsychology/objectification. Dealing with the situation that led to self-harming behavior.

Severity. Occasional minor damage to potentially life-threatening actions.

Specifications:
a) Physical, non-physical self-harm,
b) Influencing factors:
  – In a state of excitement (also e.g., sexual excitement),
  – In a dissociative state,
  – wrong action in productive psychotic symptoms (beware of imperative voices).

Neuroscientific/cognitive neuroscientific models
- Learning history: experience of a tension reduction in the situation of acute physical impairment, in injury or in self-harm.

Suicidality

Definition.
Intentions, tendencies to act, and actions directed towards one's own death.

Example
- Upon admission to the clinic a patient in a severe depression suddenly climbs onto the windowsill of the examination room and is about to jump out of the window.
- A patient interrupts the interview and runs out of the examination room, saying that everything is pointless. After being stopped, he states that he intended to throw himself in front of a moving car. ◀

Position in psychopathology. AMDP 95.

Related terms. Concrete, acute risk of self-harm, (problematic term self-murder).

Psychopathological interactions. Despair, loss of joy, hopelessness, aggression.

Differential diagnostic distinctions:
- Parasuicidal action as psychotic wrong action with only potential or actual life danger, no clear intention to die
- Self-harming behavior (see above) not directed towards death.

Self-/other person's judgment. Introspection and other person's judgment.

Interview for rating: Question about thoughts of dying, a desire to die, and the development of the intention to act,

- Questions about future orientation
- regarding the presuicidal syndrome (Ringel 1953):

Disengagement with loss of future orientation, desire to die, and death fantasies with narrowing, glorification of dying, devaluation of previously valued persons, activities, social instances, and general devaluation of previous values, concreteness of death plans, turning aggression against oneself.

Neuropsychology/objectification: Currently not possible,

- Attempt to asess the engagement with the question of why the person wants to continue living,
- is the person open in communication? etc.

Severity. Thoughts of death, unspecific statements of not wanting to live anymore up to current immediate suicide risk.

Specifications: Type:

1. Depressive suicidality,
2. Impulsive reaction in despair, e.g., current severe situation of shame,
3. Ending of objective suffering in a somatic or social emergency situation.

Personality influences. Risk is greater in active, assertive personalities

- also in impulsivity

Conceptual problems of the feature:
- Due to the significance of suicide, the tendency is already highly important and has legal consequences, but it is difficult to capture—therefore, suicidal tendencies are included in the construct.
- The person decides (except in impulsive actions and impulsive behaviors) about the end of the person
- not to be diagnosed without reference to the examination of all aspects of the person.

11.5.6 Obsessive Thoughts and Actions

Obsessive thoughts, compulsive impulses and actions have a close relationship to emotions. This relationship will be explained in more detail below. In the English-speaking world, "obsessions" refer to thoughts ("being obsessed with a thought") and "compulsions" refer to actions ("feeling compelled to perform an action"). The distinction between obsessive thoughts and compulsive actions is particularly important due to the different therapeutic approaches (see textbooks on behavioral therapy). The compulsive actions are performed consciously; in contrast, the obsessive thoughts usually come uncontrolled and uncontrollable. There is a connection to the so-called automatic thoughts (see thought disorders). Compulsive actions and thoughts differ in terms of the person's intervention possibilities: With the compulsive actions, the person can try to refrain from the action, but with obsessive thoughts, the person cannot suppress the occurrence of the thought.

Obsessive phenomena affect certain areas such as cleanliness/contamination, control, aggression/guilt, order and collecting. Additionally, there are sexual and religious themes. Certainly, obsessive disorders are a heterogeneous group of mental disorders.

The person must during the interview provide information about the actions, but especially about the thoughts, the accompanying circumstances, and above all, how they relate to the phenomena, for example, how they try to suppress the thoughts or impulses (Purdon 1999; Bürgy 2005).

An ego dystonia has been demanded in the German psychopathological tradition, i.e., the person must have a distance from the obsessive phenomena, e.g., not wanting the action but feeling compelled to do it. Consider the love of order. There are certainly compulsively orderly people who state that they want to behave in such a way, as it corresponds to their expectations of oneself. However, an obsessive patient would have to feel compelled to perform ordering actions, actions they do not want to perform, and perform because otherwise, they would experience anxiety. This example explains why ego dystonia has recently been abandoned as a diagnostic criterion, i.e., even compulsive actions to which the patient is not distanced can be diagnosed as such.

Why can't the person refrain from the action?

a) For example, it is performed because, in the person's imagination, otherwise, a disaster would occur. There are connections to overvalued ideas or delusion. Many obsessive patients feel a sense of responsibility to prevent a disaster; they believe they are responsible for protecting their family from harmful influences through the compulsive actions.
b) It is performed for tension reduction or defense against anxiety .

Models have been developed for the emergence of obsessive phenomena for tension reduction.

1. A thought or impulse gains—for reasons still unknown—an intrusiveness that is abnormal (Reinecker 2005).
2. Thinking the thought, performing a ritual or an action results in a reduction of anxiety, which, although incomplete, still means relief. This relief conditions the affective system.

The pathophysiology of obsessive symptoms is still unclear. In many, but not all, studies on resting metabolism in the prefrontal cortex, specifically the orbitofrontal cortex of obsessive patients, a pathological increase in activity was found (Baxter et al. 1987). The currently preferred interpretation of imaging findings in obsessive symptoms (overview Kordon et al. 2005) assumes a disinhibition of thalamic cortex activation.

Neuropsychology has shown that obsessive patients can perform abstract sorting tasks like the Wisconsin Card Sorting, but they apparently have problems with decision-making under risk (Cavedini et al. 2002).

Ritual actions are etiologically nonspecific; they are often observed in conditions following brain damage (Grados 2003). They seem to take on a rather behavior-regulating function after brain damage ("to order the inner chaos").

The aspect of distraction from topics that represent unbearable issues for the person is widely accepted. In other words, the content fixation on the distracting content and engagement with it prevents attention to certain critical, subjectively unbearable topics ("throwing oneself into work to distract oneself"). This model of distraction engagement could be seen as a disposition in the face of quite high genetic transmission of obsessive phenomena.

Further aspects of obsessive symptoms initially concern impulsivity. Many obsessive phenomena are related to impulse control (Chap. 7 drive). The patients are partly occupied with the defense of aggressive acts or ideas.

Obsessive Thoughts

Definition:

a) Certain thoughts, ideas, or memories repeatedly intrude and disrupt the course of the person's intended (mental) activity. They can, for example, hinder the ability to work. The person is unable or refrains from immediately pushing the thoughts away. In many cases, the patients consider the thoughts to be nonsensical.

b) The unbearable thought led to anxiety, and the anxiety recurs when the ritual thinking is omitted or interrupted.

Examples:

- A person must repeatedly think about death, which spontaneously comes to mind, or is associated with words like "ambulance", etc. that he reads. He has the fantasy that a serious illness will break out in his family if he does not ritually think these thoughts to the end.
- A person must repeatedly think about confessing, whereby trivial "impure" intentions are considered necessary to confess. This makes him unable to work and he loses his job.

Position in Psychopathology. AMDP 30.

Related terms. obsessive thinking, obsessive ideas, obsessive fears, obsessive rumination.

Psychopathological interactions. Other obsessive phenomena, anxiety, excessive worries, and strict self-relationship with self-commitment. Anxiety, for example, in obsessive fears.

Differential diagnostic distinctions:

- reflective brooding with thoughts intended by the person, which are considered necessary contemplation of a problem,
- ego disturbance with thought insertion, where an instance is suspected of transmitting the thoughts.

Further characterization. Uncontrollable ideas (thoughts, imaginations, memories) lead to a very unpleasant emotional state.

Self-/other person's judgment. Introspective statements are central.

Interview for rating: Questions about the course of the development of obsessive thoughts in the person, with the attempt to learn the significance of the thoughts for this person; what the person is anxious about.

Neuropsychology/objectification. Behavioral observation, inexplicable delays in actions or daily work prompt inquiries; or clarifying the characteristics of obsessive thoughts after the patient describes repeated disturbing thoughts.

Severity. From rare, clearly identifiable obsessive thoughts to complete preoccupation with the thoughts, which suppress any meaningful activity.

Personality influences. Conscientious persons, perfectionism, aggressive potential in the personality, strict self-relationship.

Conceptual problems of the feature: Transitions to so-called automatic thoughts that occur to a person , thought insertion and brooding.

Neuroscientific/cognitive neuroscientific models

1. It is fundamentally impossible to strive not to think about something, as this something is already a thought, a content that is mentally pre-activated. This is all the more the case when affects are linked to it,
2. emotionally charged content (affective-cognitive complex) asserts itself against normal mental activity—for example, during rest phases or meditation—"it thinks me" in automatic thoughts.
3. The person previously experienced tension reduction when certain thoughts were thought, thereby reinforcement (also distraction from even more tension-filled thought areas),

Compulsive Impulses

Definition.
Certainintentions to act repeatedly impose themselves on the person and disrupt everyday activity. They cannot be pushed away by the person or come back unexpectedly. They can hinder the ability to work. The occurrence and the possible consequences of carrying out the intention lead or led to anxiety.

Examples:

- A patient repeatedly has the idea and feels the urge to push a person in front of the subway and is frightened by it. Therefore, he avoids taking the subway.
- A person feels the intention to shout a curse, a terrible and unforgivable blasphemy.
- A person cannot see a knife without feeling the intention to hurt someone with it.

Position in Psychopathology. AMDP 31.

Related Terms. obsessive thoughts.

Psychopathological Interactions. Other compulsive phenomena, anxiety.

Differential Diagnostic Distinctions:

- imperative phonemes,
- delusional thoughts—especially those with action consequences,

see also obsessive thoughts.

Further Characterization. Uncontrollably occurring, subjectively not certainly suppressible impulses to act—although the person can actually be sure that he will not carry out the intention if he does not want to.

Self-/other person's judgment. Statement of the person necessary.

Interview for Rating. Questions about the development of anxiety in connection with the impulses.

Neuropsychology/objectification. Behavioral observation, characteristic: inexplicable delay in actions in everyday work, give reason to inquire.

Severity. From clearly identifiable isolated compulsive impulses to the preoccupation with the symptom that suppresses any meaningful activity.

Personality Influences. Conscientious persons.

Conceptual Problems of the Feature. Speech act in communication: "I feel pressured by the intention," "I have anxiety about having to do xyz."

Neuroscientific/Cognitive Neuroscientific Models
1. obsessive thoughts see above—with an emphasized action component,
2. Lack of confidence in executive control
3. impulse control is efficient

Compulsive Act

Definition:
Certain actions repeatedly impose themselves on the person, must be carried out, disrupt the progress of the activity previously intended by the person, and cannot be suppressed without the person experiencing anxiety or severe discomfort; they hinder the ability to work or the activities of daily life.

Examples:

A patient has to shower for hours because he is never sure if he has really removed all the dirt from his body—he showers so rarely that he becomes a nuisance to others due to his smell.

- A person has to check many times (e.g., well over 10 times) whether he has locked the store he runs in the evening. Each time he thinks he were not careful enough when locking it and become very agitated with each subsequent attempt.
- A female patient has to repeatedly perform a bizarre ritual of hand movements. She explains that she has to do this to prevent a feared misfortune from befalling her relatives.

Position in Psychopathology. AMDP 32.

Related Terms. Reassurance seeking often occurs together with compulsive act.

Psychopathological Interactions. Other obsessive phenomena, comorbidity with schizophrenia.

Differential Diagnostic Distinctions:
- Actions due to imperative phonemes or delusional thoughts,
- Hyperkinesias, tics—Tourette syndrome, mannerisms (can be temporarily suppressed, for example), no anxiety when suppressed
- Perseverations of actions,
- Consciously intended repetitions (of actions whose omission would lead to real unpleasant consequences) and rituals (e.g., religious),
- Utilization behavior in frontal lobe disorder (see Reischies 2005),
- Orderliness (often colloquially described as compulsiveness, but not to be evaluated psychopathologically), only to be evaluated as pathological if the time spent on it results in a restriction of everyday functions and/or the person has a distance from it, e.g., would suppress the actions if he could,
- Normal control behavior: people say they check again whether they have, for example, locked up but "once is enough",
- Impulse control disorder.

Further Characterization. Repeated disturbing actions—after exclusion of differential diagnoses. Also rituals that occur after brain damage, as they bring order to a chaos of internal states.

Interview for Rating. Question about symptom development, what consequence of omission is feared, history taken from other persons.

Neuropsychology/objectification. Behavioral observation, reaction to the attempt to prevent the compulsive act.

Severity. From clearly identifiable isolated compulsive acts to preoccupation with compulsive acts that prevent any meaningful activity (time loss in hours per day).

Specifications. Type of compulsive act, differences between control compulsions and compulsive acts with cleanliness aspect.

1. Contents
   - Cleanliness,
   - Safety,
   - Other contents,
2. Reassurance behavior

Personality Influences. Conscientiousness and aggression potential in personality.

Conceptual Problems of the Feature: Is the person's distance from the compulsive act necessary for the diagnosis?

Neuroscientific/cognitive neuroscientific models

1. Compulsion to control: failure of executive control and monitoring over the already completed control action,
   - Completion of actions in the CNS not properly processed, efference copies not deleted, etc.
2. Basal ganglia: orbitofrontal interaction disturbed (orbitofrontal overactivity, underactivity in the basal ganglia postulated).
3. like obsessive thoughts but with an action level—tension reduction experienced through control action,
4. the repetition of an impulse control failure, for example an outburst of aggression, is feared and this is to be suppressed by massive control maneuvers, which are, however, insufficient,
5. in individual cases limited to one action script—within a routine, certain actions must be repeated to avoid anxiety and a state of negative valence.
6. The person feels compelled to perform symbolic actions that promise to avert negative developments or events,
7. Low impulse control must be compensated.

References

Adolphs R, Gosselin F, Buchanan TW et al (2005) A mechanism for impaired fear recognition after amygdala damage. Nature 433:68–72

Anderson MC, Ochsner KN, Kuhl B et al (2004) Neural systems underlying the suppression of unwanted memories. Science 303:232–235

Bandura (1999) Moral disengagement in the perpetration of inhumanities. Pers Soc Psychol Rev 3:193–209

Baxter LR Jr, Phelps ME, Mazziotta JC (1987) Local cerebral glucose metabolic rates in obsessive-compulsive disorder. Arch Gen Psychiatry 44:211–218

Benson DF (1994) The neurology of thinking. Oxford Univ Press, Oxford

Bleuler E (1979) Lehrbuch der Psychiatrie, 14. edn. Springer, Berlin

Borod JC (2000) The neuropsychology of emotion. Oxford Univ Press, Oxford

Bronstein CJL (2001) Neuropharmacology of frontal-subcortical circuits. In: Lichter DG, Cummings JL (Eds) Frontal-subcortical circuits in psychiatric and neurological disorders. Guilford Press, New York, pp 92–113

Buechel C, Dolan R (2000) Classical fear conditioning in functional neuroimaging. Curr Opin Neurobiol 10(2):219–223

Bürgy M (2005) Psychopathology of obsessive-compulsive disorder: a phenomenological approach. Psychopathology 38:291–300

Bush G, Luu P, Posner MI (2000) Cognitive and emotional influences in anterior cingulate cortex. Trends Cogn Sci 4:215–222

Carlsson A (2001) A paradigm shift in brain research. Science 294:1021–1024

Cavedini P, Riboldi G, D'Annucci A et al (2002) Decision making heterogeneity in obsessive-compulsive disorder: ventromedial pre frontla cortex function predicts different treatment outcomes. Neuropsychologia 40: 205–211

Dalgleish T (2004) The emotional brain. Nat Rev Neurosci 5:583–589

Damasio A (1994) Descarte`s error. Putnam, New York (deutsch 1995, List Verlag, München)

Davis M, Walker D, Lee Y (1997) Amygdala and bed nucleus of the stria terminalis: differential roles in fear and anxiety measured with the acoustic startle reflex. Phil Trans R Soc London B 352:1675–1687

Deng W, Rolls ET, Ji X, Robbins TW, Banaschewski T, Bokde ALW, Bromberg U, Buechel C, DesriviÃ¨res S, Conrod P, Flor H, Frouin V, Gallinat J, Garavan H, Gowland P, Heinz A, Ittermann B, Martinot JL, Lemaitre H, Nees F, Papadopoulos Orfanos D, Poustka L, Smolka MN, Walter H, Whelan R, Schumann G, Feng J (2017). Separate neural systems for behavioral change and for emotional responses to failure during behavioral inhibition. Hum Brain Mapp. 38:3527–3537.

Dolan RJ (2002) Emotion, cognition, and behavior. Science 298:1191–1194
Drevets WC (2003) Neuroimaging abnormalities in the amygdala in mood disorders. Ann N Y Acad Sci 985:420–444
Ekman P (1999) Basic emotions. In: Dagleish T, Power MJ (Eds) Handbook of cognition and emition. Wiley, Chichester, pp 45–60
Frijda NH (1986) The emotions. Cambridge Univ Press, Cambridge
Gainotti G (2000) Neuropsychological theories of emotion. In: Borod JC (Ed) The neuropsychology of emotion. Oxford Univ Press, Oxford, pp 214–236
Gao WJ, Krimer LS, Goldman-Rakic PS (2001) Presynaptic regulation of recurrent excitation by D1 receptors in prefrontal circuits. Proc Natl Acad Sci U S A 98:295–300
Gao WJ, Goldman-Rakic PS (2003) Selctive modulation of excitatory and inhibitory microcircuits by dopamine. Proc Natl Acad Sci U S A 100:2836–2841
Gloor P (1997) The temporal lobe and limbic system. Oxford Univ Press, Oxford
Grados MA (2003) Obsessive-compulsive disorder after traumatic brain injury. Int Rev Psychiatry 15:350–358
Grillon C (2002) Startle reactivity and anxiety disorders: aversive conditioning, context and neurobiology. Biol Psychiatry 52:958–975
Gündel H, O'Connor MF, Littrell L (2003) Functional neuroanatomy of grief: an FMRI study. Am J Psychiatry 160:1946–1953
Haaga DA, Beck AT (1995) Perspectives on depressive realism: implications for cognitive theory of depression. Behav Res Ther 33:41–48
Hancock JA (1996) "Depressive realism" assessed via confidence in decision-making. Cogn Neuropsychiatry 1:213–220
Hariri AR, Mattay WS, Tessitore A (2003) Neocortical modulation of the amydala response to fearful stimuli. Biol Psychiatry 53:494–501
Hariri A, Bookheimer S, Mazziotta J (2000) Modulating emotional responses: effects of a neocortical network on the limbic system. NeuroReport 11(1):43–48
Hikosaka O (2010) The habenula: from stress evasion to value-based decision making. Nat Rev Neurosci 11:503–513
Holstege G, Bandler R, Saper CB (1996) The emotional motor system. Prog Brain Res 107:113–126
Hornak J, Bramham J, Rolls ET et al (2003) Changes in emotion after circumscribed surgical lesions of the orbitofrontal and cingulate cortices. Brain 126:1691–1712
Houk JC (2001) Neurophysiology of frontal-subcortical loops. In: Lichter DG, Cummings JL (Eds) Frontal-subcortical circuits in psychiatric and neurological disorders. Guilford Press, New York, pp 92–113
Koch M (1999) The neurobiology of startle. Prog Neurobiol 59:107–128
Kordon A, Leplow B, Hohagen F (2005) Zwangsstörungen. In: Förstl H, Hautzinger M, Roth G (Eds) Neurobiologie psychischer Störungen. Springer, Berlin Heidelberg New York Tokio, pp 545–575
LaBar K, Gatenby J, Gore J et al (1998) Human amygdala activation during conditioned fear acquisition and extinction: a mixed-trial fMRI study. Neuron 20(5):937–945
LeDoux J (1996) The emotional brain. Simon & Schuster, New York
Marschner A, Mell T, Wartenburger I, Villringer A, Reischies F, Heekeren H (2005) Reward-based decision-making and aging. Brain Res Bull 67:382–390
Matsumoto M, Hikosaka O (2007Jun 28) Lateral habenula as a source of negative reward signals in dopamine neurons. Nature 447(7148):1111–1115
Middleton FA, Strick PL (2000) A revised neuroanatomy of frontal-subcortical circuits. In: Lichter DG, Cummings JL (Eds) Frontal-subcortical circuits in psychiatric and neurological disorders. Guilford Press, New York, pp 44–58
Milad MR, Quirk GJ (2002) Neurons in medial prefrontal cortex signal memory for fear extinction. Nature 420:70–74
Moles A, Kieffer BL, D'Amato FR, (2004) Deficit in attachment behavior in mice lacking the μ-Opioid receptor. Gene Science 304:1983–1986
Morris SE, Sanislow CA, Pacheco J, Vaidyanathan U, Gordon JA, Cuthbert BN (2022) Revisiting the seven pillars of RDoC. BMC Med 20:220
New AS, Hazlett EA, Buchsbaum MS et al (2002) Blunted prefrontal cortical 18-fluoro-deoxyglucose positron emission tomography response to meta-chlorophenylpiperazine in impulsive aggression. Arch Gen Psychiatry 59:621–629
Panksepp J (1998) Affective neuroscience. Oxford Univ Press, Oxford
Panksepp J (2003) Feeling the pain of social loss. Science 302:237–239
Paton JJ, Belova MA, Morrison SE, Salzman CD (2006) The primate amygdala represents the positive and negative value of visual stimuli during learning. Nature 439:865–870
Phan KL, Wager T, Taylor SF, Liberzon I (2002) Functional neuroanatomy of emotion: a meta-analysis of emotion activation studies in PET and fMRI. Neuroimage 16:331–348
Phillips ML, Senior C, Fahy T, Davis AS (1997) Disgust—the forgotten emotion of psychiatry. Br J Psychiatry 172:373–375
Pietrini P, Guazzelli M, Basso G et al (2000) Neural correlates of imaginal aggressive behavior assessed by positron emission tomography in healthy subjects. Am J Psychiatry 157:1772–1781
Pissiota A, Frans O, Michelgard A (2003) Amygdala and anterior cingulate cortex activation during affective

startle modulation: a PET study of fear. Eur J Neurosci 18:1325–1331
Price DD (2000) Psychological and neural mechanisms of the affective dimension of pain. Science 288:1769–1772
Price JL (1999) Prefrontal cortical networks related to visceral function and mood. Ann N Y Acad Sci 877:383–396
Purdon C (1999) Thought suppression and psychopathology. Behav Res Ther Nov 37(11): 1029–1054
Reinecker H (2005) Grundlagen der Verhaltenstherapie. Beltz Psychologie Verlags Union, Weinheim
Reischies FM, Baum K, Bräu H (1988) Cerebral magnetic resonance imaging findings in multiple sclerosis—relation to disturbance of affect, drive, and cognition. Arch Neurol 45:1114–1116
Reischies FM (1990) Emotionalitätsfragebogen, Erfassung des emotionalen Zustands, der emotionalen Ansprechbarkeit und Ausdrucksfähigkeit mit Hilfe von visuellen Analog-Skalen. Diagnostika 36:359–365
Reischies FM (1999a) Pattern of disturbance of different ventral frontal functions in organic depression. Ann N Y Acad Sci 877:775–780
Reischies FM (1999) Pattern of disturbance of different ventral frontal functions in organic depression. In: McGinty JF (Ed) Advancing from the ventral striatum to the extended amygdala. Ann N Y Acad Sci 877: 775–780
Reischies FM (2005) Psychopathologie des Frontalhirns. In: Förstl H (Ed), Frontalhirn, Funktionen und Erkrankungen, 2. edn. Springer, Berlin, pp 83–101
Reischies FM (2021) Leid-Erleben—ein Fundament der Psychopathologie. Papst Scientific Publishing, Lengerich.
Ringel E (1953) Der Selbstmord. Maudrich, Wien
Rolls ET (1999) The brain and emotion. Oxford Univ Press, Oxford
Ross ED (1981) The prosodias: Functional-anatomical organization of the affective components of language in the right hemisphere. Arch Neurol 38:561–569
Scherer KR (2003) Introduction: cognitive components of emotion. In: Davidson RJ, Goldsmith H, Scherer KR (Eds) Handbook of the affective sciences. Oxford Univ Press, New York, pp 563–571
Scherer KR (2004) Feelings integrate the central representation of appraisal-driven response organization in emotion. In: Manstead ASR, Frijda NH, Fischer AH (Eds) Feelings and emotions. Cambridge Univ Press, Cambridge, pp 136–157
Schultz W (1998) Predictive reward signal of dopamine neurons. J Neurophysiol 80:1–27
Siegel A, Roeling TA, Gregg TR, Kruk MR (1999) Neuropharmacology of brain-stimulation-evoked aggression. Neurosci Biobehav Rev 23:359–389
Taylor GJ, Bagby RM (2004) New trends in alexithymia research. Psychother Psychosom 73:68–77
Tremblay L, Schultz W (1999) Relative reward preference in primate orbitofrontal cortex. Nature 398:704–708
West AR, Grace AA (2000) The role of frontal-subcortical circuits in the pathophysiology of schizophrenia. In: Lichter DG, Cummings JL (Eds) Frontal-subcortical circuits in psychiatric and neurological disorders. Guilford Press, New York, pp 372–400
Whalen PJ, Rauch SL, Etcoff NL et al (1998) Masked presentations of emotional facial expressions modulate amygdala activity without explicit knowledge. J Neurosci 18:411–418
Whalen PJ, Kagan J, Cook RG (2004) Human amygdala responsivity to masked fearful eye whites. Science 306:2061
Wild B, Rodden FA, Grodd W, Ruch W (2003) Neural correlates of laughter and humour. Brain 126:2121–2138
Wise RA, Rompre PP (1989) Brain dopamine and reward. Ann Rev Psychol 40:191–225
Wundt WM (1874) Grundzüge der physiologischen Psychologie. Engelmann, Leipzig

12 Illusions and Hallucinations

Contents

12.1 Introduction

Hallucination as a false perception has been known to humans since ancient times; it has gained many cultural meanings, including for shamanism and religions. Hallucinations as psychopathological features have been defined in the course of the development of psychiatry, whereby the distinction between hallucinations, illusions, and ego disturbances could be clearly determined: Hallucinations were regarded as perceptions without a corresponding stimulus, while illusions were defined as misinterpretations of perceived objects—for example, perceiving a grotesque face in a harmless wall drawing. Ego disturbances (see next chapter) generally do not have sensory qualities, unlike hallucinations—ego disturbances that could be confused with hallucinations are, for example, of the type of inserted thoughts.

Example

A woman with a poorly adjusted hearing aid has been caring for her 90-year-old mother for many years. Her own performance is now declining over time. She suddenly hears the voices of acquaintances and her mother. They insult her. During the examination in the clinic, she appears hard of hearing and absent-minded. She is severely depressed with a delusion of guilt and acutely suicidal. ◄

F. M. Reischies, *Psychopathology*, https://doi.org/10.1007/978-3-662-70293-2_12

For the person, a hallucination is a perception: A hallucination is a sensory experience with a reality character. Only the external observer can recognize that the patient's perception occurs without corresponding external stimulation. The person who hallucinates may learn from others that there was no stimulus source for their perception. Many people then react with incomprehension and rejection. Others may have already noticed that something might not be in order with their "voices".

The reality character of the hallucination makes it understandable that a person tries to make sense of the unusual perceptions. Many contents and circumstances of hallucinations are "extraordinary". The person who has a hallucination must explain what they hear or see—for example, that the deceased mother is speaking to him. This circumstance often leads to the development of a delusional explanation (see below). The diagnostic difficulty, on the other hand, is significantly higher with very realistic hallucinations.

Thus, there are two fundamentally different perspectives on hallucination: that of the hallucinating person and that of other persons. From an objective standpoint, hallucinations are a perception that occurs even though there is nothing to perceive, no stimulus for it. In other words, from the observer's perspective, a process in the patient's central nervous system must apparently lead to a perception—with the quality of a "real" sensory experience—without a real object of sensory stimulation that could be perceived as such (the observer can rule this out).

Thus, a mental content with reference to the environment is classified by the person as a perception. The erroneous experience that the hallucinated contents are perceptions is considered by the patient as evidence of the reality of what is perceived. Patients report, for example, "But I did hear that!". Since the external observer knows that the hallucinated information must have originated in the person's head, it follows: Hallucinations are mentally activated contents in the brain, which—in a state of disturbed processing of the source of information—are considered perceptions, as real. This model will be discussed further below.

Early psychopathological definitions (since Esquirol 1838) focussed on the perception, which must be false. Alternatively, it could be argued that no perception took place because a mental content was activated internally: Especially in schizophrenia, the perceptual character of thoughts is often less prominent: It is not about voices perceived as coming from outside, but voices in the head. In some patients, they are not easily distinguishable from thoughts that have been "inserted" (see below: ego disturbances).

A two-step process must be assumed for hallucination: If we assume the absence of the object of perception, we assume

(1) in the first process that the mental object was activated in the CNS. The perceptual error consists in it being falsely registered as perceived:
(2) In the second process, the source of the perception is identified, this process can be intact or faulty.
    (2a) If it is intact, the person recognizes the erroneous perception (e.g., when pressing on the eye, we see "stars").
    (2b) If the process of source identification is disturbed, the activated mental object can appear as a perception, it is hallucinated.

This process in a dream is easily understandable: A mental content has perceptual qualities and is sometimes considered a correct perception of an event that must have just happened when suddenly waking up.

In the next chapter on ego disturbances, we will discuss the case that the activated mental object is determined to be a thought that was inserted from outside.

▶ For hallucination, it is further required that the person has the subjective certainty that it is a real sensory perception, i.e., a perception of the environment. If the person considers the character as a false perception, it is called pseudohallucination.

Influence by the person: Hallucinations are mentally neither avoidable nor modifiable by the person with a schizophrenic psychosis. Hallucinations cannot be pushed back, e.g. by directing attention to the perception. The person initially perceives something that captures his attention. Concentration on the perception (listening carefully: "am I hearing this correctly?") or turning attention to something distracting cannot change the hallucination in schizophrenia. However, this is the case with other forms of hallucinations. These are, for example, forms of hallucinations that are related to falling asleep, i.e., sub-vigil phases.

12.1.1 Distinctions

Hallucinations must first be distinguished from simple perceptual distortions, such as simple optical illusions, where sensory-physiological laws have an effect. A wealth of related but differentiable perceptual disorders are presented below, i.e., psychopathological symptoms such as illusions, metamorphopsias (micropsia, macropsia), palinopsia.

Pseudohallucinations. They differ from hallucinations primarily in that the person recognizes the perception as a deception. The psychopathological term "pseudohallucinations" is, however, controversial and is not used uniformly: It is understood as a perception that is generally paler than a hallucination— and for example, it involves the misjudgment of highly emotional ideas as perceptions. A patient in a state of extreme anxiety claimed to see corpses on the floor, over which he felt compelled to step. Often, these are "as if" perceptions (the person feels as if there is a corpse lying there).

Direct, non-physiological stimulation of sensory cells leads to perceptions—for example, pressure on the eye leads to "seeing stars." The perception is recognized by the person as a sensory deception. The same applies to the stimulation of neurons in the primary cortical representation areas—it regularly leads to sensory impressions. These sensory impressions are closely related in time/space to the triggering situation and are usually elementary perceptions that do not fit into the context. The person knows that it is a misperception due to stimulation.

12.1.2 Hallucinations as So-Called "Psychotic Symptoms"

Hallucinations are currently often referred to as psychotic symptoms in psychiatry. This classification is unfortunate. For example, hallucinations also occur as pontine hallucinations in neurological disorders, which are by no means to be referred to as psychotic symptoms in the same sense as in schizophrenia. Moreover, the prevalence of hallucinations in the population is apparently much higher than that of psychoses. Additionally, the term psychosis is less defined by the characteristics of hallucinations and delusions than by a characteristic that Jaspers (1942) emphasized—a break in the development of personality. A patient with a psychosis (of any etiology) is described by relatives as "he has completely changed" or "we don't recognize him at all any more."

12.1.3 Dimensions of Hallucinations

Hallucinations differ clinically in many properties. The most important dimensions are:

1. Modality (auditory, visual, tactile, olfactory, gustatory, bodily hallucination) - spatial aspects
2. Complexity,
3. Specific stimulus quality (e.g., acoustic quality, visual characteristics)
4. Subjective meaning, relevance of the content for the person
5. Intensity,
6. Emotional congruence,
7. Subjective certainty that it is a real experience,
8. Attention.

Table 12.1 Classification of various clinical forms of hallucinations according to modality and complexity

Modality	Elementary	Complex
Acoustic	Acoasma	Hearing voices, verbal acoustic hallucination
Optical	Geometric; moving point in the visual field	Scenic
Physical	Tactile, elementary pain	Coenesthetic, e.g., sexual perception
Olfactory	Simple smell	"Poison," own smell as stench
Gustatory	Simple taste	"Poison"

A first overview of various clinical forms of hallucinations results in a classification according to modality and complexity Table 12.1 .

Specific Stimulus Quality

Some auditory verbal hallucinations are perceived very precisely describable. For example, they are the voices of people known to the patient, coming from a specific corner of the room, which the patient also looks at when the voices occur. Other hallucinations do not have this differentiated stimulus quality but are described as, for example, voices "in the head" that hardly seem to exhibit any acoustic stimulus parameters.

Subjective Importance

The hallucinations that are clinically reported often have a high emotional significance for the person. A patient considers a perception worth reporting. Then there is usually also an emotional component. However, he may also perceive other things that are to be considered hallucinations and about which he does not report (Sect. 12.4 Diagnostics). This is one of the reasons why the frequency of hallucinations in the population is unknown. For example, emotionally insignificant hallucinations are not expressed in the clinical context.

Hallucinations represent content errors of perception that are related to the person's life; less often, insignificant things are perceived in schizophrenia. The contents of the hallucination are usually affect-coupled, whether they correspond to the person's affective state or also trigger affects. The contents can appear bizarre and unrelated to the person's everyday life, like dream contents. The high subjective significance of the hallucinations is related to the content, which refers to existential problems or important people for the patient.

In deafferentation hallucinations (see below), people are often surprised by the perception of insignificant visual scenes. In this form of hallucinations, the content and affective reference to the person's life is much less or not present at all. The important affect is only the surprise and alienation. In Charles Bonnet syndrome, for example, vivid, usually small figures are seen (on the basis of afferent disturbances), which can be completely insignificant. The same applies to hearing music as a hallucination in the hearing impaired.

Intensity

The intensity of hallucinations can be very low. For example, the person must close their eyes to see the hallucinations (as if on the back of the eyelids), which can be the case with peduncular hallucinations.

In another example, a person only hears a murmur that is indistinct. When background noises like running water are added as a stimulus source, the person can hear the murmur more clearly. The term functional hallucination has been used for this, i.e., in cases where misperceptions occur only in connection with unspecific disturbing real sensory stimuli. This perceptual disorder has relationships to both deafferentation hallucinations and to illusion (see below).

The intensity of hallucinations can be high, for example, in volume (screaming voices) or in the brightness or clarity of visual hallucinations.

The intensity of coenesthetic pain, for example in the genitals, can also be significant.

Regardless of the intensity, the clarity of the hallucinations must be considered. This refers to the richness of detail and the abundance of perceptual qualities, in the auditory domain the frequency, location, dynamic course, etc., and in the visual domain the color, shape, proportion, and relation to the environment, etc. In general, the clarity of hallucinations is significantly higher than that of an imagination.

Subjective Certainty

Although hallucinations must be considered real by definition, clinically there is a transition to pseudohallucinations with insight into the perceptual distortion. On the one hand, people are absolutely certain that they have perceived something real and seek the source of the sensory impressions they consider real. They assume that their perceptions would also be perceptible to others. In other forms of hallucinations or after long experience with "their" hallucinations, patients know that their fellow humans in the environment probably do not share the perceptions. In most cases, they then do not speak or do not like to speak about these perceptions.

Emotional Congruence

In some cases, hallucinations occur in connection with emotions, with the contents of the hallucinations matching the emotion. For example, a patient has anxiety and sees grimaces, perceives pursuers, and hears their voices, e.g., threats, or sees a fire blazing. A patient with a depressive syndrome heard insults, e.g., she was called a whore or scolded by her mother. Hallucinating persons believes they are emotionally reacting to the perception; in this case, the hallucination and the activation of the emotional syndrome belong together in the pathological process.

However, hallucinations also occur without accompanying emotions. Especially in the case of deafferentation hallucination, as mentioned above, figures, scenes, or music are perceived without the contents being coupled with emotions. Also, in schizophrenia—typically in chronic courses of the disease—there are verbal auditory hallucinations with trivial contents, e.g., "there he sits again." However, the schizophrenic patient concludes from this that the people he hears as voices know everything exactly about him. He then usually suffers from the loss of privacy.

Attention/Working Memory/State of Consciousness

Some patients are captivated by their hallucinations, and the examiner notices an almost complete focus of attention on the hallucination. It does not affect the perception of the hallucinations to what extent the affected person consciously directs his attention to the hallucination. The independence of hallucinations from the conscious directing of attention in schizophrenia could be considered an argument that the person's attention processes are disturbed (see below).

Action-Accompanying Hallucinations, Sleep-Related Hallucinations

According to clinical experience, hallucinations occur on the one hand accompanying actions, for example, during the execution of an activity. In other cases, hallucinations occur during the reduction of alertness in rest phases in the evening or during tiredness in moments of dozing off—this is referred to as hypnagogic hallucinations. In the morning upon waking, sleep-related hallucinations are referred to as hypnopompic hallucinations. In these circumstances, an improvement in hallucinations can be observed when attention is awakened and directed to the hallucinations. In delirium, hallucinations occur with a clouding of consciousness, whereby delirium as a psychiatric syndrome itself is coupled with a fundamental disturbance of attention and attention control.

Control over Information Processing

In this section, a disturbance of an area of "self-consciousness" in the sense of Dennett (1984) is to be mentioned (Stanghellini and Cutting 2003). Here, a disturbance in the functions is assumed, which enables a person to actively involve themselves in their own mental life. While healthy individuals can (1) distinguish well between classes of mental activities and (2) control them, in schizophrenic patients, a disturbance is assumed (1) in the experience of differentiation and (2) in the active interaction with mental processes, such as perception, imagination, daydreaming, or thinking. This is about the disturbance of the sovereignty of the person over their mental processes in a broader sense. However, this psychopathological model formation has not yet been well studied.

Differential Diagnostic Aspects of Hallucinations

- Sporadic hallucination in healthy individuals
- Hallucinations after the loss of a partner after decades of living together
- Hypnagogic/hypnopompichallucinations, e.g., in narcolepsy
- Epileptic hallucinations:
  a) ictal hallucinosis in epilepsy
  b) hallucination in the aura of an epileptic seizure
- Deafferentation hallucinations:
  a) in disturbance of the visual afferent systems: Charles Bonnet syndrome (Podoll et al. 1989)
  b) In amputation: phantom phenomena
- Peduncular hallucinosis, in brainstem lesions (Manford and Andermann 1998)
- Hallucinations as part of a brain damage- or brain degeneration syndrome, e.g., in delirium, e.g., in dementias (Lewy body dementia)
- toxic/withdrawal
  a) Acute/chronic alcohol hallucinosis
  b) Acute hallucinogen intoxication
- Hallucinations in Parkinson's syndrome
- Hallucinations in schizophrenic/affective psychosis

12.2 Clinic

Hallucinations occur in a variety of pathophysiological contexts. If any indications of the circumstances summarized in the following overview arise, intensive efforts must be made in diagnostics to detect or exclude hallucinations. Hallucinations are not uncommon. Examples include: A high percentage of elderly people who lose their long-term partner hear their voice in typical everyday situations. Practically all patients who have suffered damage to the primary visual cortex have visual hallucinations. Many patients with hearing impairments suffer from auditory hallucinations, and many people experience hearing voices when waking up or falling asleep. In delirium, hallucinations occur. Due to social stigmatization, reliable epidemiological figures are not available.

Hallucinations are particularly important in the diagnosis of schizophrenia and exhibit some special characteristics (see Bentall et al. 1991).

Hallucinations in Schizophrenia

1. Auditory hallucinations
   Acoasms (e.g., in a delusional mood)
   verbal auditory hallucinations (hearing voices, phonemes)
   a) "Voices" in dialogue and counter-dialogue
   b) imperative phonemes
2. Somatic hallucinations
   bizarre, coenesthetic symptoms
   erotic (including painful misperceptions)
3. Olfactory hallucinations (e.g., smell of poison)
4. Gustatory hallucinations

Verbal auditory hallucinations are particularly closely associated with thought disorder, thought pressure, and compulsions to repeat in schizophrenia (Klosterkötter et al. 1988)—here, a relationship to disorders of thought control (see there) emerges. The peculiarity of schizophrenic "hearing voices" is also seen in the pathological objectification of the inner dialogue (Stanghellini et al. 2003), where this concerns the "foreign" role of the dialogue. The person in the foreign role "says" something in many cases that the person cannot accept as their own idea. Examples include sexual ideas, blasphemies, etc. Some researchers assume that defense mechanisms or coping strategies are additionally involved in this.

12.3 Diagnostics

The diagnosis of the psychopathological feature hallucination depends on the information provided by the person. Hallucinations cannot be diagnosed without the cooperation of the examiner with the affected person.

The person may either be surprised that the perception of bizarre things is happening, or they report the experience that they have found no cause for the perception.

If, on the other hand, someone hears something that is possible, nothing improbable, this event will not be reported and will only become the subject of psychopathological considerations in, for example, court reports. Although the examiner may suspect the presence of hallucinations from clinical observations—for example, if patients behave in such a way that it can only be explained by perceiving something that is not perceptible to the examiner. Examples include looking at a particular place, listening to something, inexplicable "startle response," or reacting with fingers (fidgeting), or talking to someone who is not recognizable. Among the examples mentioned are inexplicable attention-accompanying movements. They suggest hallucinations, but as long as a patient does not openly talk about these perceptions, it cannot be confirmed that a hallucination is present (in the findings, "not assessable" would be documented). Behavioral observation can therefore only be indicative.

In many cases, some noticeable remark arises during the psychopathological examination, which can be inquired about whether it could be, for example, hearing voices. However, even without indications, a statement from the patient about possible hallucinations must be requested in any case, for example: "Have you heard, seen, or smelled anything strange? For example, perceived something that surprised others when you mentioned it?"

Insight disorder

A lack of insight is part of the symptom hallucination, as it is required by definition that the falsely perceived is considered real. Diagnostically, it is often difficult to determine whether the patient did not report the hallucinations because they did not perceive the strange perceptions as hallucinations, whether they are ashamed to disclose the information (e.g., because hallucinations justify the diagnosis "psychotic"), or whether the voices forbid them to speak about it. The patient may suspect that it is unfavorable for them to talk about the "voices." There is a spectrum from lack of insight into the hallucination on one side to denial of the symptom hallucination on the other side.

Clinical experience is that hallucinations or ego disturbances, which are otherwise not reported, are often reported in psycho-educational groups. This usually happens in sessions where these features are discussed, and patients experience that fellow patients also talk about them. In self-experience groups, there are repeated discussions about the question, "Where should the information of the hallucination come from?" Patients reported hearing voices of familiar people and could not explain how these people could know something very personal about them, or the patients could not imagine that the contents of the voices they hear originated in their own heads.

Some patients believe there must be sensor chips under the scalp, special antennas, or some technical devices that communicate their private thoughts to others. The others then talk to the voices that the patients perceive about these private contents.

When a person is just beginning to experience hallucinations, it may happen that they cannot provide conclusive answers to such questions, even if they are cooperative. This is because they have not yet experienced the discrepancy with the perception of other people. The diagnosis is also related to the dissonance between the false perception and the person's expectations:

If the perception completely matches the expectation, it is usually not reported. It may then be that the person only mentions it in passing. In such cases, further inquiry is necessary. For example, people report comments from colleagues at work, at meetings, or in the choir. When many people are gathered together, these perceptions are not easily noticed as unusual. They are reported not as hallucinations but because of their content. The examiner must ask whether, for example, other choir members also heard this statement or whether a hallucination might be the underlying cause.

Many hallucinations are not detected in psychopathological examinations. For example, a patient explained only at the request of his mother during outpatient follow-up care after several inpatient stays that he had been hearing voices of people who frightened him, whom he had seen on a vacation, since the onset of clinical symptoms. The hallucination is not reported. This occurs, for example, when the patient has recognized the abnormal and inexplicable nature of their perceptions but does not talk about it, mainly because hallucinations, such as hearing voices, are socially stigmatized or associated with the diagnosis of "insanity."

Clinically and diagnostically, a transition series from perception to thought insertion must be considered.

a) perception:

Physiologically, there are

- optical illusions that suggest additional sensory information and
- gestalt completion: e.g., content fixation in ambiguous images.
- Physiologically, vivid imagination is also included.

b) Close to perception:

Likewise, vivid healthy imagination can be considered the "earworm". Additionally, the imagination of the sound of a voice: Some people can vividly imagine the speech melody and voice when reading a letter from a familiar person.

Pareidolia: images can be seen in clouds (illusion). The same mechanism is presumably responsible for the imagination of music in the loud rhythmic noise of a train, which many people can experience.

Affective illusions: children imagine a person in the bedroom curtain at night full of anxiety.

Transition to functional hallucination: a voice is heard only in the noise of the faucet (illusion).

Hypnagogic hallucinations: in sub-vigilant phases and in the transition from dream experience.

Deprivation hallucinations are common in the hearing impaired,

after the loss of a partner after decades of living together—often in a lonely situation.

c) Transition to thought insertion:

Phonemes of schizophrenic patients without consciousness or attention disorders; the phonemes can occur without sensory characteristics (voices in the head).

Thought insertion: A patient with schizophrenia claims to be able to receive and perceive thoughts from other people, i.e., he identifies thoughts as foreign (disturbed perception as actor - see below).

12.4 Neuroscience

The diversity of clinical manifestations of hallucinations cannot yet be explained neuroscientifically. There are only a few hypotheses about the fundamental mechanisms of the development of hallucinations.

Factors in the development of hallucinations include abnormal electrical activity according to the epilepsy model (Sect. 12.4.1), a disturbance of afference with a predominance of imagination (Sect. 12.4.2), and disturbed attentional functions; in addition, there are model concepts of abnormal information transmission (Sect. 12.4.3) of imagined stimuli to the primary sensory brain areas.

12.4.1 Neuronal Networks and Hallucinations

First a finding from the application of neuronal networks should be reported. Already in the chapter on language, implicit rule learning in neuronal networks was reported (LeCun et al. 2015). It has now emerged that the trained neuronal networks “hallucinate”: They are trained to fill gaps and find the most likely continuations for incomplete statements (Friston 2005). In the operation of these functions, false solutions occur, for example, in face recognition, a wrong person is identified, and in large language models, a false statement is issued (Suzuki et al. 2024). In the various intermediate layers of the network models (deep learning), information about regularities, such as language rules, or, in the image area, information about classes of living beings in the recognition of animals, etc., can be found. If information from these intermediate steps of information processing becomes accessible to a person, misrecognitions occur, which have typically certain similarity to the correct classification. This can serve as a model to explain illusions.

If it is further assumed that the linguistic processing of thoughts and the visualization of statements from other people, along with the acoustic qualities, are also performed via neuronal networks, then in the next step, a hallucination with a spontaneously completely new statement and acoustic qualities from the person’s experience can also arise.

12.4.2 Abnormal Electrical Activity

Experimental data show that perceptions, even of a complex nature, can be provoked by direct brain stimulation. This has been demonstrated in experiments, for example, with epileptic patients. Clinical experiences exist regarding elementary visual hallucinations, for example, after strokes, which are observed in the peripheral areas of vascular-induced visual field defects (e.g., epileptic, Kölmel 1985). These hallucinations are assumed to be caused by abnormal neuronal activity in higher cortical association areas that process sensory information.

Abnormal activity of individual neurons does not always lead to a perception because object encoding by populations is assumed, or gestalt recognition via the discussed neuronal networks—as presented in the section on elementary perception. In other words, the probability that stimulation will activate exactly the pattern of neurons that belongs to an object or situation encoding is very low. There was a discussion about the “grandmother neuron” with two groups of scientists, those who believed such a neuron could be found and those who believed such a thing could not exist in the CNS. Certainly, there is no grandmother neuron in the strict sense of the word—i.e., a neuron that encodes exactly one object—but there is a multitude of neurons that represent partial aspects of the “grandmother” in small ensembles. Partial aspects mean, for example, the face, posture, typical movements and sound of a voice, the smell, etc. A model would be that stimuli bring the neuronal networks (Chap. 9 language and Chap. 10 thinking) to pre-activate the representation of the “grandmother” in individual elements and then, in the second step, bring the complete image of the grandmother above the perception threshold through the mechanism of gap-filling (see below).

12.4.3 Disturbance of Afference and Monitoring

According to the clinical data and experiments with sensory deprivation, the disturbance of sensory afference must be considered as a possibility for the emergence of hallucinations. One can speak of weak-input models, where due to this weak input, neuropsychological errors occur. The CNS tries to find a plausible solution based on the insufficient sensory data. At this point, it must be emphasized that

- perception always involves an active reconstruction according to an environmental model (Chap. 2). It is important to note that this contradicts the immediate healthy experience in perception, because we experience the control of what we perceive through the objects and events in our environment. In other words, we experience, for example, visual perception as passive reception of the image of the environment.
- When insufficient sensory data are present, expectation and imagination necessarily play a greater role than with sufficiently determining sensory information. This indicates (1) a complementary role of imagination in hallucinations and (2) again shows a role of "gap-filling" by neuronal networks.

Deafferentation Hallucinoses

A number of hallucinations fall under this category:

Charles Bonnet syndrome, hallucinations in the disturbance of elementary visual information processing,

Anton syndrome after damage to the primary visual cortical areas - with intact secondary representation areas; auditory hallucinations in hearing impairment; experiments with healthy individuals who are kept in a situation where they have no perceptions (for example, looking at a gray ceiling for days).

After amputation—phantom phenomena—retained central representation, potentially this also applies to peduncular hallucinosis, as brainstem influences on the corpus geniculatum of the thalamus are discussed as gatekeepers of incoming sensory information.

In a certain relationship to deafferentation, hearing the voice of the deceased long-term partner can also be listed here. In this case, the existing multiple memory traces, which are strongly overlearned, may be reactivated by a situational context, where the usual perception did not occur and the processing (via neuronal networks) can supplement what was usually heard—"He always said that in this situation." A generative network as a model of deafferentation hallucination in Charles Bonnet syndrome has been developed (Reichert et al. 2013).

Role of Increased Imagination Functions

In the case of deafferentation, a compensatory predominance of imagination is explainable. The same applies to hallucinations in affective agitation. Limbic "overload" has been mentioned (Benson 1994). This is particularly evident when the contents of the hallucination represent wishes or fears. Also in hallucinatory wish fulfillment in childhood, e.g., imaginary playmates, increased imagination plays an important role.

An imagination leads to an imagination of the sensory experience, which can be very realistic (as when hearing the voice of the letter writer when reading a handwritten letter, or also with an "earworm" of a popular music recording). Thus, it can be, on the one hand, only the activation of the semantic unit, without perceptual features, or on the other hand, the detailed sensory imagination with all details—including the sensory qualities—that can be perceived in the real perception. This applies to both visual and auditory imaginations.

Imagination disrupts the competing perception of external stimuli. This was already described by Perky at the beginning of the 20th century for lines and tones (see Craver-Lamley and Reevers 1992, see Ford et al. 2012). Studies by Kosslyn's group have provided clear evidence, through imaging techniques and transcranial magnetic stimulation, that the primary sensory areas are activated during imagination. On the one hand, it was shown that imaginations in the primary visual cortex can be disrupted by transcranial magnetic stimulation, and on the other hand, the activation of identical specific perception areas could be shown for both perception and imagination of the same stimuli (Kosslyn et al. 1999; Slotnick et al. 2005).

Thus, we can assume an overactive realistic imagination of sensory stimuli, which are not present, as processes in the emergence of hallucination. If, in addition, the sensory input is disturbed as in deafferentation situations, imagination could represent the decisive input for the erroneous perception.

Monitoring-Deficit—Identification and Recognition of the Source of Mental Contents

There is a fundamental problem with the explanatory approaches to hallucinations as a result of dominant imagination: Why can't the person recognize that they have just imagined something themselves?

Firstly, it must be said that in human perception, something is always and constantly being imagined. Perceptions are expected. This follows from the model of active perception and preditive coding (Chap. 2). In hallucinations, imaginations can therefore have occurred unconsciously. What is crucial is what happened in information processing before the hallucination, what the ideas, expectations, imaginations, and thought contents were.

Models have been developed to explain why an imagination in hallucinations is mistaken for a perception. One was proposed by Frith 1992: He assumes a disturbance of self-monitoring, the efference copy or its processing (see reafference principle, by von Holst and Mittelstaedt 1950). The efference copy is produced, for example, with every initiation of action; it enables the comparison of the consequence of the action with the expectation based on the action planning and initiation. For example, when grasping an object from the table, "the fingers will touch the table during the action," etc., with the feedback from the fingers when the table is actually touched and the skin sensors report a touch. In self-generated actions, the anterior cingulate cortex is active alongside the dorsolateral prefrontal cortex (Frith et al. 2001). The model is that these brain areas inhibit the sensory activation of the posterior cortex areas, which provide feedback on the executed movement, so that the person does not think an independent external stimulation has occurred (Farrer et al. 2003).

According to this model, hallucinations are imaginations that become conscious in a state of lacking control over the source of information and are mistaken for perceptions. The source: "self-initiated" is confused with the source: "perception of an external stimulus."

Another related model assumes a disturbance in the intermediate storage of thoughts and percepts. Monitoring of mental processes in working memory is assumed (Goldman-Rakic and Selemon 1997). In the context of hallucinations, it is a working memory function of intermediate storage of mental contents along with their sources. Such monitoring of one's own thoughts occurs in healthy individuals—and according to the model, this instance is disturbed in hallucinations.

An indication for the described explanatory approach for auditory hallucinations in schizophrenia is that patients are not disturbed by the hallucinations in many cases. They are not as surprised by the hallucination as, for example, patients with Charles Bonnet syndrome after a disturbance of visual afference. The reason for the lack of surprise could be that they can recognize a certain familiarity with the thoughts expressed in the phonemes—they are therefore not so unfamiliar to them, almost because they have just thought them themselves.

Imaging Studies

The methods of functional imaging have made progress in explaining hallucinations (Kircher and Thienel 2005). Imaging findings have been obtained that showed both structural changes in the temporal cortex in hallucinating schizophrenic patients (Gaser et al. 2004) and a series of functional activations that can help explain the complex phenomenon.

In imaging studies, for example, it was examined whether the activation in specific brain areas can differentiate between the imaginations from hallucinations. Individuals were asked to think of words but not to speak them. In the imaginative verb generation on the one hand and in verbal auditory hallucinations on the other hand, a comparable regional activation was shown (Shergill et al. 2003). This concerned areas of speech production and speech comprehension. The data from these complex results suggest that the speech production areas, the dominant inferior frontal cortex, have insufficient functional connection with the speech comprehension areas. The model assumes that self-generated speech leads to a suppression of activity in the speech comprehension areas (Curio et al. 2000). This top-down interaction in self-generated speech could be disturbed in schizophrenic patients who are prone to verbal auditory hallucinations.

In the mediofrontal brain regions, especially the anterior cingulate, there are neurons that are active in self-initiated movements but not in externally induced movements (Shima and Tanji 1998). Disturbances in this brain region could disrupt the monitoring of whether a mental process is self-initiated or originates from a perception (see, for example, Christoff et al. 2003). Findings of disturbances in this region in schizophrenia and in delirium (Reischies et al. 2005) are consistent with the observation that hallucinations are particularly common in these disorders.

The results have been achieved in the effort to find regions whose activation allows a distinction between the imagination of words and the perception of phonemes. If there were such a function-specific region, the person could, for example, rely on the fact that words are only imagined when this additional brain region is active. Of course, other groups of neurons that cannot be represented in imaging studies may also participate in this differentiation and monitoring, and the resolution of imaging studies is still not high enough.

If groups of neurons that represent differences between self-generated mental activity and perceived content are disruptable, then this can bring us closer to answering the question of why the patient does not notice that it is only an imagination (see below). For example, if there is a disturbance in the "supplementary motor area," the person can no longer make this distinction and might mistakenly assume they heard the thought as a voice. The term comparator regions has been used. It should not be further discussed here that other areas also seem to be involved in the differentiation of feedback and efference copy, for example, the cerebellum (Blakemore et al. 2001).

Neuropsychological Findings on the Monitoring Deficit in Hallucinations
Studies on the identification of the source of consciousness contents that could support the Frith model have been widely noted. In many studies on the monitoring deficit, "source discrimination" was studied, i.e., the question of whether the source of mental contents can be identified, whether a content of consciousness was perceived or imagined. In a disturbance of source identification, it cannot be distinguished whether a content of consciousness originates from one's own intention or from sensory data.

It is a general experience that one cannot tickle oneself. This is not possible because the CNS knows from the movement planning which skin areas will be touched. This may be related to the fact that in one's own movement, the efference copy predicts the touch on the skin and thus prevents the indeterminate necessary for tickling. We had hypothesized that patients who hallucinate can tickle themselves. If the efference copy or the expectation of feedback is disturbed in schizophrenic patients, they should be able to tickle themselves. This was confirmed in later studies. It has now also been shown in imaging studies that schizophrenic patients exhibit altered sensorimotor feedback (Blakemore et al. 2000a, b).

12.4.4 Imagination and the Activation of Primary Sensory Areas

The model of a pathological activation of the primary sensory representation areas has been proposed (Dierks et al. 1999). In auditory hallucinations, the primary sensory auditory area is activated, which is not the case with imaginations. These results could be partially confirmed by further investigations (van de Ven et al. 2005).

A model of the pathological transmission of imaginations into the primary sensory areas could be postulated. It assumes a disturbance in the delimitation of brain areas that can be used or influenced by imagination. This delimitation applies to healthy individuals. However, patients with schizophrenia pathologically activate the primary cortical association areas.

Follow-up studies by Shergill et al. 2000 did not yield a clear picture. Nevertheless, consistent with Silbersweig (Silbersweig and Stern 1996), thalamic and parahippocampal activation was found.

In summary, no functional model of hallucinations can yet be derived from this. A possibly dispositional decisive variance exists in the imaginability of sound. There are patients who can realistically imagine a voice or music without any problems.

The decisive objection to the model of hallucinations as pathological activation of primary sensory brain areas could be the above-reported finding of the Kosslyn research group (Kosslyn et al. 1999) on the non-pathological activation of the primary sensory areas by imaginations, at least in the visual domain. Findings on the context dependency of size perceptions in the primary visual area (Murray et al. 2006) also argue against a fundamental inaccessibility of the primary sensory regions to top-down influence (see also Koch 2005).

12.4.5 Integration of Various Pathophysiological Factors

How are the pathophysiological factors presented above to be summarized into a functional model of hallucinations? Do they contradict or complement each other?

Competition Between Perception and Imagination

Based on the available data, it must be assumed that there are sensory cortex areas in which a kind of competition between sensory information and imagination can take place. From the experiences of deafferentation hallucinations, such competition is to be assumed. For when the external information fails because the afference from the sensory organs is disturbed, hallucinations are often perceived. For example, where is the information represented when I imagine a summer hit that pursues me like an "earworm" with intense acoustic qualities?

We must assume that the imagined sensory information is represented in the specific sensory areas. Findings for this are presented above. Accordingly, in hallucinations, the sensory areas are overstrained. In some cases, one can clinically observe an apparent hearing loss or speech comprehension disorder in patients who hear intense acoustic hallucinations.

Thus, we should rather assume competition at a perception matrix, the sensory representation areas, whether they are the primary or secondary areas. These can be reached "bottom-up" by sensory data and "top-down" by imagination. The metaphoric concept for this would be a projection screen that can be played from two sides—from one side by perception information and from the other by imagination. Recently, this basic model has also been accepted by other researchers (Collerton et al. 2023). According to the constructivist model of perception, we must assume that sensory information is generally embedded in pre-information by perception, which happens "top-down" - predictive coding (Fig. 12.1). The development of a reality-based construction, which is, however, error-prone, could also be explained by the properties of neuronal networks (see above).

In this "double-sided projection," the balance of input from sensory information on the one hand or from imagination on the other hand could have shifted in hallucinations, namely towards an overweight of imagination (possibly also in hypnagogic hallucination in narcolepsy and pontine hallucinosis).

Disturbance of Monitoring and Identification of the Source of Mental Content

Furthermore, the monitoring of the intention to one's own thoughts or the identification of the source of consciousness content is likely to be disturbed. In the case of a disturbance in this

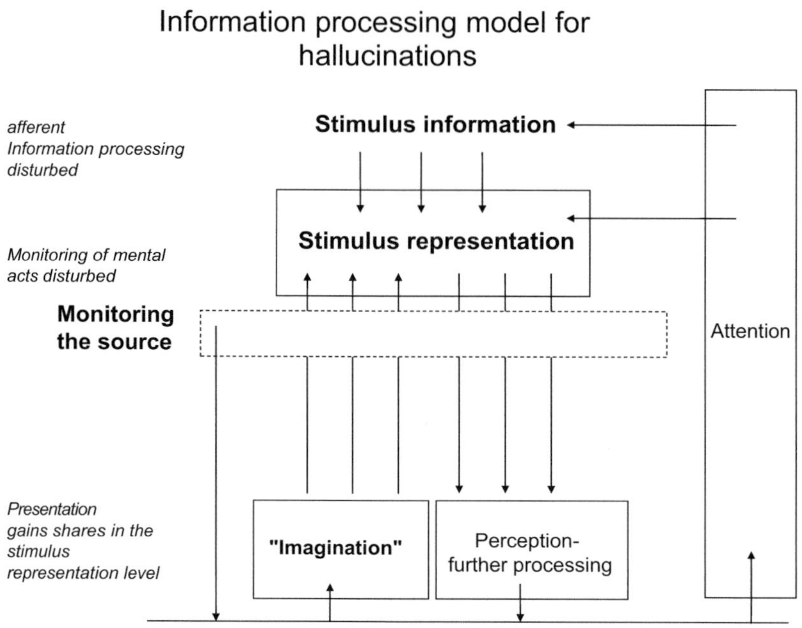

Fig. 12.1 To explain hallucinations, models such as the disturbance of source recognition are examined. One must assume a level of stimulus representation that is used by both perceptual stimuli and imagination, like a projection screen used from two sides. The monitoring of the source of information that enters this stimulus representation can be disturbed, i.e., the information about whether external, perceived stimuli or internal, imagined stimuli were present. For self-actively imagined stimuli, traces of one's own authorship should be found (equivalents of the "corollary discharge" or reafference, Chap. 7)

area, it becomes understandable that thoughts and consciousness content are not recognized as one's own, or that the person does not realize that they have imagined the hallucinated content. This factor has at least a relationship to thought control disorder in schizophrenic hallucinations (see above) and the ego disturbances presented in the next chapter.

Findings for this point are the results of "source discrimination" studies (see above). In the case of disturbed attention or consciousness disorders such as delirium, a monitoring disturbance is to be expected.

Errors in the Construction of Perception

Finally, we must return once more to the generally accepted model of the construction of perception, where errors can occur. Some findings particularly impressively demonstrate this. The entire perception is composed of elements, with some elements sometimes not being integrated or being integrated incorrectly.

Particularly impressive optical illusions have been presented: (1) The image of the politician Mrs. Thatcher, which is upside down, but with the eyes not turned upside down (in a kind of collage), leads to the perception of a completely upside-down image—the incorrectly placed eyes are not noticed. The image appears correct. (2) The error, however, becomes immediately and surprisingly apparent when the image is rotated back and now stands upright—then the eyes are upside down, in contradiction to the upright-oriented head. Upon seeing this image, one is startled by the incorrect eye area. A similar example is the adaptation to inversion glasses. After a certain time, all objects and buildings in the surroundings are seen upright, but individual elements are not integrated, for example, a clock is not turned upside down. Our perception is constructed and is partly erroneously composed of the various elements.

Primary information processing is handled in primary representation areas, which, however, should not be imagined as a complete "internal screen"—certainly not as a coherent screen, but irregularly distributed, with respective information about the retinal position of an object and recalculated external space position. The current environmental model shapes the construction of what is perceived at all times.

It is not to be assumed that an entire hallucinated object with all perceptual qualities is active in the primary representation areas or on the perception matrix. The hallucinated information contains, following this argument, gaps and will only partially retain the features of elementary perception. As an internal "pars pro toto", i.e., premature conclusion, one can consider that an (imagined) content of consciousness is then perceived as a perception when individual elements appear as perceived. In complex hallucinations, e.g., of schizophrenic patients, elements of perception and imagination are constructed into a subjective complex perception. Thus, only parts of the total hallucination are elaborated down to sensory qualities.

This corresponds to the clinical experience that in schizophrenia many patients cannot experience or provide information about all sensory aspects of their voices. When schizophrenic patients are asked to describe the voices they have perceived in detail, they report only individual elements of the perception of physical voice qualities, almost never all perceptual details: either in which direction the voices were heard or, on the other hand, what gender they were, how loud, and whether they had any accent, etc. Practically all patients can indicate that there are differences between the perceived voice and the experience with a real speaker. One patient "felt" her voices physically; otherwise, they were thoughts. Often, only "thoughts in the head" occur, with no elementary perceptual features being indicated. There is likely a variance whose clinical significance cannot currently be estimated: patients with the hearing of sound properties say they are hallucinations; others without the experience of sound properties say they are just thoughts originating from others. Additionally, there are patients who realize that they are their own thoughts—they report hearing one's own thoughts (see below).

▶ In Compliance-therapy groups, it proves useful to talk about hallucinations. Patients should be encouraged to describe the complete perception with all sensory qualities, especially the qualities that speak for the reality of the "voices." This should help the patient learn to characterize the perception as imagination.

Attention, Vigilance, Information Processing in Sleep/Dream

Many patients cannot imagine where the information they perceive in a hallucination comes from. But they are not surprised by the most vivid conversations they experience in a dream or intense visual scenes they see in a dream. Hardly anyone today assumes that dream content is somehow input from the outside. Today, it is accepted that there is a mode of fantasy or creativity on the one hand and, on the other hand, a compilation of the experiences of the last days and weeks, which is "played out" or constructed in the dream.

Hypersomnia and disturbance of vigilance are clinically observed in many cases of hallucinations, for example in hypnagogic hallucinations. Hallucinations frequently occur under drugs that affect vigilance, after sleep deprivation or in delirium with consciousness disturbances and disruptions of the day-night rhythm. Hallucinations seem to prefer hypovigilant states. Therefore, one can suspect a disturbance in the control of dream phases, possibly interspersed micro-REM phases. The hypothesis here is that dream mechanisms are activated during wakefulness. In the case of sleep deficit, hallucinations occur, which can be explained as REM intrusions.

The role of attention disorder in hallucinations is particularly supported by peduncular hallucinosis with hypersomnia. In this clinical syndrome with hallucinations, a serotonergic and cholinergic effect on the lateral geniculate body is discussed (Manford and Andermann

1998). The switching processes of sleep regulation could be desynchronized—among other things, in connection with a disturbance of the cholinergic system.

The alteration of the innervation of the geniculate body in peduncular hallucinations affects the information flow to the primary sensory brain areas, as the visual and auditory sensory information runs through the geniculate body (medial and lateral). This can lead to a promotion or a kind of unlocking of imagination on perception fields, an imbalance in the perception matrix, as outlined above. For the dream, it is assumed that there is a constellation of information processing that enters the imagination information into the perception matrix.

Various pathophysiological factors have now been presented. From the arguments presented, it becomes clear that hallucinations in most clinical pictures are embedded in a disturbed vigilance state, an altered environmental model, a source discrimination disorder, and usually also a particular emotional mood-state.

The question is whether the various neuroscientific factors of hallucinations must come together and then can explain why hallucinations occur, or whether one of the factors is sufficient and therefore different hallucinations also have different pathophysiological causal factors. They would then also need to be specifically treated. The latter assumption is initially more plausible because hallucinations are common and occur in many heterogeneous clinical pictures. This suggests that hallucinations can already occur with the disturbance of one or a subgroup of the factors.

Are Specific Transmitters or Receptors Involved in the Pathophysiology of Hallucination?

So far, there are no convincing models on how transmitter systems or their receptors are involved in the pathophysiology of hallucinations. It is certain that molecular processes at receptors can lead to hallucinations. Even traces of lysergic acid diethylamide (LSD) can induce vivid hallucinations in healthy individuals. Often, only elementary hallucinations such as colors or geometric shapes are seen, or they are illusions. With cannabis, about 15% of individuals report hallucinations. It is observed that usually a state of altered consciousness and a certain sedation are achieved.

Intensive research has been conducted on the mechanisms of the hallucinogenic effect. However, how the pathophysiological mechanism of these potential active factors can be explained remains unclear. There is only speculation about a switch function in the information flow from the sensory organs to the cortex. It is known that serotonergic neurons are particularly numerous in the cortical layers of the primary sensory areas that receive information from the thalamus. This could lead to a pharmacological alteration of the sensory "input" for perception and thus to the predominance of imaginative information (see above). Alternatively, pathophysiological mechanisms in the prefrontal cortex related to thinking could be considered, where the top-down control of perception would be altered. Visual memory images could also be mistakenly involved in the development of perception due to changes in mediotemporal memory processes.

Are there direct cholinergic mechanisms of hallucinations? This could be suspected because an anticholinergic delirium with vivid visual hallucinations occurs. The activity of the cholinergic neurons of the basal forebrain has attention-promoting functions in almost the entire cortex (Chap. 4 attention). However, the primary visual sensory cortical areas are not anatomically supplied by these neurons of the basal forebrain. An attempt is made to explain the frequency of visual hallucinations precisely by a disturbance due to the underactivation of the secondary visual areas.

Hallucinations can also occur as a result of general attention disorders in anticholinergic delirium. Specifically, in delirium, a general dysfunction of prefrontal functions is observed, which could explain the impairment of attention.

These include the above-mentioned monitoring functions, which are explained by sustained-activity neurons of the prefrontal cortex.

Furthermore, dopaminergic mechanisms of hallucinations must be considered, for example, the hallucinations in Parkinson's syndrome, especially under dopaminergic therapy. The mechanism can also only be speculated about at present. Hypothetically, it is considered a gating of stimulus-perception channels by overactive cortico-subcortical loops (the frontal loops) related to thinking, whereby imaginations could also be processed as perceptions. However, these explanations are mainly intended to demonstrate that there are now enough hypothetical pathophysiological mechanisms, but experimental or clinical data must decide which ones are correct.

How can transmitter-related or metabolic disorders explain the pathophysiology of hallucinations? Transmitters and hallucinogenic drugs could regulate the information flow as modulators in the perception matrix discussed above, which hinders the perceptual bottom-up process and allows the top-down process to take its place.

In general, regarding hallucinogenic effects, a result of psychological studies should be mentioned, which emphasizes the suggestibility of mild hallucinogenic effects. Students were given firstly cannabis or placebo and secondly were either informed that they would receive cannabis or no cannabis. Surprisingly, hallucinations also occurred in the group that only received the information that they would receive cannabis but were actually given a placebo.

12.5 Psychopathological Symptoms of Illusions and Hallucinations

Illusion
Definition. A stimulus is misinterpreted as something else—a source of stimulus is present and perceptible to others. The illusory perception is initially taken as true, but the impression of reality can be relativized later.

Examples

A child perceives a figure in the curtains, which frightens them.

A patient sees devilish grimaces in the faces of other people. ◀

Position in psychopathology.
AMDP 47.

Related terms.
Misinterpretation, illusion.

Psychopathological interactions.
Emotional activation/agitation not only triggered by the misinterpretation but also before the misinterpretation; metamorphopsia (see below).

Differential Diagnostic Distinctions:
- Hallucination—no perceived stimulus is present
- one of the known optical illusions,
- Perceptual error -see elementary perception, perceptual misidentification,
- Delusional perception: correct perception reinterpreted delusionally (see below).

Self-/other persons's judgment.
Information from the affected person is necessary, other persons's judgment based on hallucination-accompanying motor activity is uncertain.

Interview for Rating.
Question about peculiarities in perception, about frightening or surprising perceptions, history taken from other persons.

Neuropsychology/objectification.
Behavioral observation e.g. attention-related movements, hallucination-accompanying motor activity, such as looking in an inexplicable direction, which should be explained by the person.

Severity.
Mild and/or rare misidentifications without behavioral consequences up to subjectively serious, vivid experiences that cause intense emotional reactions.

Specifications:
- persistently judged as real, an error is excluded, later relativized reality judgment
- When a person misperceives contents in voices echoing from the loud street that frighten them—this is also referred to as functional hallucination, a hallucination that occurs only in close sensory connection with a real stimulus (e.g. with the sound of running water)—transition to hallucination.
- pareidolia: imaginative addition of a shape to an image e.g. in cloud formations, rocks, etc.

Conceptual Problems of the Feature:
Also simply defined as perceptual distortion of a real stimulus (Berrios 1996),

- Diagnosability also depends on the dissonance between the perception and the patient's expectation; otherwise, the illusion can remain undetected if the person does not want to talk about it (also related to the emotional valence of the illusion).

Neuroscientific/Cognitive Neuroscientific Models
1. Errors in perceptual information processing, the perception of objects, sounds, smells, etc.,
2. weak input model:
   a) Signal-to-noise ratio low,
   b) perceptual errors physiologically: imagining a melody in the loud rhythmic noise, e.g. of the train between the carriages,
      - Transition to functional hallucination (hallucination only with external stimulus see above),
3. presumably must also be present:
   a) activation of emotionally significant ideas before the illusion occurs,
   b) for personally important contents (DD overvalued ideas, delusion).

Metamorphopsia
The shape of a visual stimulus is perceived as distorted, e.g. in parietal brain damage. It is questionable whether this feature is involved in body dysmorphia.

Verbal Auditory Hallucinations
Definition. A person hears a human speaking without that person being nearby, i.e. without the acoustic stimuli corresponding to the perception—no other person in the vicinity can hear this human speaking.

Examples

- A patient receives a command from a divine voice to perform an action.
- A desperately depressed lady is insulted as a whore from a corner of the room.
- A patient hears a voice upon admission that warns him and commands him not to speak about what he has heard, otherwise he will be tortured with unbearable rays.
- A patient hears the neighbors on the toilet saying about him, "There he is sitting on the toilet again…" ◀

Position in Psychopathology.
AMDP 48.

Related Terms.
Hearing voices, phonemes.

Psychopathological Interactions:
- Check ego disturbances with commenting voices, i.e., the patient assumes that the speaking persons can read his thoughts,
- Embedded in an emotional activation before the hallucination (mood), or after the hallucination—as an apparent reaction.
- Delusion
  a) primary—as activation of contents perceived as voices, and
  b) secondary—as explanatory delusion after the primary hallucination.

Differential Diagnostic Distinctions:

- illusion—with an existing stimulus source,
- Audibility of one's own thoughts.
- pseudohallucination, the patient hears the voices and knows that he is under a misperception.

Interview for Rating.
Ask about strange, irritating noises; inquire if it could be hearing voices if any unexplainable statement or movement is observed. History taken from other persons is necessary.

Neuropsychology/Objectification.
Behavioral observation, e.g., attention-related movements, such as looking in an inexplicable direction, which should be explained by the person (looking in the direction of voices), talking to voices.

Severity.
Occasionally—behavior is dominated by the experience and especially by the contents of hearing voices.

Specifications:

a) in a schizophrenic psychosis important specification of phonemes:
   - commenting,
   - in dialogue,
   - imperative.
b) The person can build a distance to the perception of hearing voices and question the reality character—transition to so-called pseudohallucinations (see below).
c) affective relationship
   1. negative emotions, specifically: urging to suicide or self-harm,
      - other affective valence: praising, insulting, devaluing, etc., role for the person
   2. mood congruence: e.g. affectively compatible with depressive syndrome, compatible with manic syndrome.
d) sensory restriction,
e) interaction with ego disturbances,
f) with or without delusional explanation,
g) voice in the head, localization in space
   - in the middle of the head, without sound quality
   - thoughts that are considered not to be thought by the patient and are referred to as "voices" because they have a different quality than one's own thoughts, where the acoustic quality may play a role (marginally also differential diagnosis to ego disturbance),
   - from outside with sound quality (male/female, age of the speaker, volume).

Conceptual problems of the feature:

- not noticed by individuals, then also not diagnosable, or often not reported for other reasons—prevalence in the dark,
- diagnosability depends on many factors, which is why the psychopathological examination should be appropriately thorough.

Neuroscientific/cognitive neuroscientific models (see e.g. also Stanghellini and Cutting 2003)

1. An imagination, e.g. generated by an error in a neuronal network, gains reality character, pathological activation of the primary sensory brain areas by an imagination.
   - Monitoring the source of information is disturbed (see above),
2. Primary pathological activation of sensory neuron groups (epileptic, brain stimulation, pharmacogenic, genetic neuronal connectivity disorder,
3. Predominance of imaginative information; the primary sensory area is disturbed or the afference from the sensory organs (deafferentation hallucination)—or no perceptive stimuli for a long time (deprivation hallucination).

Other auditory hallucinations
Definition. Auditory perceptions without a stimulus source—except hearing voices.

Examples

- A patient anxiously hears a crackling in the heating—thinks this is a signal from a neighbor in the house.
- A nun first hears chorales, then disturbingly march music.
- A patient hears a rustling of something "like parchment paper" close to his ear. ◀

Position in psychopathology.
AMDP 49.

Related terms.
Acoasmos.

Psychopathological interactions.
see above.

Differential Diagnostic Distinctions:
- »earworm« (summer hit with lively acoustic qualities repeatedly imposes itself),
- vivid imagination in a loud rushing environment,
- pseudohallucination,
- tinnitus.

Self-/other persons's judgment.
other persons's judgment based on introspection data.

Interview for Rating.
Questions as with verbal acoustic hallucinations, any noticeable remark where it can be asked whether it could be about hearing voices, history taken from other persons (e.g., complaints about noise that cannot be traced.)

Neuropsychology/objectification.
Behavioral observation—e.g., looking in an inexplicable direction, which should be explained by the person,—likewise with incomprehensible handling of objects.

Conceptual Problems of the Feature.
Like other sensory illusions—often only reported if affectively important to the person or if a change in behavior is to be commented on.

Neuroscientific/cognitive neuroscientific models
- Elementary sounds that can be triggered by electrophysiological neuronal activation in the primary brain areas: primarily epileptic, Epilepsia partialis continua Kojewnikow,
- pharmacological: hallucinogens,
- otherwise see above (phonemes, hearing voices).

Visual hallucinations
Definition. Visual perception without corresponding sensory stimuli, or without the perceived object being perceptible to others.

Examples

- A patient sees grotesque heads in the empty shelf next to the door, which cause her to panic.
- An old woman repeatedly sees visitors in her apartment. She says they are people she knows fleetingly.
- A patient observes small people moving on the bedspread - there is a severe visual impairment.
- A young man repeatedly sees flash-like appearances on the street, which show him that he is being followed.
- A patient after a stroke sees colored rings at the edge of the visual field defect. ◀

Position in Psychopathology.
AMDP 50.

Psychopathological Interactions.
Sensory restriction/afferent disorder, sensory deprivation.

Differential Diagnostic Distinctions:
- Pseudohallucinations (seeing stars after a blow to the eye),
- known optical illusion

Interview for Rating.
Questions about irritating things the person has seen and follow-up questions; history taken from other persons.

Neuropsychology/objectification.
Behavioral observation—characteristic: focus of attention on places in the room where others do not discover anything—inexplicable attention-accompanying movements.

Severity :
occasionally indistinct to impairment of everyday life.

Specifications:
- Clarity and intensity—e.g., only visible with closed eyes ("on the back of the eyelids?")
- Complexity: a) elementary visual hallucinations; b) complex—scenic
- Contents: objects: faces, physiognomization of the environment—self: heautoscopy.

Neuroscientific/cognitive neuroscientific models:
So far, no sufficient explanations have been found for the majority of hallucinations (see e.g. Podoll et al. 1989; Kölmel et al. 1985),

- Epileptic elementary hallucinations, e.g., at the edge of cortically induced visual field restrictions,
- elementary visual hallucinations triggered by hallucinogens, partly with particularly striking colors—possibly a 5-HT receptor effect plays a role,
- Source memory disorder with weak-input/perception disorder and vivid imagination or due to errors from generative model of neural networks,
- A prerequisite may also be: activation of the imagination of emotionally charged, e.g., feared or loved objects,
- deprivation hallucination (also in healthy individuals),
- deafferentation hallucination in peripheral visual disorder, also in Anton syndrome,
- Caused by disturbed cholinergic innervation, which seems to be most easily disturbed for the secondary visual brain areas.

Body hallucinations
Definition. Body hallucinations are referred to as inexplicable perceptions within the body of the affected person that cannot be explained by information about external or internal physical changes in the body.

Perceptions from the somatosensory innervation within the body are in principle not fully comprehensible from the outside.

Examples
- A patient feels something physical in her brain, like a skin or like a wall.
- A patient feels a gelatinous mass running down her back from her neck and is disgusted by it.
- A patient suffers from severe shooting pains in the testicle, which he experiences as being caused by former schoolmates through radiation. ◀

Position in psychopathology.
AMDP 51.

Psychopathological interactions.
- Focusing attention on the body.
- Coenesthetic hallucination fantastic, inexplicable, bizarre—coenesthetic delusion, explanatory delusion,

Differential diagnostic distinctions:
- Physically explainable pain (caused by a disease), unrecognized somatic changes,

- somatization ,

Self-/other person's judgment.
Statements of the person about possible body hallucination. Degree of bizarreness of body perceptions, characteristics of the perceived appear unlikely according to medical knowledge.

Interview for rating:
Questions about strange perceptions in the body

Severity:
a) Vividness, intensity,
b) Duration,
c) Impairments in everyday life due to body hallucinations.

Specifications:
(1) Body hallucination with sensory information of interoception, transition to
(2) Coenesthetic hallucination, bizarre, not oriented to real somatic conditions (not to be confused with the person's attempt to compensate for expression problems)
  - Sexual: hallucination related to the sexual organs,
  - Pain (also in sexual organs) experienced as caused by radiation,
  - Related to a disease—relationship to hypochondriacal fears and hypochondriacal delusion.

Conceptual problems of the feature.
Like other sensory illusions see hearing voices.

Neuroscientific/cognitive neuroscientific models
- difficult to scientifically investigate: unverifiable perceptual equivalents in the body area
- anxiety about bodily changes and diseases,
- attention is directed to the body (possible pathological thalamic activation and thus activation of specific body representations in the sensory homunculi)—see also somatization disorder,

Tactile hallucinations
Definition. Tactile body misperceptions that occur without a stimulus comprehensible to others.

Examples
- A person feels a crawling and creeping on the skin, which they attribute to parasites, while others cannot detect any foreign bodies or creatures.
- A patient feels touched and sexually abused by a person at night. ◄

Related terms: tactile hallucinations, misperceptions in body schema disorder

Psychopathological interactions. – Directing attention to the body.

- Body schema disorder

Differential diagnostic distinctions:
- non-physiological skin perceptions like usual itching etc.

Further characterization: In contrast to body hallucinations, an external assessment of the stimuli for the misperception is possible.

Interview for rating: Questions (1) about strange perceptions on the skin or (2) changes in one's own appearance, e.g., in the mirror image

Severity only upon inquiry up to a subjectively severe suffering

Specifications:
- Tactile hallucinations: specifically misperception of skin innervation—hallucinations related to delusional parasitosis; e.g., a patient feels movements on the skin, which he attributes to parasites.

- dysmorphophobic fears and misjudgments possibly with misperception—relationship to body schema, body ideal

Conceptual problems of the symptom: Heterogeneity of influencing factors speaks for a further subdivision of the symptom

Hallucinatory misperception of body appearance
Misperception of an external change in one's own body, changes in body surface, shape

Examples

- A patient suffers from the misperception of her emaciated body as too fat.
- a patient perceives his nose as misshapen, too long, too crooked, and too skewed, and fears that he will not find a woman because of this

Influence of body schema and body ideal not only leads to an assessment as too fat or too ugly etc. but also to misperception. Relationship to dysmorphophobia.

Conceptual problems of the feature: difficult distinction between shameful misjudgment and misperception

Synesthesia
Perceptual process in one sensory modality (e.g., visual) causing a perceptual experience in another sensory modality (e.g., auditory perceptual change).

Reported, for example, in cases of intoxication.

A tendency towards synesthetic sensations: genetic and neurobiological explanation through altered cortical connectivity in adjacent areas of reading and color information was provided by Ramachandran (Hubbard and Ramachandran 2005).

Olfactory hallucination
Definition. Perception of a smell without a source of the smell.

Examples

- A patient reports smelling celery from time to time, even when no celery is nearby.
- A woman has been perceiving a smell of sewage in her apartment for some time, although her acquaintances do not detect any such source of odor.
- A young man smells gas at various places in the house and interprets this as a sign that he is being followed - he wants to move out of the house. ◀

Position in psychopathology. AMDP 52.

Related terms. Osmic Hallucination.

Differential diagnostic distinctions:
- very sensitive sense of smell, which perceives more than that of the examiner,
- osmic disorder, especially in the case of a disturbance of the olfactory mucosa.

Interview for rating. Question about strange smells in his environment, history taken from other persons.

Neuropsychology/objectification. Inquiries about unusual behaviors (sniffing, inexplicable avoidance of rooms or apartments, inexplicable attention-accompanying movements, etc.).

Severity. Isolated and behaviorally irrelevant misperception to the cause of severe behavioral disorder (e.g. living on the street).

Conceptual problems of the feature. Like other hallucinations, see hearing voices.

Neuroscientific/cognitive neuroscientific models: generally see above,

- afferent disorder,
- epileptic misactivation in cortical olfactory areas.

Taste hallucination

Definition. Taste perception without objective chemical influence of a corresponding taste substance on the oral mucosa.

Example

- A patient reports a strange taste in his mouth, which he interprets as poison. He believes his spouse must have mixed it into his food.
- A patient tastes a metallic flavor in the food, which cannot be explained. ◀

Position in psychopathology. AMDP 52.

Related terms. Gustatory hallucination.

Psychopathological interactions. Olfactory hallucination.

Differential diagnostic distinctions. Disorder of the gustatory sensory organs, delusional perception.

Interview for rating. Question about taste changes, history taken from other persons.

Neuropsychology/objectification. Inquiries about unusual behaviors (attentive tasting behavior with special mouth movements, inexplicable avoidance of foods and drinks, etc.).

Severity. Isolated and behaviorally irrelevant misperception to the cause of severe behavioral disorder.

Neuroscientific/cognitive neuroscientific models.

- Central misactivation of primary cortical gustatory sensory areas, epileptic misactivation in cortical taste areas.
- Afferent disorder

Pseudohallucination

The term pseudohallucinations is used in two meanings:

First, according to German psychopathological tradition, it is defined as a hallucination in which the person does not consider the misperception to be real because they realize that it is a misperception.

An example is seeing stars when pressure is applied to the eyes.

The question is whether, for example, in the case of hearing voices with and without insight into the deceptive nature, these are different pathophysiological states of the triggering brain function systems. Especially patients with chronic schizophrenia become familiar with the characteristic of hearing voices over time and can gain a certain insight into the error of perception. Therefore, the designation of hearing voices with and without insight into the misperception (as a specification) is more appropriate.

The second definition aims at pseudohallucinations in theatrical personalities, which are reported in a state of emotional exception. In this case, the perception is not described as real to the same extent as in schizophrenic hearing of voices, but rather in the sense of "as if" (it seems to me as if) or as a dreamlike pale perception of highly emotional scenes or voices.

References

Bentall RP, Slade PD (1985) Reality testing and auditory hallucinations: a signal detection analysis. Br J Clin Psychol 24:159–169

Bentall RP, Baker GA, Havers S (1991) Reality monitoring and psychotic hallucinations. Br J Clin Psychol 30:213–222

Benson DF (1994) The neurology of thinking. Oxford Univ Press, Oxford

Berrios GE (1996) The history of mental symptoms. Cambridge Univ Press, Cambridge

Blakemore SJ, Frith CD, Wolpert DM (2001) The cerebellum is involved in predicting the sensory consequences of action. NeuroReport 12:1879–1884

Collerton D, Barnes J, Diederich NJ et al (2023) Understanding visual hallucinations: A new synthesis. Neurosci Biobehavioral Rev 150208:1–14

Christoff K, Ream JM, Geddes LP, Gabrieli JD (2003) Evaluating self-generated information: anterior prefrontal contributions to human cognition. Behav Neurosci 117:1161–1168

Craik FI, Morris LW, Morris RG, Loewen ER (1990) Relations between source amnesia and frontal lobe functioning in older adults. Psychol Aging 5:148–151

Craver-Lemley C, Reeves A (1992) How visual imagery interferes with vision. Psychol Rev 99(4):633–649

Curio G, Neuloh G, Numminen J (2000) Speaking modifies voice-evoked activity in the human auditory cortex. Hum Brain Mapp 9:183–191

Dennet D (1984) Elbow room. MIT Press, Cambridge

Dierks T, Linden DE, Jandl M et al (1999) Activation of Heschl‘s gyrus during auditory hallucinations. Neuron 22:615–621

David AS, Cutting JC (Hrsg) (1994) The neuropsychology of schizophrenia—(Brain damage, behaviour and cognition series). Erlbaum, Hove

Esquirol E (1838) Des maladies mentales considérées sous les rapports médicaux, hygieéniques et médicolégaux. Baillère, Paris

Ford JM, Dierks T, Fisher DJ, Herrmann CS, Hubl D, Kindler J, Koenig T, Mathalon DH, Spencer KM, Strik W, van Lutterveld R (2012) Neurophysiological studies of auditory verbal hallucinations. Schizophr Bull. 38:715–723.

Friston KJ (2005) Hallucinations and perceptual inference. Behavioral and Brain Sciences 28:764–766

Frith C (1992) The cognitive neuropsychology of schizophrenia. Erlbaum, Hove

Frith CD, Friston K, Liddle PF, Frackowiak RS (1991) Willed action and the prefrontal cortex in man: a study with PET. Proc R Soc Lond B Biol Sci 244:241–246

Frith CD, Blakemore S-J (2003) Self-awareness and action. Curr Opin Neurobiol 13:219–224

Gao WJ, Krimer LS, Goldman-Rakic PS (2001) Presynaptic regulation of recurrent excitation by D1 receptors in prefrontal circuits. Proc Natl Acad Sci U S A 98:295–300

Gao WJ, Goldman-Rakic PS (2003) Selective modulation of excitatory and inhibitory microcircuits by dopamine. Proc Natl Acad Sci U S A 100:2836–2841

Gaser C, Nenadic I, Volz HP et al (2004) Neuroanatomy of »hearing voices«: a frontotemporal brain structural abnormality associated with auditory hallucinations in schizophrenia. Cereb Cortex 14:91–96

Goldman-Rakic PS, Selemon LD (1997) Functional and anatomical aspects of prefrontal pathology in schizophrenia. Schizophr Bull 23:437–458

von Holst E, Mittelstaedt H (1950) Das Reafferenzprinzip. Naturwissenschaften 37:464–476

Hubbard EM, Ramachandran VS (2005) Neurocognitive mechanisms of synesthesia. Neuron 48:509–520

Jaspers K (1942) Allgemeine Psychopathologie, 4. edn. Springer, Berlin

Kircher T, Thienel R (2005) Functional brain imaging of symptoms and cognition in schizophrenia. Prog Brain Res 150:299–308

Klosterkötter J (1988) Basissymptome und Endophänomene der Schizophrenie. Springer, Berlin Heidelberg New York Tokio

Kölmel HW (1985) Complex visual hallucinations in the hemianopic field. J Neurol Neurosurg Psychiatry 48(1):29–38

Koch C (2005) Bewusstsein—ein neurobiologisches Rätsel. Spektrum—Elsevier, München

Kosslyn SM, Pascual-Leone A, Felician O et al (1999) The role of area 17 in visual imagery: convergent evidence from PET and rTMS. Science 284:167–170

LeCun Y, Bengio Y, Hinton G (2015) Deep Learning. Nature 521:436–444

Manford M, Andermann F (1998) Complex visual hallucinations—clinical and neurobiological insights. Brain 121:1819–1840

Murray SO, Boyaci H, Kersten D (2006) The representation of perceived angular size in human primary visual cortex. Nat Neurosci 9:429–434

Podoll K, Osterheider M, Noth J (1989) Das Charles Bonnet Syndrom. Fortschr Neurol Psychiatr 57:43–60

Reichert DP, Seriès P, Storkey AJ (2013) Charles Bonnet syndrome: evidence for a generative model in the cortex? PLoS Comput Biol 9:e1003134

Reischies FM, Neuhaus AH, Hansen ML (2005) Electrophysiological and neuropsychological analysis of a delirious state—the role of the anterior cingulate gyrus. Psychiatry Res Neuroimaging 138:171–181

Shergill SS, Brammer MJ, Fukuda R (2003) Engagement of brain areas implicated in processing inner speech in people with auditory hallucinations. Br J Psychiatry 182:525–531

Shergill SS, Brammer MJ, Williams SC et al (2000) Mapping auditory hallucinations in schizophrenia using functional magnetic resonance imaging. Arch Gen Psychiatry 57:1033–1038

Shima K, Tanji J (1998) Role for cingulate motor area cells in voluntary movement selection based on reward. Science 282:1335–1338

Siegel RK, West LJ (1975) Hallucinations: behavior, experience, and theory. Wiley, New York

Silbersweig D, Stern E (1996) Functional neuroimaging of hallucinations in schizophrenia: toward an integration of bottom-up and top-down approaches. Mol Psychiatry 1:367–375

Slotnick SD, Thompson WL, Kosslyn SM (2005) Visual mental imagery induces retinotopically organized activation of early visual areas. Cereb Cortex 15:1570–1583

Stanghellini G, Cutting J (2003) Auditory verbal hallucinations—breaking the silence of inner dialogue. Psychopathology 36:120–128

Suzuki K, Seth AK, Schwartzman DJ (2024) Modelling phenomenological differences in aetiologically distinct visual hallucinations using deep neural networks. Front Hum Neurosci. 17:1–25

van de Ven VG, Formisano E, Roder CH et al (2005) The spatiotemporal pattern of auditory cortical responses during verbal hallucinations. Neuroimage 27:644–655

Further Reading

Benson DF, Blumer D (1975) Psychiatric aspects of neurologic disease. Grune & Stratton, Orlando

Blakemore SJ, Smith J, Steel R et al (2000a) The perception of self-produced sensory stimuli in patients with auditory hallucinations and passivity experiences: evidence for a breakdown in self-monitoring. Psychol Med 30:1131–1139

Blakemore SJ, Wolpert D, Frith C (2000b) Why can't you tickle yourself? NeuroReport 11:R11–16

Farrer C, Franck N, Georgieff N et al (2003) Modulating the experience of agency: a positron emission tomography study. Neuroimage 18:324–333

Frith C (1996) The roje of the prefrontal cortex in self-consciousness: the Gase of auditory hallucinations. Philos Trans R Soc Lond B Biol Sci 351:1505–1512

Johnson MK, Hashtroudi S, Lindsay DS (1993) Source monitoring. Psychol Bull 114:3–28

Keefe RSE, Arnold MC, Bayen UJ, Harvey PD (1999) Source monitoring deficits in patients with schizophrenia: a multinomial modeling analysis. Psychol Med 29:903–914

Shallice T (1988) From neuropsychology to mental structure. Cambridge Univ Press, Cambridge

Ego Disturbances 13

Contents

13.1 Introduction

13.2 Manifestations and Differentiation of Ego Disorders

Ego disorders refer to specific psychological disturbance characteristics predominantly in patients with schizophrenic psychosis. For example, a patient believes that a chip has been implanted under his skin, which reads his thoughts and communicates them to his persecutors.

People with ego disorders feel manipulated and monitored in their movements, thoughts, perceptions, and feelings. When a patient says he is sure "this is not my thought," everyday psychological communication fails when he tries to explain this to others. The investigators cannot comprehend what the patient means by this.

Classification

Ego disorders are partly classified as bizarre Delusion. They are treated as delusional symptoms according to the Anglo-Saxon tradition. However, the classification as bizarre delusion does not do justice to all these psychopathological features. In an analysis of the psychopathology of schizophrenic patients, the group of ego disorders emerged as a distinct factor, compared with paranoia and other delusional symptoms of the patients (Kimhy et al. 2005). In the German tradition, many arguments have been presented that justify a special status of these symptoms as a group of ego disorders. The term ego disorder may be somewhat unfortunate; perhaps it would be better to emphasize the ego boundary, which is disturbed; however, it must be immediately added that not much is known about an

F. M. Reischies, *Psychopathology*, https://doi.org/10.1007/978-3-662-70293-2_13

ego boundary either. Can we argue that the commonality of ego disorders lies in a pathological change in the boundary between the environment and the sphere of awareness of one's own person? This means that in a patient suffering from thought transmission, a kind of violation of the fundamental boundary between their personal experience and the environment must be noted.

From the area of ego disorders, the occurrence of some symptom constellations speaks against the independence of the group of ego disorders: The phenomena described as ego disorders are partly considered as delusional explanations, e.g., in body hallucinations—when pain is experienced as external influence through radiation. If a person further recognizes their thoughts in what voices say to them, they may conclude that other people have apparently read their thoughts.

Phenomena that have relationships to hallucinations can also apply to ego disorders. Often, patients only complain about thoughts in their heads that are foreign but that they do not hear (like a verbal auditory hallucination). Accordingly, one could speak of a spectrum of auditory quality, ranging from the highest sensory presence in a hallucination to the loss of quality as a sensory stimulus in ego disorders (see above). If this model of a spectrum of auditory properties were correct, then we could describe thought insertion as hallucinations without sensory quality. However, this is not the case. A crucial dimension is missing, on which mental contents differ: It is the sensation of being the actor; being the person who performed the act of thinking, remembering, perceiving, etc., the "my-ness" of these processes.

Considering the possible mental contents that a person currently has in consciousness (the source of the mental content can be perception, invention of the thought, quoting, remembering, singing along, etc.)

1. My new thought that I am currently thinking,
2. A thought that I am quoting, like my mother always said, "don't play with weapons,"
3. Expression with auditory quality, "earworm" melody with auditory quality
4. Verbal expression as auditory hallucination
5. Thought insertion

These differ in the dimensions:

a) Auditory quality: yes, no b) Source of the thought: I, others and c) sensation of being the actor (my-ness, sense of ownership as sensation): yes, no

- Auditory quality is present in 3. and 4. (possibly also the memory of a sentence from the mother)
- I as the source—author of the thought: only (1), my self-thought verbal expression that just occurred to me
- the actor sensation refers to the thinking of the current content; the sense of ownership, that I am thinking the thought, is missing in thought insertion. In hallucination, the sense of ownership refers to the perception, but the person considers the thought to be foreign.

In summary, we can characterize the sense of ownership (or conversely the sense of foreignness regarding the thought) in thought insertion as decisive, using the example of the qualities of mental contents in relation to the actor role.

13.2.1 Quality of Experience

The critical question is the immediate experience of external influence, as already mentioned above—what situation are we dealing with:

1. experience of phenomena like radiation as external influence, thought insertion, or control of the person's movements.
2. Delusional explanation for thoughts or intentions that represent contents incompatible with one's own person, or delusional explanation for unspoken, secret thoughts that the voices, experienced as coming from outside, seem to know.

13.2.2 Disturbance of the Self-Environment Boundary

Patients with thought broadcasting and thought transference suffer from a loss of their privacy. They experience themselves as being monitored by processes that involve a breach of the "barrier" between the conscious inner world and the environment. The person may develop the hypothesis that it could be possible to read thoughts through a technical device like a "sensor chip." Some technically savvy individuals speak of a science fiction machine that could read thoughts. To explain this aspect of self-disturbances, it must be asked whether people with schizophrenic psychosis have a disturbance of the boundaries of their own person to the environment. Such an approach assumes that in the schizophrenic crisis, the boundary of the self to the surroundings can be more easily overcome or collapse.

How should such a disturbance of the boundaries of the self be imagined? Today, we know too little about the self and even less about whether there is a self-boundary and how it could be determined. For this reason, it is better for now not to use the self-boundary for the definition of the symptom group.

For example, in hypnosis, we are dealing with a form of overcoming the boundary between person and environment. For hypnosis, prerequisites can be found in the personality of the hypnotized person; not everyone can be hypnotized. Following this line of argument, it can be examined what prerequisites exist in schizophrenic patients for the disturbance of the self-environment boundary.

13.2.3 Dimensions of the Experience of the Self

In the experience of one's own person by the patient, gaining knowledge about oneself, characteristic disturbances can occur (Scharfetter 1981). Some of the dimensions he describes have relationships to the self-disturbances described here. In addition to 1.) the disturbance of self-vitality, there are 2.) disturbances of self-activity, where one's own actions are not perceived as self-determined, which is also referred to as the experience of passivity. This can possibly be explained by the Frith model (see below) of a disturbed monitoring of the intention to act. As bizarre delusions, beliefs of patients who show 3.) a disturbance of ego consistencyaccording to Scharfetter were considered. They assume, for example, that they are dissolving or being divided within themselves. There is a relationship to depression, especially to the nihilistic delusion of severely depressed patients. 4.) The disturbance of ego demarcation refers more to what was described in the classical psychopathology of self-disturbances. There is the tormenting feeling of the loss of protection by the self-environment boundary. 5.) The disturbance of self-identity. Under this, a multitude of anomalies in the perception and internal concepts of one's own person, body schema, self-awareness, sexual identity, etc., are understood.

The disturbance of the monitoring of mental contents according to the Frith model initially refers to the "made" nature of actions "from outside," as many patients with schizophrenia report. An attempt is made to include the disturbance of the "self," the actor and their self-perception, as well as the disturbance of reflexive consciousness (Chap. 8 consciousness) in the explanation of self-disturbances (Kircher and David 2003).

13.3 Clinic

In the clinic of severe mental illnesses, such as psychoses, ego disturbances are diagnosed. The patients report

- a loss of privacy because their thoughts become known to enemies, or
- their thoughts are manipulated, i.e., the thoughts they are thinking are not their own thoughts,
- inexplicable, frightening changes to their body, or

- the restriction of the freedom of their own movements—they feel like puppets being controlled, etc. These changes are also accompanied by an experience of passivity—the events are no longer controlled by their own activities (see also thought control disorders)

If a person states that he has episodes in which he experiences an alienation of familiar perception, this feature can occur in isolation and possibly be diagnosed within the framework of the disease concept of a derealization-depersonalization disorder. However, it may also be that further questioning reveals an ego disturbance: The person feels in the spontaneously complained episodes of derealization that the environment was not only perceived as changed but was also staged as a theater for them.

Ego disturbances have been considered pathognomonic for schizophrenia. At least not all symptoms of ego disturbances are characteristic of schizophrenia: Ego-awareness and person-awareness are also altered in dissociation and anxiety-related depersonalization (see Berrios 1996). Specific ego disturbances, such as thought broad casting or thought transmission, have been confirmed as specific symptoms of the first rank of schizophrenia. They correspond to pathognomonic features of severe schizophrenia disorders with rather poor prognosis.

13.4 Diagnostics

Problems in the diagnostics of ego disturbances arise, among other things, due to the difficulties in communicating the complex circumstances of ego disturbances.

Psychopathological Examination

The quality of the diagnosis depends on the quality of the psychopathological questioning and observation. There are no neuropsychological examination procedures or psychological tests that can help in the examination.

Special circumstances with delusional explanation have already been pointed out: People with verbal auditory hallucinations often cannot explain the fact that the people they hear must know their thoughts in any other way. This fallacy must be separated from the immediate experience of thought transmission.

13.5 Neuroscientific Explanatory Approaches

Efference copy: The efference copy, information that a certain movement is being executed, is generated with every action initiation (Holst et al. 1950 see above, Frith 1992). The concept was initially related to motor acts with the innervation of muscles.

The efference copy allows the comparison of the consequences of the action with the expectation based on the action planning and initiation. For example, when grasping an object from the table, "the fingers will touch the table during the action," etc., with the feedback from the fingers when the table is actually touched and the skin sensors report a touch. In self-generated actions, the anterior cingulate alongside the dorsolateral prefrontal cortex is active (Frith and Blakemore 2003).

It is suspected that for the person's mental activity as well—for self-actively imagined stimuli, traces of one's own authorship should be found (equivalents of the "corollary discharge" or reafference, Chap. 7) and thus also for thoughts, information about this respective mental act should be processed. The model assumes a disturbance in the information about the initiation of thinking a thought.

In the mediofrontal brain regions, specifically the anterior cingulate, there are neurons that are active during self-initiated movements, but not during externally prompted movements (Shima and Tanji 1998). Disturbances in this brain region could disrupt the monitoring of whether a mental process is self-initiated or originates from a perception as a reactive process (see, for example, Christoff et al. 2003).

In a study (see Fig. 13.1), patients could see movements of their own hand versus a recorded hand of another person on a TV

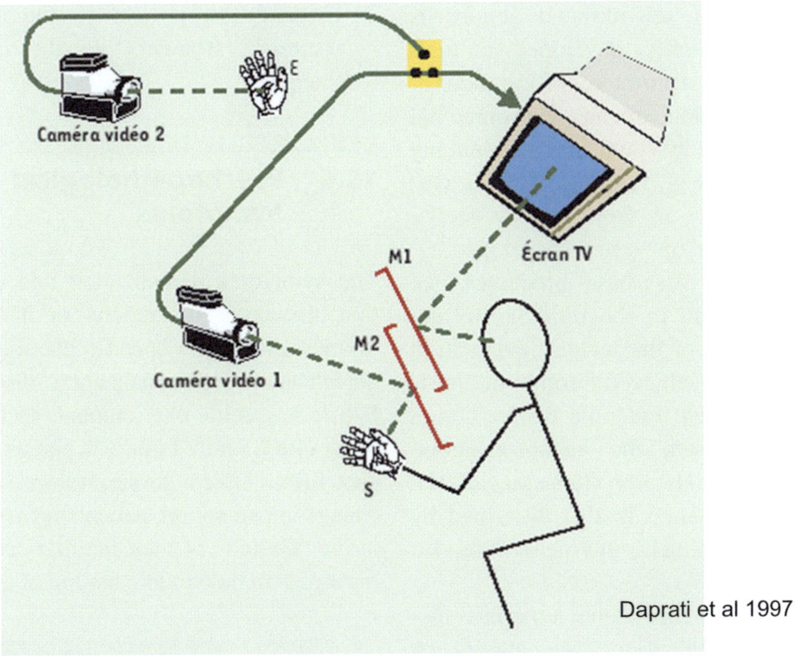

Fig. 13.1 Self-perception experiment conducted to explain ego-disorders. Schizophrenic patients make errors in recognizing whether the hand shown on a screen during manipulations is their own or that of another person performing similar manipulations. To explain ego-disorders, a disturbance of the "corollary discharge" or reafference is assumed, where the information about one's own action is either not present, lost, or incorrectly compared with the feedback from the sensory organs (Mod. after Dapatri et al. 1997).

monitor. Patients with hallucinations were unable to recognize that it was occasionally the hand of another person (Dapatri et al. 1997). Schizophrenic patients with ego-disorders were less able to recognize a technically realized deviation of the displayed movement from the performed movement than healthy individuals. For deviations up to about 30 degrees, more patients with ego-disorders said that they had performed this movement (Franck et al. 2001). Other studies showed that with a slight acoustic distortion of their own voice, their own voice could no longer be reliably identified from other voices (Johns et al. 2001; see also Knoblich and Prinz 2001).

Actor information plays a central role in the discussion of ego-disorders (Dapatri et al. 1997). The self-actor information provides source identification not only for perception but also for actions. This allows self-disorders to be classified: Only for 1) my own thoughts does the information apply that I am the actor—it is my thought (my-ness). 2) Thought insertion differs precisely here: The person does not have the self-actor information—the thought appears somehow foreign.

The feeling of external influence, i.e., performing movements like a puppet not controlled by oneself, also applies here: The self-actor information enables the differentiation of this feature. Only for one's own, self-planned, self-initiated, and self-controlled movement does the self-actor information apply, but not for externally controlled movement as a symptom of ego-disorder and not for passive movements (e.g., as part of a physical examination).

General concept of feedback processing: Concepts of an evolutionarily early development of a basal consciousness (Merker 2007) with a rudimentary control of motor functions adapted to the environment raise the question of whether less developed animals have not just a basal consciousness but can also realize self-initiated actions.

The perception of self-initiated actions is assumed for less highly developed animals because they benefit from the information of whether the perception of an environmental change was triggered by them or by an enemy in the environment (e.g., rustling in the leaves while walking—snake in front of my feet?). Thus, a signal "I-actor" must have developed.

It is assumed that these basal processes take place in the brainstem in the reticular formation up to the region of the tectum. Adaptation to the environment is achieved through the feedback of an unfavorable outcome of the action (negative valence) with the backpropagation training of neuronal networks (Reischies 2021). The self-actor information is also described by some authors as a feeling of "my-ness" (see also Metzinger 1999).

Scharfetter (1981) formulated complex disturbances of self-perception (see above). A broadly defined concept of a disturbed perception of oneself could, also because it contains complex further constructs such as a sense of identity, not determine the group of self-disorders.

The concept of passivity (see above) can be understood according to today's neuroscientific models with a disturbance of the monitoring of action initiation. The person no longer experiences themselves as thinking (see Chap. 10) or acting, he assumes that other people or foreign powers initiate or control these processes.

Alienation of Feedback Perception

It must be examined to what extent the ego disturbances can generally be explained by a) an elementary disturbance in the feedback of active processes, i.e., processes initiated by the person. It must also be assumed b) that the insecure person misinterprets this disturbed feedback as pointing the finger of guilt towards the outside world, or sees a hostile environment as the cause:

1. Effects of alienated, disturbed feedback from the periphery—eye muscles, trunk and neck muscles, speech motor skills, and the activation of thoughts—possibly with the effect of alienation of feedback during covert speech
2. Tendency to project to the outward world, assuming strangers as the cause of the changes.

13.6 Psychopathological Symptoms

The symptoms derealization and depersonalization also occur in anxiety- or intoxication syndromes and in the specific classification unit of derealization-depersonalization disorder ICD-10 F48.1. A specific environment, such as the living room of a friendly family, is perceived in its complex form. After a stroke, however, with a slight change in perception, patients report that a change in the "Gestalt" of their familiar environment has occurred, an indefinable feeling of change.

Derealization
Definition. The environment is perceived as strange, people notice an unfamiliarity, have a general feeling of change regarding the surroundings

- with a tendency towards unreality up to the feeling of being fabricated (changed for the person, pretended)

Not specifically triggered by the perception of actually changed environmental elements.

Examples

- A patient reports feeling like under a glass dome; experiences a mitigation, a seeming distance, or a veiled perception.
- An anxious person says they experience an unpleasant insecurity, dreamlike unreality.
- A patient with schizophrenia reports in the beginning delusional mood of perceptions that somehow seem strange to him; he feels that something is just being pretended to him, that everything is just being staged for him. ◄

Position in Psychopathology. AMDP 53 in ego disturbances—relationship to dissociative integration disorder.

Related Terms. dissociation, paramnesia.

Psychopathological Interactions. Memory disorder, dissociation, delusional mood.

Differential Diagnostic Distinctions:
- Ego disturbance: "everything seems unreal to me", a film is being played to me, science fiction.
- Metamorphopsia, hallucination or illusion, hypnosis,
- delusional misinterpretation of reality
- amnesic recognition error, "jamais vu" in paramnesias.

Further Characterization. Strangeness of perception in an unchanged environment.

Interview for Rating. Question about strange perceptions, experiences of alienation, history taken from other persons.

Severity. Threshold of occasionally occurring alienation up to complete misinterpretation of the environment.

Personality Influences. Histrionic, borderline personality disorder.

Specifications: a) without further ego disturbances, hallucinations or delusions, b) with features of schizophrenic psychoses ("unreal", "a film is being played to me"), c) memory disorder as a symptom of brain damage.

Conceptual Problems of the Feature:
- Purely subjective feature,
- obvious inhomogeneity, difficult to diagnose.

Neuroscientific/Cognitive Neuroscientific Models
- In addition to the models discussed above of a disturbance of the specific efference copy or generally of the feedback from actions and mental acts:
- Affects alter perception, amygdala interaction with secondary and tertiary sensory processing areas,
- Amygdala interaction with hippocampal activation during retrieval and situational orientation,
- Errors in parahippocampal recognition, signal resulting in disturbance in familiarity, the "familiarity"; also characterized as paramnesia

Depersonalization
Definition. A person experiences a strange change, an alienation in himself. His own reactions and sensations, but also his own body, is experienced as altered and unfamiliar, or something foreign is perceived within him. The naturalness of his own body or his own characteristics has been lost; self-knowledge is uncertain.

Examples

- A woman reports: "I feel like I'm standing beside myself. I no longer feel my body." The extremities of the body are perceived as shrunken or enlarged for a short time.
- A patient with severe depression says he is already dead, he can already smell the rotting of his body. ◀

Position in Psychopathology. AMDP 54 in ego disturbances, also related to dissociative integration disorder (see above).

Related Terms. Delusion of being another person, relationship to derealization, dissociation.

Psychopathological Interactions. Sense of identity of the person, body schema disturbance, experience of change, dysmorphopsia, dysmorphophobia.

Differential Diagnostic Distinctions. Metamorphopsia (e.g., micropsia), hypnosis.

Further Characterization. Perception of change in one's own person and/or body with a tendency to interpret the change as influenced from outside.

Interview for Rating. Question about change or any peculiarity in the perception of oneself, subjectively; history taken from other persons.

Severity. From the threshold of normal when paying attention to oneself and one's own body to massive change in self-perception and change in perception of aspects of one's own person.

Specifications:
What changes:

- Physical characteristics or sensations, personality
- Ego disturbance with anxious interpretation of the change as made from outside
- Dissociation-related, dissociative integration disorder.

Personality Influences.
Histrionic, borderline personality disorder.

Conceptual Problems of the Feature:

- Purely subjective,
- Inhomogeneous feature: 1) from the area of anxiety disorders with emphasis on the relationships to dissociation, 2) from the area of schizophrenic ego disturbances with relationship of the feature to delusional mood and the experience of change being made from outside.

Neuroscientific/cognitive neuroscientific models (see also Sierra et al. 2002).

Information processing of the person about themselves is disturbed, with disturbed self-perception of the change, in severe schizophrenia a lack of a sense of unity; discussion about the role of traumatic experiences

- at the onset of the disorder perplexed and anxious about it,
- e.g., noticed actions or thoughts in themselves that are not under their own control,
- »catastrophic interference« in the change of neuronal network connection weights in a psychotic process,

Thought broadcasting
Definition. A person experiences that their own thoughts become known to other people, e.g., others have telepathic abilities to read thoughts; loss of privacy of mental events.

Examples

- A patient does not speak during the interview—when asked, he says the examiner already knows everything. Upon further questioning, it becomes clear that he believes his thoughts have spread telepathically.
- A patient believes he can manipulate people around him. Upon further questioning, it becomes clear he experiences that other people can receive his thoughts.
- A patient suddenly screams desperately in the clinic: "You can all read my thoughts!" ◀

Psychopathological interactions. Position in psychopathology. AMDP 55.

Possibly a reaction to the content of verbal auditory hallucinations.

Differential diagnostic distinctions. Magical experience, esoteric experiences (common in the population).

Further characterization. "ego-environment boundary" seems to be disturbed in the direction from the person to the environment.

Interview for rating. Question about the suspicion that others know the person's thoughts; whether something like "telepathy" has occurred.

Neuropsychology/objectification. Interview behavior, follow-up questions.

Severity. Occasionally and without associated distress to severe communication disorder and subjective suffering due to the loss of privacy.

Pathognomonic for: Schizophrenia.

Specifications:
- without influence on others
- with effects on others (e.g., other people are influenced),
- thought broadcasting with/without experience of thought echo.

Conceptual problems of the feature. The privileged access to one's own experiences is questioned.

Neuroscientific/cognitive neuroscientific models
- in addition to the models mentioned above: voices of others experienced and misinterpretation of a common source of knowledge and ideas explained as thought broadcasting.
- Possibly learning history, parents had guessed intentions.
- Possibly related to symbiotic relationships with people in the environment.

Thought withdrawal
Definition. Thoughts are experienced as being withdrawn from the outside.

Example

- A patient reports, as she pauses in conversation and looks around confused, that she suddenly no longer knew what she had been thinking and wanted to say, and even when thinking about the course of the conversation, she could not find out anything more about it. She suspected that the thoughts were somehow erased by the enemies who want to kill her. ◀

Position in psychopathology. AMDP 56.

Related terms. disruption of thought, experience of external influence.

Further characterization. "ego-environment boundary" is interpreted as disturbed.

Self-/other persons' judgment. other persons' judgment based on introspection data.

Interview for rating. Inquiries when communication is interrupted.

Neuropsychology/objectification. Observing interview behavior—characteristic: disruption of thought with inquiries about the subjective perspective.

Severity. Occasionally to disabling.

Pathognomonic for: Schizophrenia.

Specifications:
- Suspicion or certainty of causation from outside.
- With or without disruption of thought,
- global: all thoughts are taken away from outside. The person does not think self, but foreign powers thinking in his head.

Neuroscientific/cognitive neuroscientific models
Two-part: a) Working-memory disorder: loss of mindset on a argumentation, b) with belief that the error does not lie with the affected person self, but is caused from outside. Conceivable as the subjective side of thought disruption, with the projection of the error's causation onto the environment,

- Loss of thought control experienced and interpreted as influenced from outside

Hearing one's own thoughts
Definition. Own thoughts become loud, they acquire a sound character. For this reason, the person explains that others can overhear the thoughts. Thought echo.

Thought insertion
Definition. Experience of external influence in the realm of thoughts: thoughts are experienced as not one's own thoughts, thought by the person self—but as inserted from outside.

Examples

- A patient explains that he does not think self, but a foreign power thinks "through him"; the thoughts are not his.
- A patient does not recognize aggressive thoughts as her own.
- A patient without religious bonding says his thoughts are inserted by God. ◄

Position in psychopathology. AMDP 57.

Related terms. telepathy.

Differential diagnostic distinctions:
- magical experience, esoteric experiences,
- obsessive thoughts: thoughts experienced as own, but with a distance to them, i.e., the desire not to think these thoughts—development of discomfort, anxiety.

Further characterization. The experienced authorship of one's own thoughts is disturbed, disturbed feeling of my-ness, the patient experiences himself as passive.

Interview for rating. Question about the experience that thoughts were felt as foreign, inserted from outside—possibly referring to telepathy, which is reported by many apparently healthy individuals as known to them.

Severity. Occasionally to disabling.

Pathognomonic for Schizophrenia.

Specifications:
- particular contents to which the person has a distance or rejects; in the case of personally unbearable thoughts.
- with grandiose ideas,
- Disturbance of formal thinking (thought chaos) interpreted as caused from outside.

Personality Influences. Mystical, esoteric interests.

Conceptual Problems of the Feature:
- unclear how the feature can be reliably diagnosed,
- unclear: mode of experience or excuse for thoughts, denialof unbearable thoughts,
- dissonance between the person's attitudes and values and their own thoughts experienced.

Neuroscientific/Cognitive Neuroscientific Models
- source perception disturbed: the distinction of the source of information; i.e., thoughts are no longer identified as one's own ideas or as information from outside.
- thoughts incompatible with one's own person are experienced as caused from outside and thus "defused" for self-knowledge.
- Change in the experience of "my-ness," the belonging of thoughts to one's own person—possibly as a disturbance in brainstem networks that process basal actor information (see above).

Experiences of External Influence
Definition. Experience of external influence—on emotions, intentions, or actions, or control of intentions and actions as well as the influence on emotional sensations (excluding thought insertion and thought withdrawal).

Example

- A patient feels manipulated, determined in actions by other people, he is just a puppet.
- A patient reports that she is under hypnosis all the time.
- A patient reports that her sexual sensations are experienced as being made from outside. ◀

Position in Psychopathology. AMDP 58.

Differential Diagnostic Distinctions:
- Exclusion of ordinary, everyday influences on behavioral decisions (through campaigns, advertising, parents, politics, etc.),
- hallucinations, e.g., somatic hallucinations,
- "unio mystica" in religious experience, hypnosis

Further Characterization. Loss of privacy in intention formation and self-determination, organizing one's own person, passivity.

Self-/Other Person's Judgment. Other person's judgment.

Interview for Rating. Question about the feeling of losing control over actions, so that others determine the actions—explain the difference to generally meant (social) external determination.

Severity. Occasionally to severely disabling.

Pathognomonic for: Schizophrenia.

Specifications:
- intentional, motor
- emotional.

Personality Influences. Suggestibility, hypnotizability.

Conceptual Problems of the Feature:
- purely subjective feature,
- differentiate: mode of experience of being a puppet or excuse for wrong actions or distancing from one's own actions.

Neuroscientific/cognitive neuroscientific models
- The experience of external control is particularly difficult to understand (see Stirling et al. 1998). A). It is questionable whether faulty initiation of actions, which the person intends, plays a role—as shown in models of neuronal networks, the activation of units is faulty when system properties are altered, e.g., the computational units (hidden units) are disturbed. The faulty activated action is then experienced as unintended. B) This faulty activation of motor functions will additionally alter the feedback, which then contrasts with the expected feedback of the person's original intention.
- Questionable: the experience of the real dependency of consciousness states, the mood is interpreted as being directly influenced from the outside—without the normal illusion of one's own authorship and the connection in the subjective concept of identity.
- Actions considered incompatible with the personality are declared as made from the outside (as self-not-caused faults in action selection).

References

Christoff K, Ream JM, Geddes LP, Gabrieli JD (2003) Evaluating self-generated information: anterior prefrontal contributions to human cognition. Behav Neurosci 117:1161–1168

Dapatri E, Franck N, Georieff N (1997) Looking for the agent: an investigation into consciousness of action and self-consciousness in schizophrenic patients. Cognition 65:71–86

Franck N, Farrer C, Georgieff N et al (2001) Defective recognition of one's own actions in schizophrenia. Am J Psychiatry 158:454–459

Frith CD, Blakemore S-J (2003) Self-awareness and action. Curr Opin Neurobiol 13:219–224

von Holst E, Mittelstaedt H (1950) Das Reafferenzprinzip. Naturwissenschaften 37:464–476

Johns LC, Rosseli S, Frith C et al (2001) Verbal self-monitoring and auditory verbal hallucinations in patients with schizophrenia. Psychol Med 31(4):705–715
Kimhy D, Goetz R, Yale S et al (2005) Delusions in individuals with schizophrenia: factor structure, clinical correlates, and putative neurobiology. Psychopathology 38:338–344
Kircher T, David A (2003) The self in neuroscience and psychiatry. Cambridge Univ Press, Cambridge
Knoblich G, Prinz W (2001) Recognition of self-generated actions from kinematic displays of drawing. J Exp Psychol Hum Percept Perform 27:456–465
Merker B (2007) Consciousness without a cerebral cortex: a challenge for neuroscience and medicine. Behav Brain Sci 30:63–81
Metzinger T (1999) Subjekt und Selbstmodell. Die Perspektivität phänomenalen Bewusstseins vor dem Hintergrund einer naturalistischen Theorie mentaler Repräsentationen. Mentis, Paderborn
Reischies FM (2021) Leid-Erleben, ein Fundament der Psychopathologie. Pabst Scientific Publishers, Lengerich
Scharfetter C (1981) Ego-psychopathology: the concept and its empirical evaluation. Psychol Med 11:273–280
Sierra M, Senior C, Dalton J et al (2002) Autonomic response in depersonalization disorder. Arch Gen Psychiatry 59:833–838
Stirling JD, Heileweil JSE, Quraish N (1998) Self-monitoring dysfunction and the schizophrenic symptoms of alien control. Psychol Med 28:675–683

Further Reading

Farrer C, Franck N, Georgieff N et al (2003) Modulating the experience of agency: a positron emission tomography study. Neuroimage 18:324–333

Delusion—Content-related Thought Disorders

14

Contents

14.1 Introduction

In psychopathology, delusion is traditionally described as 1. a false firm conviction that a person has adopted and 2. whose truth is immediately evident to the person, i.e., requires no justification. The person does not perceive the delusional thought as knowledge but as a personal belief. 3. Their environment does not share the belief, and in the cultural context, the opinion is considered false. 4. The person has no insight into the erroneous nature of the conviction.

In the development of psychopathology, this definition of delusion has been proposed, which

F. M. Reischies, *Psychopathology*, https://doi.org/10.1007/978-3-662-70293-2_14

is clear and clinically applicable. However, many researchers and neuroscientists argue that a logically unchallengeable definition of delusion is not helpful.

The conventional definition probably represents only a part of the whole, which is not appropriate for the underlying problem. The delineation by the psychopathological definition may be arbitrarily related to the definability for clinical purposes. Thus, there is a risk that the clinically psychopathological definition, while practical, does not do justice to the underlying conditioning factors.

Specifically, it is assumed: The neuroscientific factors affect a larger group of psychopathological symptoms associated with delusion.

In the case of delusion, which is psychiatrically diagnosed, we are dealing with the tip of an iceberg. Among the clinically clear cases of, for example, paranoia, there is thus a base of the iceberg in the population with many cases of irrational assumptions that are more or less relevant to everyday life. In addition, there is a plethora of other false beliefs that people hold on to. Fears are usually irrationally based, such as fears of confined spaces or standing at great heights—anxiety about blood or injections (Kendler et al. 1983, Sutherland 1992). These fears are based on false assumptions or beliefs. Not only are irrational fears common, but epidemiological studies have also found a high number of people with delusional thoughts (van Os et al. 2001).

Accordingly, we are dealing with a continuum of irrationality—a spectrum of false considerations, a transition from harmless irrational fears and more or less dysfunctional personal beliefs, convictions, and ideologies, as well as a boundary to "overvalued ideas" and delusion. We construct a boundary, but the definition of delusion as a false firm conviction that is uncorrectable could thus represent an artificial subdivision in this continuum.

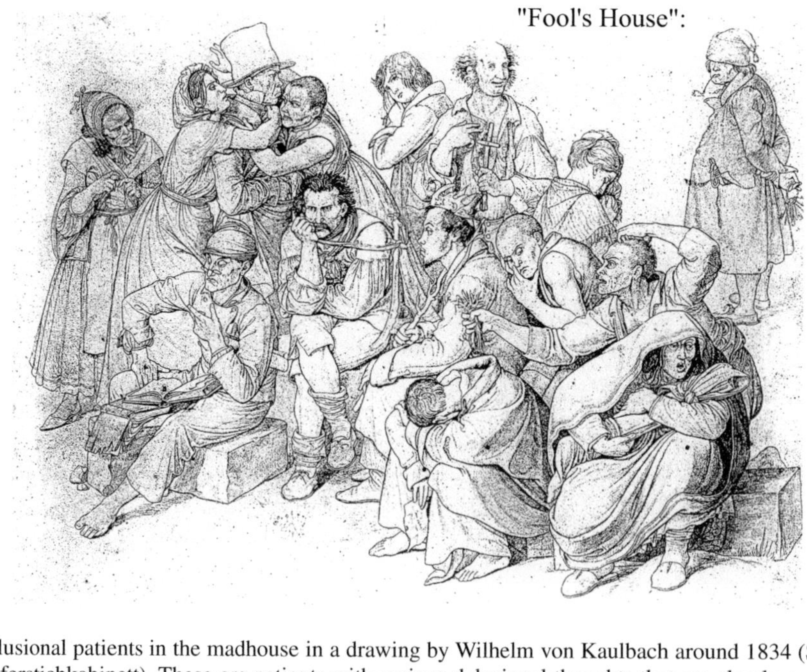

Fig. 14.1 Delusional patients in the madhouse in a drawing by Wilhelm von Kaulbach around 1834 (State Museums in Berlin, Kupferstichkabinett). These are patients with various delusional thoughts that are clearly manifested externally. Additionally, the lack of social interaction between the individuals is depicted. (Note: Public domain)

14.1.1 Defining Elements of Delusion

Falsity of the Belief
Not every false thought is a delusional idea: e.g., a mistake. Predominant delusional themes are threats from enemies, poverty, illness and guilt etc., or enhancements of one's own person through a special mission, power, love, or lineage, etc.

The delusional idea can stem from the usual ways of thinking in the person's environment. However, it is required that the delusional belief must stand in contrast to the belief in the patient's cultural environment. This has, among other things, to do with the very diverse cultural, religious, and political irrationalities, about which we judge psychiatrically with caution. It is difficult to distinguish delusion from superstition and political ideologies, especially fanaticism. The situation is diagnostically clear when the patient is in contrast to the prevailing opinion.

Self-Reference
A reference of the delusional thought to one's own person is obvious. The delusional ideas usually concern an autobiographical theme and not a general societal issue like foreign policy, taxes, or unemployment. There is a reference to the person, their development in the family, partnership, or professional sphere.

Occasionally, one can speak of an "abnormal relationship positing" when a person in the illness experiences relationships of their own person to people and institutions; however, these relationships are not real.

Incomprehensibility
Jaspers (1942) demanded incomprehensibility, i.e., an examiner cannot reconcile the development of the person into the delusion, cannot comprehend the origin; the examiner does not "understand" the patient's delusional development. This characteristic refers to the attempts of fellow humans or the family to understand the delusional thought. A "break in the pathway of life" becomes evident when the biographical context is illuminated. The "break" is caused by the development of the delusional thought in the person, e.g., it is not understandable why a person suddenly quits a long-term employment contract after successful and mutual satisfaction. Attempts to understand the delusion are limited to understanding the "how" of the delusion, not the "whether," i.e., the "being so" not the "being there" of the delusion (Schneider 1992).

This refers to the perspective of the outsider; for the question of the meaning of the delusional thought for the person self, research has been conducted, see below (Ritunnano et al. 2022).

Uncorrectability
Uncorrectability is at the center of the definition of delusion. Delusion is, first of all, a false opinion that is maintained in discussion. The delusional person does not let themselves be dissuaded from the false thought in discussion.

It is an essential aspect of delusion that the person also opposes their own cultural environment with the delusional belief. The social component, which consists of the patient separating from the consensus of their social context with their opinion, plays a role in the description of delusion that is often overlooked. Usually, the person suffers consequences from the environment after the development of the delusion. Fellow humans are alienated by the actions and discussions and often have a rejecting attitude.

Most of the time, the person with a delusion does not even engage in a discussion. The reason for this is an experience of evidence.

Experience of Evidence
For the patient with a delusion, the delusional ideas are "evident." The feeling of evidence is a criterion for delusion. One speaks of a feeling of evidence in the case of subjective conviction, without the need for proof, without the person having to think about justifications. Usually, the person states that they "have experienced it" and what someone self has experienced is—without doubt—true.

Patients with the paranoid-hallucinatory form of schizophrenia often suffer from very poorly substantiated delusional thoughts—the arguments for their assumptions, which are "evident" to them, are not sufficient for the examiner. For example, a patient explains that the same man has repeatedly stood on the corner of the street, opposite their own house. That is the proof that he is being shadowed by the secret police.

The patients are considered "gullible." In the Anglo-Saxon world, one has spoken of "jumping to conclusions" (see below).

Inability to "Transcend"
Transcendence in this context means that a person should consider the counter-position of the delusional thought, to step over to the other perspective, as a trial. This is not possible for a person with a delusional thought; they reject it, and it seems that the free choice of the other position, even as a trial, is denied to them.

Besides the defining elements of delusion, there are a number of conditioning factors and other influencing factors such as emotionality and personality variables. The complexity of the clinical phenomenon of delusion is great (Kendler et al. 1983).

14.2 Forms of Delusion

In the introduction, it was stated that the definition of delusion has been framed too strictly on the one hand. On the other hand, it is suspected that the definition of delusion is again too unspecific and needs specification. The differences between primary and secondary delusion or between emotion-congruent and emotion-incongruent delusion are presumably neurobiologically significant. Accordingly, there are serious differences between the delusional phenomena of the various psychiatric disorders (Scharfetter 2002). These differences relate to the conditioning factors, the course, the prognosis, the treatment, etc.

14.2.1 Influencing Factors on Delusional Themes

There are many different delusional themes. They are practically always derivable from the individual living conditions The usual delusional themes such as persecution, impoverishment, guilt, illness, grandeur are, as has been said, the great motives of human life.

In different stages of life, we find the predominance of different delusional themes (Fig. 14.2). The delusion of poverty was less common among younger patients in the Berlin clinic than among older ones. This can be related both to the frequency of delusional depression in old age and to life fate and cultural influences. The same applies to the delusion of guilt. In the case of the delusion of guilt, the cultural change regarding the acceptance of religious morality is also important; it has led to a reduction in cases with delusion of guilt.

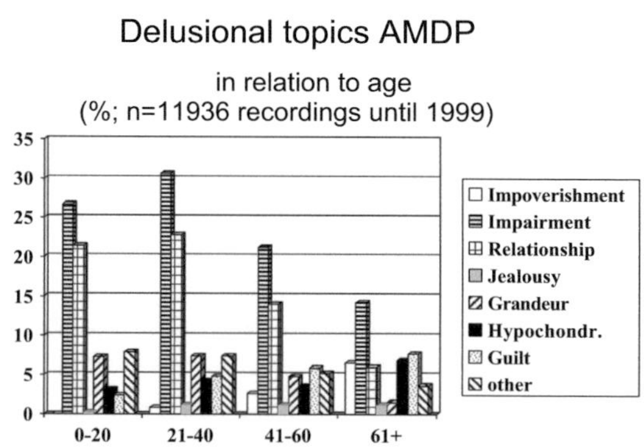

Fig. 14.2 Delusional themes of younger adults are different from those of older patients. In younger adulthood, more patients with delusion of persecution, impairment, and delusions of reference are admitted to the clinic. In older age, the delusion of impoverishment, hypochondria, and delusion of guilt in the context of depressive affective psychoses increases. Here, cohort effects, i.e., different life experiences, for example, in the case of the delusion of poverty, could also have an impact (data from 2 decades up to 1999). Overall, the proportion of patients with delusional symptoms is high (multiple delusional thoughts of various kinds occurred)

In stark contrast, younger people are more likely than older people to have a delusion of an impairment or paranoia and a general delusions of reference .

The frequency of persecution delusion can probably be explained by the frequency of schizophrenia in young adulthood. It can be seen that delusional thoughts are overall very common in different psychiatric disorders.

14.2.2 Secondary Delusion

May the uncorrectability of a false belief be explainable by a disturbance in the understanding of counterarguments? Must delusion exist with clear consciousness and preserved judgment ability? If not, then the false beliefs or delusional ideas of demented and delirious patients would not be considered delusional thoughts. It is to be discussed whether it is sensible to demand for the definition of delusion that the delusional ideas would be maintained despite the person's ability to judge counterarguments.

Secondary delusion has been spoken of when, for example, a primary brain disease causes the judgment disorder, and delusional thoughts arise on this basis. However, practically all psychiatric diseases are associated with brain changes. The distinction between primary and secondary loses significance the more neurobiological disorders are found that can explain delusion formation.

14.2.3 Insight Disorder Due to Cognitive Deficits

Delusion in Brain Damage- or Brain Degeneration Syndromes

Many patients with dementia exhibit fleeting delusional thoughts. These often revolve around themes of being stolen from or jealousy. In the case of something being stolen, the misplacement of items and forgetting storage locations are often the reasons for the development of these delusional thoughts. This leads to a projection: the problem that an item cannot be found immediately is turned into a suspicion directed outward—with the patient speculating that other people come into the apartment to steal. The patient does not understand the counterarguments that others present against the possibility of a burglary. These types of delusional thoughts are usually fleeting because the patients themselves forget the problem, the theft ideas —or find the sought item, or are shown it by helpers.

Initially, the fleeting delusional idea is discussed; in many families with a dementia patient, the development of delusions with the persistence of false beliefs is perceived as a particular burden, for example, when the patient suspects that the family or neighbors are after the money he needs for his future life. In the case that the patient is led to wrong actions by his delusion, conflicts arise that often end in the protected accommodation of the patient (Rabins and Lucas 1982).

Delusional thoughts in dementia have been associated with changes in the brain's transmitter systems due to neurodegeneration. Because the degeneration of the brain affects not only the cortex and the hippocampus but also the brainstem nuclei responsible for the control of dopamine and noradrenaline release in the brain (Zarow et al. 2003). Cholinergic neurons also degenerate. This can lead to an imbalance, where, for example, a relative predominance of the dopaminergic system exists (role of dopaminergic function in schizophrenia symptoms see Abi-Dargham 2004).

14.2.4 Influence of Emotion on Delusion

Delusion with Mood-congruent delusion—Delusion in depression and mania

The delusional idea can develop out of an emotional exceptional situation. There is—with exceptions, see below—a relationship between delusion and emotion—which perhaps can already be derived from the mentioned self-reference of the delusional thought.

One of the important specifications of delusion is mood-congruence, i.e., the connection of the delusional thought with an emotional exceptional situation such as anxiety, grief, anger, hatred. A delusion with congruent mood usually disappears when the affective symptoms have remitted.

In affective psychoses, depression and mania, we see a form of delusion that is clearly different from that in dementias. Both in depression and in mania, mood-congruent delusion occurs. Patients with depression often suffer from delusions of poverty, guilt, or insufficiency.

Some patients with depressive delusion do not show a typical depressive syndrome. For example, a patient with a stony expression said he was not in a depressed mood and did not suffer from depression, but he suffered from the guilt of ruining his family. As a reason for a depressive delusion, a supposed financial misjudgment is cited, for example. The people around and also the examiner try to explain the development of the delusion from the patient's despair. However, this is not easily possible. In very severe depressive syndromes, there are even completely incomprehensible, bizarre delusional assumptions, such as the delusion of no longer being alive.

Some researchers see the depressive delusion at least partially as an attempt at rationalization, whereby the pseudo-rational delusional arguments distract from the enormous emotional pressure and suffering—into cognitive processes, into thoughts and brooding .

In contrast to the forms of delusion in a depressive affective psychosis, mania is accompanied by increased self-confidence, and some patients develop megalomania. They believe themselves to be geniuses and capable of immense achievements; they think they have made a grand invention, a promising business idea, etc. Often, however, they ultimately plunge the family into financial ruin.

The mood congruence of the delusion corresponds to the phase dependency. The depressive delusion disappears when the depression lifts. The person with mania can distance themselves from their grandiose ideas when the mania subsides. If a delusion persists beyond the affective phase, an additional existing delusional disorder is usually suspected.

Does the schizophrenic delusion also have to do with the affective system? Especially the anxiety and eeriness in the delusional mood of schizophrenic patients point to a role of affect in the formation of delusion, especially in paranoia, also in schizophrenia. Conversely, with the loss of delusional dynamics, the belief in delusional thoughts also decreases in schizophrenic patients, enabling distancing and gradual correction, see below.

In addition to the explanatory delusion (see below), delusional systems occur in schizophrenic patients that can no longer be differentiated in their conditional constellations. However, it often becomes clear that behind the delusional thoughts lies an explanation for a special role of the patient, a mission, etc. Even the paranoia in most cases in schizophrenia has a background of assumptions about the patient's own great importance, for which they are persecuted (unless, on the other hand, there is, for example, persecution due to supposed transgressions in depression).

In some cases, delusional development occurs without depression, dementia, or schizophrenia being present. A delusional disorder is usually diagnosed. Often, the delusion of love is present. This delusion is also closely linked to emotions.

Mood-incongruent delusion

The mood-incongruent delusion could have other conditioning factors and a different course than the mood-congruent delusion. In chronic schizophrenia, delusional symptoms are often observed that do not seem to be directly related to emotions.

Explanatory delusion

Some of the delusional thoughts in mood-incongruent delusion can be illustrated with the concept of explanatory delusion. Patients experience verbal auditory hallucinations of contents that they are astonished by and try to explain. They ask themselves: "How does my neighbor know about my intentions, which I have not told anyone about?" Or they experience bodily hallucinations, which they try to make sense of. The close temporal coupling to other psychopathological symptomats, such as hallucinations or ego disturbances, is given in explanatory delusion .

Aggressive actions in Delusion

One of the specifications of delusion is the degree of practical relevance in terms of delusion-driven actions.

People with delusion can commit aggressive actions when they feel compelled to act out of the perceived necessity of their delusional conviction. The people with delusion act subjectively rational. Additionally, there is a loss of empathy, of compassion for fellow human beings, who can be the sufferers of the action.

14.2.5 Course of Delusion

The abnormal process of generating beliefs has already been addressed.

Let us consider the further time-course How long can a delusional idea be uncorrectable?

1. Fleeting delusional ideas, for example in delirium,
2. Delusional thoughts that a person clings to for a certain period and
3. chronic and more or less systematized delusional systems are distinguished (Table 14.1).

It may not be so much a false idea—the idea of a delusional thought—that is decisive, but rather the maintenance, especially against the resistance of the environment.

The fate of a delusional thought is characteristic in the development of delusion in schizophrenia (Conrad 1958): the delusional idea occurs in a triggering situation, e.g., in a delusional mood, in which the person is emotionally tense, anxious, experiences everything as uncanny, and has an abnormal experience of meaning (see below). It can be an isolated delusional idea or a delusional reinterpretation of a correct perception of the environment, the delusional perception.

Once the patient has had the delusional idea, the effort to rationalize the delusion begins. In the past, it was more common to elaborate a comprehensive delusional argumentation, as in the case of Daniel Paul Schreber, who wrote a book about his delusional thought structure, which is still available (Schreber 1903). Today, the effort to rationalize the delusion with the systematization of a delusional structure is often interrupted by the psychiatric treatment of the psychosis.

It is particularly important to consider that there are factors that favor the maintenance of the delusion. Many patients with schizophrenia lose their delusional thoughts at the end of the acute episode. On the other hand, chronically schizophrenic patients often also suffer from persistent delusional thoughts. These additionally lead to isolation from the environment.

Let us first consider the recovery from a delusional thought. The improvement of the delusion begins 1) with a distancing. 2) The delusional dynamic, the emotionality coupled with the delusional thought, reduces. Later, the patient can 3) have a double bookkeeping, in which he argues both according to the logic of the delusion and according to the realities of the environment. In the transition from delusional certainty to acceptance of counterarguments, there can be alternating states of delusional

Table 14.1 Temporal aspects of irrational assumptions

	Irrational fear	Overvalued idea	Delusion
Fleeting	Assumption is situationally corrected	e.g., recurring in anxiety or anger	e.g., in delirium
During an emotional exceptional situation	Situationally corrected during a calm phase	e.g., hypochondriacal assumptions	Depressive delusion
Persistent	Dysfunctional assumptions	e.g., thoughts about neighbors' intentions	e.g., delusional disorder

conviction and distancing or corrective thoughts. From perception, the oscillation between two contrary viewpoints is known from the Necker cube. It is the flipping and reverting of spatial perception in the wire model of the Necker cube. As a thinking model, this can help to illustrate the fluctuating states in the gradual correction of the delusion. 4) Finally, the correction of the delusion takes place. The patient still remembers the delusional thought, but he can clearly express that he had become entangled in this false thought.

14.2.6 Transitional Forms

Content-related thought disorders differ in the extent of their detachment from reality.

A) Irrational fears are, for example, known from phobic anxieties and compulsive acts. They can each be corrected if the emotion is not as strongly pronounced, as in acute panic, for example. However, they tend to return. These are often described as automatic thoughts. In meditation, these automatic thoughts, intrusions, often occur, and patients can experience that their thoughts do not always appear to be intentionally and voluntarily controlled by them, but rather unintentionally, they say: "It thinks me..".
The practically important difference is thus a) the person in panic, with the certainty of dying, e.g., from a circulatory crisis, and b) the bizarre delusion that an X-ray assistant came at night to irradiate the brain. Because in the first case, it is about unrealistic fears that are fleeting and can affect almost anyone. In the second case, we have one of the signs that it is a schizophrenia with a poor prognosis.
B) Overvalued idea. A transitional form from irrational thinking to delusion is the overvalued idea. In this case, the person is usually convinced of the (false) thought over a longer period and is affectively fixated on the idea. An example is the belief of a person that the neighbor harbors a hostile attitude towards him and occasionally expresses it in disputes.
The emotions are triggered when the topic is addressed. The thinking revolves around this idea. It determines his behavior. But (1.) the person can also intellectually engage with the possibility of error—there is the possibility of overcoming it—and (2.) the overvalued idea is not immediately evident. The false statement can even be questioned, and the person may admit that some of the cited evidence could be based on coincidental circumstances.

14.3 Clinic

Content-related thought disorders, i.e., delusional thoughts, pathological beliefs, and overvalued ideas, are very common in psychiatric conditions, such as schizophrenia, depression, dementias, obsessive-compulsive disorders, and also in some anxiety disorders.

Delusional themes differ between psychiatric conditions or the age of patient groups. For example, delusional thoughts about abnormal relationships to another person and persecution are more common in young adults, while themes like impoverishment and guilt are more common in older patients with depression. For the delusion of guilt or ideas of impoverishment, the specific experiences of the generation, such as deprivations during and after the world wars, must be considered (s. also Fig. 14.2).

14.3.1 Delusion in Schizophrenia

Delusional thoughts in patients who hear voices partly relate to the explanation of how these voices can occur. Other thoughts try to provide an explanation for the fact that the voices spread content that can only be known to the patient (see above). In the English-language literature, the group of ego disorders is considered part of the delusional symptomats of schizophrenia, with the factor structure seeming to be complex (Kimhy et al. 2005).

Another group of delusional thoughts in schizophrenia includes ideas of grandeur. Thus, delusions of descent and the delusion of having a special function are classified as megalomania, for example, being the new Messiah. They are to be considered differentially diagnostically in terms of the fate of a narcissistic personality or an accompanying manic syndrome. In many of the persecutory delusions of schizophrenic patients, themes of grandeur can be identified in detailed exploration. In most cases, the patient explains that they are being persecuted by powers that perceive them as an equally powerful opponent. Sometimes the question of who would take the trouble to shadow, observe, or eliminate the patient is helpful.

Particularly revealing in patients after a prolonged effort to rationalize the delusion is the painful gap that arises when the delusion disappears due to neuroleptic therapy. Patients with a delusion of grandeur or delusion of love, but also, as explained above, after paranoia, go through a crisis with mostly depressive mood, in which they have to adapt to the new life situation.

14.3.2 Delusion in depression

Especially in depression, the entire spectrum of anxiety thoughts, dysfunctional beliefs, pathological beliefs, and clearcut delusion must be considered. A) In some cases, the delusional nature of guilt thoughts is not immediately apparent and must be explored. B) On the other hand, patients come to the clinic who agitatedly present delusional thoughts, for example, not being able to pay for the hospital stay, increasingly falling into debt, or being arrested and taken away or killed at any moment due to their own guilt.

The emotionally distressing delusional thoughts disappear completely under neuroleptic medication or—as a last resort—under electroconvulsive therapy. After some time, the patients no longer mention the thoughts and may state that they were apparently mistaken. This reversibility of the delusion at the end of the phase or due to the successful therapy, which was started quickly after the onset of the illness, explains why there is no effort to rationalize the delusional thought. In depression, the systematization of delusional thoughts is practically not seen, as it is impressively observed in schizophrenic patients and patients with delusional disorder.

The psychopathological identification of depressive delusion is often of vital importance. Although certainly psychotherapy is indicated in severe depressive episodes, psychotherapy is generally contraindicated in delusional depression. For the patients recognize the therapist's efforts but cannot notice any subjective change in their suffering. This often only puts them in an even more desperate mood (see textbooks of psychotherapy).

14.3.3 Delusion in obsessive-compulsive syndromes

Clinically, all transitions from dysfunctional thoughts to overvalued ideas and delusional thoughts are observed in obsessive-compulsive patients: A patient reports irrational assumptions, for example, that contamination would lead to illness and infection of the entire family. This can become an overvalued idea, which takes on bizarre irrational traits. For instance, a patient is convinced that the infection could somehow be transmitted over hundreds of kilometers, even if there is no contact between the patient and the family.

14.3.4 Capgras syndrome

A patient encounters a person known to him and thinks the person seem somewhat changed. Another person must be hidden behind him, merely acting as if he is the person known to the patient. Attempts have been made to explain this disorder neuroscientifically with altered facial perception or altered emotional reaction to the perception (Ellis and Young 1990, Ellis et al. 1997). The change in facial processing leads to a "dissonance" that the patient believes can only be interpreted as another person being behind it. For example, a patient sees a strange change in a known Catholic priest, who otherwise had no contact with her, and interprets it as another man playing this priest.

14.3.5 Delusional disorder

A delusional idea without further psychiatric symptoms, i.e., isolated delusional symptoms, is often diagnosed as sensitive delusions of reference. Patients report about mobbing, about discrimination by colleagues, etc. A personality disorder is present in many cases, e.g., a querulous personality.

14.3.6 Delusional Symptoms in Dementia

In the early stages of some dementia diseases, paranoid symptoms are triggered, which have been classified as late schizophrenia or paraphrenia. The mechanism of this "triggering" is not yet explainable in detail. It is based on Bonhoeffer's concept that the brain, given a certain predisposition, tends to develop one of several reaction types, including the paranoid reaction.

The delusional symptoms in dementia do not develop as in schizophrenia, as described above. In dementia, there are also different types of delusional thoughts that are not observed in any other disease. These include the delusional forms described in more detail below, such as theft delusion, special types of confabulations that are adhered to, and misidentification symptoms.

Brain damage from Alzheimer's dementia is often used as an explanation. It is likely to be a specific brain damage syndrome. Currently, attempts are being made to learn more about the mechanisms of delusion from the neuropsychiatric symptoms of dementia.

Theft delusion: The common delusional belief of having been stolen from, when the patient has merely misplaced something and cannot find it again, is explained by memory disorders. Attention disorders are also used to explain this (Fukuhara et al. 2001).

Delusional misidentification: A clear example is mirror image self-misidentification. For this reason, it is sometimes necessary for relatives to cover all mirrors in the living areas—then the patient is not startled every time they do not recognize themselves and believe they see a stranger in the room. They may feel justified in aggressively attacking this perceived stranger.

In addition to person-related misidentification symptoms, there are also location-related symptoms. A patient developed the delusion that her husband was being held in the clinic's basement. Not only was this surprising because he had long since passed away, but particularly that the patient confused parts of the house she lived in with the clinic and was firmly convinced that the doctor only needed to take her to the basement so she could find her husband again.

People with dementia believe that the vivid and large images of modern televisions bring the depicted famous politicians into their home in person. Some dementia patients consider their stuffed animals to be alive. Such animistic beliefs are found to be associated with right frontoparietal degeneration (Shanks and Vennerici 2004).

Patients can report imagined content as subjective truth. In doing so, relationships to spontaneous confabulations should be considered (see Schnider et al. 2003). Patients report false autobiographical data with conviction.

14.4 Diagnostics

How can the examiner suspect that a person has become involveded in a delusion, and how can this diagnosis be confirmed? The patient is not aware of the pathological nature of his assumption; otherwise, it would not be a delusion. Therefore, many delusional thoughts remain undiagnosed. They are not mentioned, not inquired about, or the delusion concerns areas that are not covered in the standard psychopathology interview and are thus initially inaccessible. They are only diagnostically illuminated when a person presents the delusional thoughts during the examination or when behavioral consequences prompt questions about the reasons.

For the diagnosis of delusion, it is necessary to inquire every time something in the person's statements is inexplicable or even just peculiar, i.e., does not align with the rational expectations of the person's cultural environment. Since these are thoughts that are generally important to the person in their social contexts, peculiarities in comments, statements, and behaviors will raise suspicion. Then it helps to ask questions to crystallize and substantiate a suspicion.

In the history taken from other persons, relatives can report that the person's interests have changed, becoming more or less focused on religion, politics, or neighborhood relations. While this is almost always a healthy shift in interests, it can indicate a developing delusional topic in the context of a mental illness.

In the interview, it is necessary to ask about common delusional themes. These include questions like: What are you worried about—e.g., money, illnesses? Are there problems with superiors or neighbors? Are other people talking more about you now—are they speaking ill of you, is there bullying? Other questions include whether the person feels he has a special task to fulfill, a mission etc.

Listing these questions makes it clear that to share such very personal information, the greatest possible trust between examiner and patient must be achieved. The delusional ideas, which the person already anticipates that it would be difficult to explain to relatives and friends, will otherwise not be mentioned. Therefore, many patients with chronic delusional symptoms have a certain partial insight into the problem of the specific delusional thought—it relates to the incomprehension of the environment. Delusional diagnostics also demonstrate the dependence of psychiatric diagnostics on the qualities of the examiner.

14.4.1 Delusion-Driven Behavior

Delusional thoughts can lead to aggressive actions that are executed brutally and unpredictably. They are motivated by the specific delusional thought—for example, the patient believes he is acting in self-defense, from which he "must strike," or he thinks he is being hindered in his mission and must now proceed with all his might.

At this point, it is important to emphasize: A delusion cannot be diagnosed solely based on behavior. If a person behaves incomprehensibly, suspicion of a delusion can be raised—to explain the behavior. But the examiner must, in a second step, ensure through discussion with the person that it is indeed a delusion.

Please imagine a conversation during a confrontation. A confrontation in the case of a delusion of love would proceed as follows: The person with a delusion of love will affirm the question "Is this your love partner?" while the other will not. Often, the delusional person later says that the partner could not publicly declare his love for her in that situation. But she could perceive certain signs again that he is indeed in love with her and will soon reveal it.

If you imagine a situation where you ask a person about their belief of being followed by a neighbor and let them describe specific situations of the confrontation, you will notice how many assumptions come to your mind about the thoughts of the conversation participants in this confrontation. These assumptions about the intention of a conversation partner are further discussed in the section on the Theory of Mind. Discussing a confrontation is often helpful in conversations with patients to clarify whether the belief is uncorrectable.

A reliable delusion diagnosis via questionnaire or computer-based interview is excluded based on the aforementioned. To be sure whether it is really a delusion, the examiner must 1. let the situations be described, 2. discuss with the person.

Regarding uncorrectability, an attempt at correction, a test of transitioning to the alternative belief, must be undertaken to check how subjectively evident the person's belief is. Is the person able to even consider the counterposition? In many cases, such a discussion will not be possible because the delusional thought appears immediately evident to the affected person ("but I saw it") and they therefore reject a discussion. Additionally, the patient may want to avoid annoying arguments from previous experiences discussing their delusional topic—for example, within their family. The tendency of patients with delusions is to expose themselves as little as possible to arguments against their delusional belief.

Exclusion of Chance

In some cases, the patient provides a justification during the exploration. For example, they perceived something specific, something strange. When the examiner then argues that the observation could also be explained differently or occurred by chance, the patient will reject this possibility outright. The "exclusion of chance" in this context is one of the delusion criteria that can be helpful in diagnostics. The criterion of "exclusion of chance" is associated with a procedure noted in recent literature: The discussion with the patient about a hypothetical refutation of the delusional thought proves to be clinically useful (Hurn et al. 2002). A hypothetical event that would refute the delusional thought is described, and the patient is asked how he would react to it, i.e., to what extent a patient is willing to accept or reject the hypothetical event as possible.

14.5 Neuroscientific Explanatory Approaches

In the past, it was believed that while the delusional themes were explainable to others, the fact that the patient developed a delusional thought at all, the "whether" of the delusion, was not. Today, we know more about the mechanisms of delusion formation in some forms of delusion. Subsequently, the question of explaining the frequency of delusion will be addressed, and general mechanisms that favor the formation and maintenance of the delusion will be examined.

Delusion is usually successfully treatable in schizophrenia, depression and mania using neuroleptics. This has led to speculation that the psychopathological phenomenon is caused and thus explainable at the level of transmitter-dependent cell and network functions.

Today, delusion is more likely attributed to matters at the level of representations and semantic processing. The factors described above, especially emotional factors, apparently influence this in a specific way, so that the complex phenomenon of delusion clinically manifests. Through these influencing factors on delusion development, which can be explained by molecular or cellular mechanisms, secondary influences on transmitters or electrophysiological elementary processes occur. This will be presented below.

14.5.1 Specific Mechanisms Explaining Delusion Formation

Judgment Disorder, thought error

Cognitive deficits as a factor in the development of delusion in dementia—as an explanation for one of the forms of delusion—have already been described. With the approach of delusion development arising from thought errors, delusional thoughts in schizophrenia have been explained. In the meantime, a mechanism for improving the prediction of the next events has been identified (Clark 2013). The Bayesian characteristic of information processing in the human brain was presented as an optimization of prediction probability; in other words, (1) at a basic level, feedback from actions is used in neuronal networks for adaptive optimization (see ego disturbances). In the cortical functioning of predictive coding (2) there is optimization and also acceleration of actions—through prediction and adaptive correction of the prediction. Errors in deep learning have already been reported in hallucinations. In the area of delusion, a source of "fake news" can lie in the predictive nature of cognitive working methods of learning and cortex representation (Weilnhammer et al. 2020, Sterzer 2022).

Attribution Styles, black-and-white thinking, jumping to conclusions
Not only can attention be altered with regard to certain contents, but also the attribution of values and potential dangers. In general, patients with paranoid delusion tend to attribute good qualities or events to themselves, but bad qualities or mishaps to others.

Black-and-White Thinking
Another characteristic is black-and-white thinking. Delusion patients are less able to relativize—they usually evaluate in extreme categories. Many patients with delusional symptoms cannot assess gradations; a person is either a friend or an enemy, supportive or dangerous.

Jumping to Conclusions
Additionally, there is a peculiarity in information processing in acute schizophrenia, which is referred to as jumping to conclusions, or making conclusions without sufficient evidence. People with acute schizophrenic psychosis often have false assumptions about the intentions of others and tend to make hasty conclusions. The spontaneous confabulation, which is adhered to, and the "jumping to conclusions" should be mentioned here (Garety and Hemsley 1994, Gilleen and David 2005).

In this context, the disorder of judgment of complex issues should be mentioned: The clinically frequent observation of the inability of schizophrenic patients to explain proverbs; the understanding of metaphors is impaired (de Bonis et al. 1997). Some studies also showed that patients have difficulty understanding contradictions (de Bonis et al. 1992).

Theory of Mind:
Another approach attempts to explain the specific situation in paranoia. First, a basis should be presented: In communication between two people, complex conclusions about the underlying goals of the other person's actions are the norm (Fig. 14.3). A controller of the linguistic utterances of the counterpart is suspected: "Why is he saying this now?"—in other words, people always have assumptions about what controls the utterances of our counterpart, i.e., their intentions, expectations, fears, and also the distortion of this person's perspective. These assumptions about the intentions of the counterpart are incorrect in paranoia.

The theory about the thoughts of others has been referred to as "Theory of Mind." The theory about the thoughts of others particularly concerns social situations. For example, we experience how someone is deceived. We assume that this person must have a false assumption because he has been deceived. An example is the marriage swindler. The deceived person believes that the partner loves her.

Patients with autism and schizophrenia apparently have a significant disturbance in social information processing, which is evident in assumptions about the thoughts that others have. For example, they cannot empathize with the deceived person and express the assumptions that this person has formed. Despite otherwise high intelligence, they are unable to comprehend a deception situation in the mental representations of those involved. The information about the theory of the thoughts of others is presumably processed primarily in the medial frontal lobe (Frith and Frith 1999; Förstl 2007). This performance has been attributed to the "social brain". Imaging findings in patients with delusional symptoms have shown less mediofrontal activation when activated by stimuli that concern themself (Blackwood et al. 2004).

Attention Control
Especially in anxiety-laden delusional themes such as paranoia, but also in sensitive delusions of reference, influences from a disturbed attention control could become effective. It is about the patient's attention being fixed on the delusional object. The patient practically thinks exclusively about the delusional object. It is not a general disturbance of attention, but a disturbance of the flexibility of directing attention. The patient cannot detach their attention from

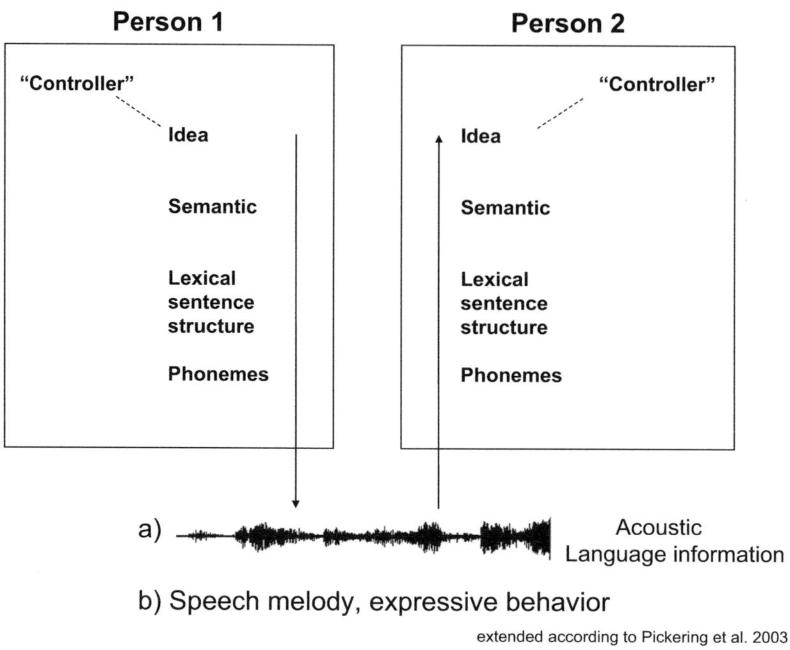

Fig. 14.3 Delusional thoughts about the "controller" of other people's utterances. In indirect speech acts, the intention of the speaker must be inferred ("it is cold" can, for example, be expressed as a request to close the window). A model assumption of delusion formation, especially relationship and paranoia, assumes a disturbance in this information processing. Generally, a disturbance of the "Theory of Mind" is assumed, the model that every person has at all times about the inner motives of other people in the social environment. (Extended after Pickering and Garrod 2004)

the delusional topic, and conversely, they cannot direct their attention to possible indications that contradict the delusion (Bentall 1989).

Therefore, studies on the attention of paranoid patients have been conducted. It turned out that the patients hold their attention sparsly on the feared object (Phillips et al. 2000, Green and Philipps 2004). This finding has also been observed in phobia, where anxiety patients particularly look at the objects they are anxious about very little. The evidence is not yet satisfactory, but a role of attention on thought content that generates fear, whether initially in the form of increased attention to critical stimuli or later in the form of diverting attention away that prevents the delusional belief from being refuted, seems to be involved.

Delusion of Explanation

One starting point for the explanation of delusional thoughts concerns the general difficulty of individuals to perceive and explain changes within themselves. Usually, internal processes are related to changes in the environment. When something inexplicable occurs, such as hallucinations, unusual explanations must be found to explain the perceptions from outside—for this, the term delusion of explanation has been coined (see also Maher 1988). A surprising experience of physical, emotional changes or alienation of perceptions, the occurrence of hallucinations, and generally explaining a situation that is unbearable for the person can apparently be the reason for developing a delusion. For example, when schizophrenic patients interpret bizarre experiences bizarrely, the development of the delusion could be related to the pressure the patient feels to make the special experience understandable to himself. The cognitive explanation model that the delusion provides to the patient for the unnatural experiences reduces unbearable emotions, tensions, and inexplicability.

A longitudinal study on the development of delusional symptoms in children who reported verbal auditory hallucinations showed a worse prognosis for voices heard outside the head (Escher et al. 2002). Additionally, a predictor was whether the phonemes seemed to have a subjective influence on the person.

For Capgras syndrome, it is assumed that a dissonance arises between correct face recognition and a non-corresponding emotional attitude towards the person. This could occur due to errors in the information processing of faces. The dissonance is then "explained" by the assumption of an actor imitating the person known to the patient.

Such an initial situation is depicted in the following schema Fig. 14.4. A patient is in an emotional exceptional state of anxiety, despair, or even mania, where this state relates to an experience of change. He is perplexed and insecure. The delusional idea is able to explain the change, i.e., to provide a rationalization for the emotional exceptional state. In many cases, it also manages to strengthen his self-esteem.

14.5.2 General Mechanisms

Corrective for thought error

A general approach of neuroscientific explanations of delusional symptoms concerns the attempt to explain the frequency of irrationality. In the information processing of the human brain, in contrast to sensory accuracy, for example, the sharp visual image of the environment, a correction can only be found with difficulty in the conceptual-categorical domain. In other words, sensory errors can be corrected immediately; however, in the realm of statements, a correction of an error sometimes succeeds only for intellectually honest people. Although there are also optical illusions and only these resist correction: we fall for them again and again; but the correction of conceptually vague and false conclusions is much more problematic.

Some facts are easy to verify for their truth, such as the number of corners of a triangle or the dependence of living expenses on the income and savings of a household. But the truth about the mental attitudes of other people, intentions, and emotions cannot be obtained

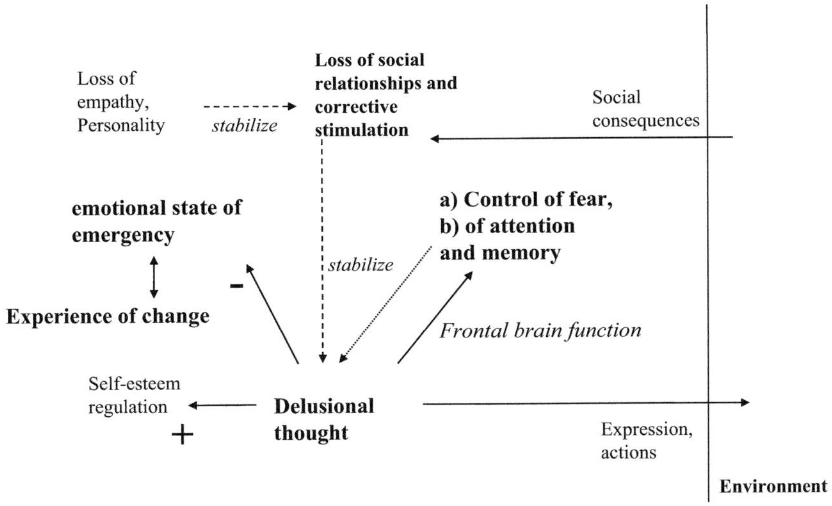

Fig. 14.4 Delusional thoughts can have functions for the person of the patient, which usually only become clear when the patient is cured of the delusion; then something is missing. Delusional thoughts can initially be a help in emotional exceptional situations, they seem to create clarity, raise self-esteem, or manage to reduce anxiety. However, this happens at the expense of social feedback from fellow humans, who withdraw because of the delusion or are actively avoided because they could contradict the delusional thought. The patient also avoids remembering facts that contradict the delusional thoughts.

with absolute certainty. This becomes evident, for example, in many cases in court. Thus, delusional thoughts can more easily form and be maintained, for example, about a person's love, about the hatred of people, and hostile intentions of organizations.

The question of when a person changes his opinion helps in this context. Thus, we hear of "bitter recognition," having been deceived in a person, or of "making peace with it," when it comes to limitations that come with age, for example. Just as people misjudge loved ones, as well as in the assessment of their own person, a misjudgment can easily arise. One speaks of "delusion" regarding grossly exaggerated self-assessment, or someone has "fallen into delusion," seeing a person as their savior, who turns out to be someone who exploits the person for others.

The misjudgment of people has to do with the constructive character of the human conceptual inner world, i.e., the level of elementary propositions about all important objects: Even the visually-perceptive environment is constructed (see perception); in addition, there is the error susceptibility of predictive coding (see above). For delusion, the crucial point is that the person forms a conceptual construction of our social world. This mental-cognitive construction of the environment is very abstract and, crucially, less sensorily or through experience controllable. While in perception only the well-known optical illusions can deceive us, there is no such effective, self-perceivable corrective for a false world-model. The mental-cognitive construction of the environment consists of the elementary propositions about everything the person knows about the environment: e.g., Kurt is a teacher, the apartment is 86 square meters, Lisa is left-handed, etc. In doing so, possible and true facts can be confused, especially when the statements refer to unverifiable facts. Examples of this are assumptions about mental states such as: Lisa likes me or Lisa does not like me (Fig. 14.5).

What is the basis for correcting a false "assessment"? Generally, people change their opinion only when the pressure of evidence against the assessment becomes very high. This applies especially when an emotional attitude exists for the assessment. Conversely, in a negative direction, in the case of suspicion, the initially neutral assessment of a fellow human being is very quickly changed into that of an enemy. This is observed in suspicious paranoid patients, for example, in clinical everyday life on the ward.

14.5.3 Emotional Influences on Delusional Thoughts

Emotionality in Thought Processes becomes evident when you compare a chess player with a computer as his partner: The player's thinking is coupled with various emotions—hopes, for example, for the decisive role of a piece in the further course of the game, anger at oneself and the opponent when losing pieces, etc. In our context, hope and the defense of anxiety are particularly noteworthy. People spend a lot of money to be allowed to hope, for example, in lotteries. Just as "being allowed to hope," the positively perceived self-image is a general goal of actions and mental operations. Thus, threats to the positive self-image must be avoided and disappointments cognitively devalued.

In the delusional mood, which in many cases of schizophrenia initiates the formation of delusions in acute psychosis, the patient usually has anxiety about something uncanny, something changing. However, it is also common for an old delusion of a chronically schizophrenic patient to be presented emotionlessly—it is a delusion whose emotional contexts are decoupled. Mood incongruence in schizophrenic delusion, which is not merely an explanatory delusion of hallucinations, is rather rare. The delusional themes are usually emotion-related.

Delusion induced disorganized thinking

The so-called "delusion induced disorganized thinking," i.e., the finding that a formal thought disorder becomes more apparent when addressing the delusional topic, is also in most cases associated with agitation—and often with emotional agitation. Formal thought disorders, such

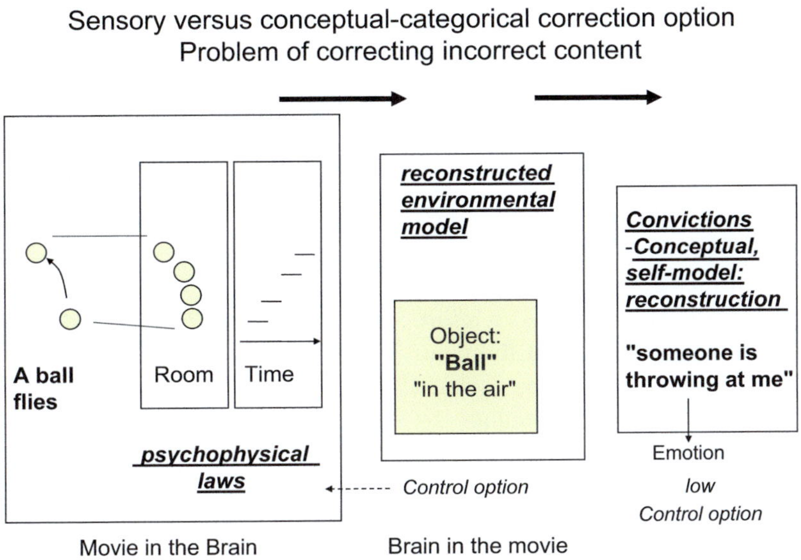

Fig. 14.5 Error possibilities in complex statements for which no sensory feedback is possible. In psychophysical correlates, i.e., the assessment of perceptual images of the environment, only a few illusions occur (e.g., optical illusions). However, the sensory information is further reconstructed into an environmental model: From a passive "movie in the brain" it becomes an active "brain in the movie" when the person, for example, looks around and interacts with the environment. The integration of interpretations and emotional conclusions is more error-prone because there are fewer or hardly any feedback possibilities. In doing so, the quality and certainty of the judgment foundations are not perceived in many cases

as a sudden appearance of incoherence, could become particularly evident when addressing the delusional topic (Haddock et al. 1995). This can be explained by the fact that emotional components are addressed in the patient with the delusional topic. It is recurrently astonishing to find that patients with a chronic delusion become agitated and exhibit formal thought disorders when the delusional topic is broached. This is a sign of a continuing delusional dynamic (see below). At the same time, the formal thought disorder can hinder a rational approach to the matter and the insight.

Some researchers consider whether the development of delusions, analogous to obsessive phenomena, serves positive emotions, the defense of anxiety. It is known from the study of affective actions that a person cannot act rationally controlled in emotional exceptional situations (Saß 1993). In this sense, it is assumed that a patient is brought by the emotional pressure in an affect storm to adopt a distortion of the cognitive world-model. An analogous approach is based on the positive emotion. The reward of a certain belief can be the cause of irrationally holding on to this opinion (see also Watzlawick 1981). This applies not only to chances of winning in gambling or the effect of advertising on the assessment of brands but also to the assessment of people who reward their subordinates.

Conclusion
First, we can state that, on the one hand, there is a susceptibility to errors in the conceptual sphere, which, secondly, in emotional situations of distress and a limitation of the ability to think logically in affect, gives rise to delusional thoughts.

14.5.4 Maintenance of the Delusion

So far, only neuroscientific explanations for the emergence of a delusion have been presented. What factors are responsible for its maintenance? What distinguishes the fleeting delusional thought from the persistent delusion of a delusional patient? What, in contrast to a quickly corrected thought error, leads to the maintenance, systematization, and chronicity of the delusional thought?

Usually, the delusional ideas are at first expressed by the person to people in their surroundings: The environment reacts with incomprehension and social consequences. As a result, the communication connection about the delusion breaks off. Once a patient has isolated themselves from their social connections by expressing their delusional thoughts, a loss of correction suggestions occurs.

Presumably, personality traits of patients with chronic delusion support the further course: Especially in people with relationship disorders, such a situation stabilizes, i.e., a delusional idea can solidify through effort to rationalize the delusion. These individuals cannot empathize with the emotions of others like healthy people and continue the exchange about their problems.

Functions of the delusional thought for the patient

In chronic delusion, it is necessary to ask whether the delusion has a specific function for the person that stabilizes the delusional thought, for example, in the control of anxiety. Emotion regulation and affect control is supported by specific frontal lobe functions (Chap. 11 emotion and affect). The frontal control of amygdala functions involves a cognitive-emotional "interface." It allows at least a certain, albeit imperfect, but still partially efficient control of anxiety.

In addition to specific anxiety control, the regulation of attention and other behavioral functions can also achieve a diversion from anxiety-inducing content. In this context, the diversion from correcting false assumptions is particularly interesting, as it exerts an anxiety-defensive or self-esteem-stabilizing effect. If anxiety-inducing thoughts and objects are not attended to, anxiety or confrontation with events and thoughts that could undermine self-confidence can also be avoided.

▶ Clinically, it must be clarified whether a personality disorder is present that favors a patient isolating themselves in their delusional world. This way, they evade the pressure of the environment, which demands correction and urges them to abandon their false belief.

14.5.5 Other Influencing Factors

It has long been known that schizophrenic patients have difficulty flexibly searching for new solutions. The flexibility of evaluations, as required in the Wisconsin Card Sorting Test, is reduced in schizophrenia (see, e.g., Bersani et al. 2004), as well as in Alzheimer patients with delusional development (Jeste et al. 1992). This could be used as an explanation for why patients remain with the belief they once reached in an emotional exceptional situation, because they cannot flexibly consider different aspects of a matter, or because no correction of thought patterns can be achieved in the brain through plasticity of network connections. There have also been speculations that the right, non-language-dominant hemisphere is responsible for a rather irrational access to the experience of the environment and is involved in the genesis and maintenance of delusional phenomena (Ramachandran and Blakeslee 1998).

Particularly in schizophrenic patients with a delusion, brain imaging studies have been conducted—less so in delusional individuals. The findings of the many studies are not yet consistent, and most findings are likely to be state-dependent. In other words, they provide an explanation for the prerequisites for the emergence or chronic persistence of a delusion, but not for the differential consideration of the various phases of the delusion. Only comparative studies over time could provide insights into differential neuroscientific explanations of the manifestations of delusion.

An overactivity in the ventral striatum showed an association with delusional symptoms (see Blackwood et al. 2001). The finding is consistent with the concepts of therapy for schizophrenic psychoses with neuroleptics, which reduce dopamine function—this particularly affects the ventral striatum (Abi-Dargham 2004). The role of the dopaminergic system in signaling the rewarding significance of stimuli has been discussed (see "incentive salience", Berridge and Robinson 1998, Pankow et al. 2012). In this context, schizophrenia is thought to involve a false attribution of significance due to the disturbance in the dopaminergic system.

This is related to the neuroscientific explanation of delusion as due to a misguided reward for a false conviction. This explanatory approach assumes that the delusional ideas are rewarding, for example, by warding off anxiety or increasing self-esteem. The plastic neuronal activity triggered by the reward in the ventral striatum (Montague 2005) could explain why a plastic change in connectivity in the brain is achieved through the recurring reward as a consequence of the delusional thought, which in turn stabilizes the delusional thought. To what extent semantic networks can also change in schizophrenia (see Spitzer 1990, 1995) is conceivable but not proven.

14.6 Psychopathological Symptoms

Delusional Mood
Definition A person experiences a tense, uncanny mood, a change within himself and/or in the environment, and in his affected state he does not know what is happening to him. Attempts at interpretation and abnormal experiences of significance "seem" to occur.

Anxiety and perplexity but also emerging feelings of happiness are possible.

Example

A person anxiously experiences a strange atmosphere with eeriness, unusual sensory impressions—associated with attention to small details like the cracking in the wall, which seem to have some significance for him. ◀

Position in Psychopathology AMDP 33.

Related terms. Relationship to apophenia (Conrad 1958).

Psychopathological Interactions Emotional disturbance: anxiety, suspicion, euphoria; increased undirected attention.

Differential Diagnostic Distinctions Anxiety syndrome, dissociative disorder, "I am anxious about going crazy" -possibly even with anxiety-laden pseudo-hallucinations.

Further Characterization Described as one of the developmental stages of delusion in schizophrenia (Conrad 1958). Uncertainty, emotional involvement, emotional exceptional situation, and attempts at interpretation. Also in existing delusion in renewed florid delusion development.

Interview for Rating Question about uncanny moods.

Neuropsychology/objectification Emotional expression of insecurity, of perplexity or also anxiety—observation of the confrontation with it.

Severity Only upon questioning, mild to incapacitating.

Pathognomonic for Schizophrenia.

Personality influences Esoteric tendencies, anxious personality.

Conceptual problems of the feature In some cases, the phase of the onset of delusional symptoms is described retrospectively in this way.

Neuroscientific/cognitive neuroscientific models Not clarified:

1. anxiety due to the feeling of unfamiliarity in a familiar environment—e.g., amygdala dysfunction and recognition dysfunction in the

mediotemporal cortex, possibly abnormally initiated amygdala activity in the first psychotic episode—with anxiety equivalents,
2. no delusional ideas yet, no effort to rationalize a delusion, which seemingly explains the phenomena as caused externally.

Delusional thought

Definition A person expresses a belief that holds great significance for him but is false—and incompatible with the beliefs in the culture of his environment.

The thought is accompanied by (1) emotional involvement. (2) The content is evident to the person, requires no explanation; (3) there is a lack of insight; the belief is uncorrectable in conversation. (5) not comprehensible in the context of life history, a break in biographical development,

Examples

paranoia, delusions of grandeur, delusion of love, delusional jealousy, delusion of poverty etc. ◀

Position in psychopathology AMDP 36. Lack of insight (Falret and Berrios 1996), not empathizable (Jaspers 1942),

Related terms paranoia; delusional idea, delusional imagination

Differential diagnostic distinctions
- fleeting thoughts that are immediately corrected: ideas of persecution, hypochondriacal ideas, ideas of guilt or ideas of grandeur,
- Overvalued ideas that are behaviorally relevant, that generate long-term emotional tension but are not uncorrectable: e.g., "the neighbor hates me and is trying to harm me."
- dysfunctional cognitions, e.g., "I can't succeed at anything" to "I am a failure."

Further characterization Uncorrectability by evidence; false, new belief that resists correction (Griesinger 1845); no effort is apparent to justify the delusional thought to others; exclusion of coincidence in events that seem to justify the delusion, e.g., being observed by pursuers.

Self-/other persons' judgment. other persons' judgment.

Interview for rating Address potential areas for delusional themes (e.g., opponents, enemies, are there special assignments the person has, etc.), inquire about incomprehensible decisions and plans, history taken from other persons. An attempt should be made to challenge the person's belief, i.e. that the thought is false.

Neuropsychology/objectification There are no delusion-specific tests. Observation of the confrontation with counterarguments. With perfect double bookkeeping not diagnosable.

Severity
- Significance of the delusion for everyday life: non-existent to life-dominating,
- Proportion of time spent on delusional thoughts.

Specifications Bizarre Delusion

Objective delusion—delusional ideas refer to general, e.g., social matters, which do not necessarily have an immediately recognizable relation to the person with the delusion.

Problematic areas:

a) A person in the GDR felt persecuted by the "Stasi" and, as a mentally ill person, was also under observation by the state security agency. Nevertheless, the symptomats are to be classified as delusion, as the delusion relates to the characteristic of feeling persecuted and included one's own great importance to the "Stasi" and the life-threatening danger, which did not actually exist.
b) A person developed the hypochondriacal delusion of dying from a heart disease, who actually had a milder, benign heart disease.

However, the hypochondriacal delusion with life-threatening danger did not refer to this.

- **Delusional themes**:
- delusions of reference (AMDP 39) none of the other delusional themes—only abnormal relationship setting
- Delusion of impairment or persecution (AMDP 40); delusion of hostility with fear of harm from others,
- delusional jealousy (AMDP 41)—often in alcoholism and dementia,
- delusion of guilt (AMDP 42)—e.g., in depression,
- delusion of impoverishment (AMDP 43)—in depression,
- Hypochondriacal delusion (AMDP 44)—see above, additionally relationship to delusional parasitosis, dysmorphophobia,
- Megalomania (AMDP 45)—often in mania and schizophrenia,
- other delusions (AMDP 46)—fantastic, bizarre delusion etc.,
- Cotard's syndrome: nihilistic delusion; e.g., delusion of already being dead,
- Delusion that something is being played to the person, the person is involved in a game; relationship to ego disturbances (being manipulated), derealization,
- Capgras phenomenon—people in the surrounding are replaced or entire situations are not authentic to deceive the patient etc.—often in schizophrenia (see also delusional misidentification).

4. Delusion-driven actions—actions determined by delusional thoughts—also with dangerous aspects
5. Recovery: In characteristic stages: a) Distancing from delusional thoughts: The delusional content demands less attention, has less behavioral relevance, but is still held onto, b) Correction of delusional thoughts: The person still thinks about the delusional topic (not the false firm conviction reappears, but memories of the time when the patient believed it), but can recognize that the thought was wrong.

Personality influences

- paranoid personality,
- schizotypal personality,
- Tendency towards magical, esoteric content.

Conceptual Problems of the Feature

- possibly so-called life lies,
- spectrum from dysfunctional beliefs to delusion,
- question whether less important delusional thoughts are not diagnosable? Or are there no "unimportant" delusional thoughts due to the necessary affective component?

Neuroscientific/cognitive neuroscientific models

1. Deficit model:
   - Neuropsychological findings:
     a) initially: in schizophrenia a subtype: paranoid schizophrenia without massive thought disorders,
     b) judgment disorder,
     c) affective pressure in depression with explanatory delusion, which seemingly helps to understand the unbearably bad condition,
     d) counter-evidence is not understood,
   - Alzheimer's dementia, neuropsychologically justifiable lack of insight into counter-evidence,
   - problems with logical thinking.
2. Abnormal imprinting:
   Imprinting as particularly extinction-resistant learning:
   - model of early childhood imprinting, e.g., of greylag geese by K. Lorenz,
   - possibly amphetamine-induced delusional symptoms: bomber pilots in World War II; addicts (Abi-Dargham 2004).
3. Explanatory pressure:
   - e.g., hallucination, ego disturbances

   Reward aspect of the delusional thought: simple solution (explanation, relief, higher self esteem), turning away from counter-evidence: selectivity of attention; lack of correction pressure.

4. Capgras delusion—model: correct perception, but disturbed amygdala processing leads to an unusual emotional activation that does not match the percept. The person therefore assumes that there must be something wrong with the percept.

Delusional Perception
Definition Misinterpretation of a correct perception in the sense of a delusion.

Examples

- In delusional mobbing, an employee interprets a public statement by the superior as a sign that he will now be dismissed.
- A man sees his mother, who has passed away and whom he believes was kidnapped, in an unknown woman (not otherwise explainable—he has no prosopagnosia or other perceptual disorder, etc.).
- A wave of one's hand from a person at the bus stop is interpreted by the patient as the signal to his enemies that his enemies will now strike. ◀

Position in Psychopathology AMDP 34.

Related terms. Delusional memory, where a memory is misinterpreted in the sense of the delusion.

Psychopathological Interactions anxiety.

Differential Diagnostic Distinctions Explanatory delusion of a hallucination.

Further Characterization A) Existing delusion and reinterpretation of correct percepts; inclusion of a current perception into the existing delusion. The person realizes that their perception can be explained by the delusion. b) As a sudden new idea that this new (delusional) thought explains the observation of uncanny change, it is described as one of the developmental steps of delusional development in schizophrenia (see below delusional idea).

Interview for Rating Question about strange perceptions, follow-up on unusual evaluations.

Pathognomonic for Schizophrenia.

Personality Influences Sensitive personality.

Conceptual Problems of the Feature In the delusion formation in schizophrenia: From the delusional mood, a person interprets a perception delusionally.

Transition from dysfunctional cognition in the perception of social interaction—"they don't like me" etc.

Delusional idea
Definition A person suddenly has a delusional idea during the florid delusion development.

Example—A patient interrupts the admission interview and says: "You are in cahoots with them!"

Often from a delusional mood, in which no delusional idea has yet clearly crystallized. Possibly feeling emotional relief that the person finally "understands."

Position in Psychopathology AMDP 35.

Delusional dynamic
Definition degree of emotional activation by the delusional thought in a conversation.

Example

A patient, with whom an orderly interview was possible, develops intense emotional agitation when the delusional topic is touched upon, the thinking becomes disorganized – "delusion induced disorganized thinking" with incoherence when talking about the delusion. ◀

Severity From lack of affective involvement (e.g., old delusional thoughts) to strong emotional turmoil, e.g., anxiety or despair.

Position in Psychopathology AMDP 38.

> **Systematization of Delusion**
> **Definition**: Degree of argumentative relations supporting the delusional construct that a person has considered and presents.

How strongly a delusional argumentation has already been built; in conversation upon follow-up questions or under pressure to correct. Generally interpreted as a product of the effort to rationalize the delusion. The person strives to make the argumentation seamless in discussions with others. He has clarified everything for himself, everything is clear to him.

Position in Psychopathology AMDP 37.

> **Overvalued Idea**
> **Definition** A belief that is false (and incompatible with the beliefs in the culture of the environment) affects a person's emotions or is evident in behavior; however, unlike a delusion, the person can consider doubts about the idea and can admit that the situation might be different.

Examples

- A person is convinced that the neighbors have something against him and approaches them overly cautiously, suspiciously. This additionally prevents the development of a good-neighborly relationship.
- A patient washes compulsively. When asked about the reasons, it becomes clear that he has anxiety that an infection could destroy him and his family, even though the family lives far away and only has contact with him via telephone.
- A person is unsure whether the railings of a bridge would hold if he has to hold on to them. This thought occurs together with phobic anxiety about crossing a bridge. This belief persists even though it has been demonstrated to him several times that these railings are safe. ◄

Position in Psychopathology Included as an additional item in the AMDP.

Interview for Rating Questions as with delusional thoughts. Check whether a challenging thought or temporary correction in the argumentation about the thought is possible (see above).

Severity To what extent are everyday experiences and behaviors influenced by the irrational assumption.

Specification:

- irrational beliefs—coupled with emotion
- ideas of reference.

A person thinks that certain events refer to him, where it is not just a one-time accidental misjudgment of a situation, but these thoughts occur frequently.

Personality influences Paranoid, sensitive personality.

Conceptual problems of the feature Transition from dysfunctional cognition in the perception of social interaction—"they don't like me" etc.—to overvalued idea and delusion.

Neuroscientific/cognitive-neuroscientific models (see above).

> **Delusional misidentification**
> **Definition**
> 1. Belief of being in another place—misidentification of a place, an object.
> 2. In person-related delusional misidentification, the patient believes that a person he sees is actually another person who is only disguised and moves like the person known to the patient. The delusional ideas specifically concern the identification of persons.

Examples

- A dementia patient is convinced that his own house is not the old house, but another one, or that he is at home when he has just been admitted to a clinic.
- belief that a family member is another person. ◀

Position in psychopathology Not in AMDP.

Related terms. Person-related misidentification symptoms are also referred to as Capgras syndrome (see above) or Fregoli syndrome: e.g., a person appears as several other people.

Psychopathological interactions Perception, judgment, memory disorders, hallucinations, metamorphopsias, phonemes, intense affective involvement (anxiety, infatuation).

Differential diagnostic distinctions Many of the delusional misidentifications of persons have so far been classified as illusion, but the typical feature of misidentification is a perception of change in persons and delusional interpretation—not a delusional misrecognition, for example, as a devil, etc.

Further characterization More common with sensory restriction (see hallucination with sensory restriction), possibly as explanatory delusion.

Interview for rating Ask about peculiarities in the perception of persons, have the current location explained.

Severity Fleeting, delusional misidentifications versus persistence, high behavioral relevance of misidentification.

Specifications:

a) Person-related—also occurring in schizophrenia,
   - a person known to the individual is replaced by an actor : Capgras syndrome,
   - related to the Fregoli syndrome

b) Place-related—mostly occurring in dementias,
   - reduplicative paramnesia: objects and entire environments are falsely recognized
   - self/other: self-duplication, heautoscopy;

Conceptual Problems of the Feature Misidentifications form a characteristic symptom group, usually in degenerative brain diseases, which exhibit pathophysiological peculiarities.

Neuroscientific/Cognitive Neuroscientific Models

a) Person-related misidentification symptoms are partly attributed to a disturbance in the various parallel perception pathways, leading to inconsistencies. The "incongruity," the error in identification, can be, for example, an altered emotional reaction of the perceived person, which causes the person to perceive something different than usual and interpret it as a change in the person.
b) Location-related misidentification is attributed to a disturbance in hippocampus functions. The current location is confused with the experience of another location. The location map is incorrectly created, so that, for example, in the hospital, a patient searches for people who are at his home. In both forms, a primary recognition dysfunction is assumed, and the person considers their perception as proof of the truth of the assumption.

References

Abi-Dargham A (2004) Do we still believe in the dopamine hypothesis? New data bring new evidence. Int J Neuropsychopharmacol 7(Suppl 1):1–5

Blackwood NJ, Howard RJ, Bentall RP, Murray RM (2001) Cognitive neuropsychiatric models of persecutory delusion. Am J Psychiatry 158:527–539

Blackwood NJ, Bentall RP, Ffytche DH et al (2004) Persecutory delusions and the determination of self-relevance: an fMRI investigation. Psychol Med 34:591–596

Bentall (1989) Content specific processing and persecutory delusions: an investigation using the emotional Stroop test. Br J Psychiatry 62:355–364
Berridge KC, Robinson TE (1998) What is the role of dopamine in reward: hedonic impact, reward learning, or incentive salience? Brain Res Rev 28:309–369
Bersani G, Clemente R, Gherardelli S, Pancheri P (2004) Deficit of executive functions in schizophrenia: relationship to neurological soft signs and psychopathology. Psychopathology 37:118–123
de Bonis M, Epelbaum C, Feline A (1992) Cognitive processing of contradictory statements: an experimental study of reasoning on proverbs in schizophrenia. Psychopathology 25:100–108
de Bonis M, Epelbaum C, Deffez V, Feline A (1997) The comprehension of metaphors in schizophrenia. Psychopathology 30:149–154
Clark A (2013) Whatever next? Predictive brains, situated agents, and the future of cognitive science. Behav Brain Sci 36:181–204
Conrad D (1958) Die beginnende Schizophrenie. Thieme, Stuttgart
Ellis HD, Young AW (1990) Accounting for delusional misidentifications. Br J Psychiatry 157:239–248
Ellis HD, Young AW, Quayle AH, De Pauw KW (1997) Reduced autonomic responses to faces in Capgras delusion. Proc R Soc Lond B Biol Sci 264:1085–1092
Escher S, Romme M, Buiks A (2002) Formation of delusional ideation in adolescents hearing voices: a prospective study. Am J Med Genet 114:913–920
Falret J, Berrios G (1996) Delusions. In: Berrios G (Ed) The history of mental symptoms. Cambridge Univ Press, Cambridge, pp 85–139
Förstl H (2007) Theory of mind. Springer, Berlin Heidelberg
Frith CD, Frith U (1999) Interacting minds—a biological basis. Science 286:1692–1695
Fukuhara R, Ikeda M, Nebu A et al (2001) Alteration of rCBF in Alzheimer's disease patients with delusions of theft. NeuroReport 12:2473–2476
Garety PA, Hemsley DR (1994) Delusions: Investigations into the psychology of delusional reasoning. Oxford Univ Press, Oxford
Gilleen J, David AS (2005) The cognitive neuropsychiatry of delusions: from psychopathology to neuropsychology and back again. Psychol Med 35:5–12
Green MJ, Phillips ML (2004) Social threat perception and the evolution of paranoia. Neurosci Biobehav Rev 28:333–342
Griesinger W (1845) Die Pathologie und Therapie der psychischen Krankheiten. Krabbe, Stuttgart
Haddock G, Wolfenden M, Lowens I et al (1995) Effect of emotional salience on thought disorder in patients with schizophrenia. Br J Psychiatry 167:618–620
Hurn C, Gray NS, Hughes I (2002) Independence of „reaction to hypothetical contradiction“ from other measures of delusional ideation. Br J Clin Psychol 41:349–360
Jaspers K (1942) Allgemeine Psychopathologie, 4. edn. Springer, Berlin
Jeste DV, Wragg RE, Salmon DP (1992) Cognitive deficits of patients with Alzheimer's disease with and without delusions. Am J Psychiatry 149:184–189
Kendler KS, Glazer WM, Morgenstern H (1983) Dimensions of delusional experience. Am J Psychiatry 140:466–469
Kimhy D, Goetz R, Yale S et al (2005) Delusions in individuals with schizophrenia: factor structure, clinical correlates, and putative neurobiology. Psychopathology 38:338–344
Maher BA (1988) Anomalous experience and delusional thinking. In: Oltmanns EF, Maher BA (Eds) Delusional beliefs. Wiley, New York, pp 15–33
Montague RP, Hyman SE, Cohen JD (2005) Computational roles for dopamine in behavioural control. Nature 431:760–777
van Os J, Hanssen M, Bijl RV, Vollebergh W (2001) Prevalence of psychotic disorder and community level of psychotic symptoms: an urban-rural comparison. Arch Gen Psychiatry 58:663–668
Pankow A, Knobel A, Voss M, Heinz A (2012) Neurobiological correlates of delusion: beyond the salience attribution hypothesis. Neuropsychobiol 66:33–43
Phillips ML, Senior C, David AS (2000) Abnormal processing of ambiguity in paranoid schizophrenia: a visual scan path study. Psychol Med 30:157–167
Pickering MJ, Garrod S (2004) Toward a mechanistic psychology of dialogue. Behav Brain Sci 27:169–190
Rabins NL, Lucas MJ (1982) The impact of dementia on the family. J Am Med Assoc 248:333–335
Ramachandran VS, Blakeslee S (1998) Phantoms in the brain: human nature and the architecture of the mind. Fourth Estate, London
Ritunnano R, Kleinman J, Whyte Oshodi D, Michail M, Nelson B, Humpston CS, Broome MR (2022) Subjective experience and meaning of delusions in psychosis: a systematic review and qualitative evidence synthesis. Lancet Psychiatry 9:458–476
Saß H (1993) Affektdelikte. Springer, Berlin Heidelberg New York Tokio
Scharfetter C (2002) Allgemeine Psychopathologie. Thieme, Stuttgart
Schneider K (1992) Klinische Psychopathologie, 14. edn. Thieme, Stuttgart
Schnider A (2003) Spontaneous confabulation and the adaptation of thought to ongoing reality. Nat Rev Neurosci 4:662–671
Schreber DP (1903) Denkwürdigkeiten eines Nervenkranken. Neuausgabe Kulturverlag Kadmos, Berlin; Schreber, Daniel Paul (1903). Memoirs of My Nervous Illness. New York: New York Review of Books
Shanks MF, Venneri A (2004) Thinking through delusions in Alzheimer's disease. Br J Psychiatry 184:193–194
Spitzer M (1990) On defining delusions. Compr Psychiatry 31:377–397

Spitzer M (1995) A neurocomputational approach to delusions. Compr Psychiatry 36:83–105
Sterzer P (2022) Die Illusion der Vernunft. Ullstein, Berlin
Sutherland S (1992) Irrationality: The enemy within. Constable, London
Watzlawick P (1981) Die erfundene Wirklichkeit. Piper, München
Weilnhammer V, Röd L, Eckert AL, Stuke H, Heinz A, Sterzer P (2020) Psychotic Experiences in Schizophrenia and Sensitivity to Sensory Evidence. Schizophr Bull 46:927–936
Zarow C, Lyness SA, Mortimer JA, Chui HC (2003) Neuronal loss is greater in the locus coeruleus than nucleus basalis and substantia nigra in Alzheimer and Parkinson diseases. Arch Neurol 60:337–341

15 Judgment Ability

Contents

15.1 Introduction

In addition to the characteristics of psychiatric disorders, the ability to judge must be considered in the psychopathological examination, if only because of its importance for consent to examination and treatment.

Impairment of judgment is a common consequence of various psychiatric syndromes, i.e., a number of psychopathological dimensions affect a person's insight, (1) the ability to assess a situation—for example, the group of formal and content-related thought disorders, affective exceptional states, attention and working memory disorders, consciousness disturbances, etc. Furthermore, there are psychiatric effects (2) on the ability to express the decision appropriately.

How can the ability to judge be defined for practical clinical diagnostics? For what is the ability to judge to be considered in clinical everyday life?

A) On a pragmatic level, the ability to judge concerns the ability to make appropriate decisions and express them, with appropriateness being considered regarding the situation and the involved person. In clinical everyday life, the ability to consent and the capacity to contract must be assessed.

B) On a neuropsychological level, one asks about the individual abilities that can be disturbed: the ability to judge is a complex function composed of many different components. In this presentation of psychopathology, the basis of insight and control processes was described in the preceding chapters.

Insight

1. Understanding complex situations,
2. activation of all relevant knowledge elements, subjective attitudes, and memories,
3. Processing the situation in terms of relevant objective and subjective aspects,

F. M. Reischies, *Psychopathology*, https://doi.org/10.1007/978-3-662-70293-2_15

Control Ability

4. Elaboration of decision alternatives,
5. Keeping the arguments for the alternatives available,
6. Decision behavior that is appropriate (decision algorithm),
7. Act of decision and
8. Communication or implementation.

A valid treatment contract requires the ability to consent of the patient; strictly speaking, this requirement even applies to consent to the psychopathological examination of insight and control ability itself. The complexity becomes clear with consent to medical treatment, which may carry the risk of undesirable side effects:

Understanding the situation requires (1) language comprehension and (2) sufficient intelligence. It is often required for the assessment of insight that the person can provide an appropriate verbal description of the situation. In the discussion about decision options, it should become clear that the person has understood the problem. Certainly, there are people who cannot verbally express everything they have understood by far (e.g. aphasia).

In addition, there should be the principle availability (or current activatability) firstly of all decision-relevant objective aspects of the situation, and secondly of personal attitudes and decision reasons. The person should be able to recall memories of comparable decision situations. The correct representation of the situation usually also indicates the availability of decision reasons.

For the mental processing of the problem, sufficient premorbid intelligence is necessary; this concerns a prediction of whether the person could have understood the situation at best. Premorbid intelligence can be considered a competence—this competence can be limited or even nullified on the performance side due to psychopathological disorder. A reduction in the current performance of intellectual ability can exclude the ability to judge for certain problems.

Generation and Evaluation of Decision Alternatives:
The development of decision options can be derived on the one hand from the memory of options in comparable decisions from the past and from the experience of decisions made by other people. Specific options are developed from the logical analysis of the situation in the concrete situation.

Availability of thought content regarding options

(1) The current free availability of all possible "ideas," i.e., mental entries that are potentially available to the person and decision-relevant, is impaired in many psychopathological syndromes, for example in delusion.
    For adequate decision capability, the logical development of the tableau of decision options is necessary, as well as the current options space. Fodor (1983) demanded for thinking the availability of all CNS functions that can contribute to the respective topic. Thus, every act of thinking and decision-making becomes an irreducible act of complex utilization of all theoretically available CNS entries on a topic—world knowledge and self-knowledge of the person.
    The verbal description of decision options in the psychopathological interview provides (as mentioned above, the presentation and discussion of the matter) a certain indication of the extent to which the person has solution options available. However, this only applies to linguistically representable options and reasons.
    In principle, however, it cannot be ensured in the examination whether a person cannot evaluate a group of options because they are, for example, obstructed by anxiety, defense or delusional thoughts.
(2) Retaining availability of options: When the execution of the decision is pending, some of the options must not already be forgotten, as is the case with patients with dementia. Retaining alternatives and the arguments

developed for them in memory is necessary for the choice. Episodic memory is necessary for recalling comparable situations that the self has experienced (or knows from stories).

Decision criteria, or decision algorithms

Adequate decision algorithms must be available. This means,

1. that the person decides, for example, based on risk, chances, emotional preference, or personal experience, which is related to the "statistics" of experienced consequences in comparable situations ("gut feeling decision").
2. An adequacy of the decision algorithm is not given for many people in everyday life. If a person decides on consent to psychotherapy or medication purely emotionally based on their possibly negative prior experiences, although an overweight of arguments would enable the person to make a different decision based on a rational decision algorithm, then they are not judging according to appropriate criteria.
3. Psychiatric symptoms such as impulsivity, anxiety, etc., impair rational decision-making.

(3) Execution of a decision

In everyday life, the anxious delay of decision-making repeatedly plays a significant role. Patients with thought disorders can be completely incapable of making decisions.

The act of decision-making is a performance of executive functions, which—like any conscious motor action—also controls the complex mental decision. Decision criteria are practiced in upbringing and education, depending on the type, e.g., of family decision-making models and the quality of education.

(4) Expressing the decision

The decision is first mentally available to the person and must be expressed to the environment or shown through actions. Communication may fail due to severe communication disorders.

From the listing of components of the complex process, it becomes clear that various psychopathological mechanisms presented in the previous chapters play a role in the limitation of judgment ability.

Intervening variables:
General or specific judgment ability

Using an example like that of a blind fashion critic, we must point out peculiarities: A limited impairment of judgment ability can consist in the specific area of the matter to be judged being disturbed: The visual impairment does not affect the judgment ability, but only everything related to visual perception.

However, the example also makes it clear how judgment ability can be specifically impaired in psychiatric illnesses: Above all, a delusional topic can affect a group of judgments. If a person with delusional poisoning fear rejects an intravenous injection of a medication in the therapy situation, this is usually due to the delusion. It is a judgment incapability that usually encompasses more than just the fear of poisoning, but also the insight into the illness, etc.

It does not help in jurisprudence to formulate a natural will that is immune to delusion—and immune to psychiatric or neurological illnesses. This natural will would have to be regarded as lying outside the natural insight and control ability.

Low intelligence

Although 50% of the population, by definition, have an intelligence quotient (IQ) of below 100, only a few percent have a pathologically low intelligence, which, according to common intelligence tests (such as the HAWIE-R), lies below two standard deviations under the norm, i.e., below an IQ of 70 (one standard deviation in IQ corresponds to 15 points). This degree of impairment is referred to as mild intellectual disability. Patients with an IQ of below 4 standard deviations under the norm are very rare. They have a developmental age of approximately 6 to under 9 years, i.e., they achieve only a maturity comparable, e.g., to that of a 6-year-old child.

The severity classification of low intelligence is shown in Table 15.1.

Table 15.1 Intellectual Disability: Quantitative Gradation (ICD)

IQ	Standard Deviation	Definition Limits	Designations	Max. Achievable Developmental Age	Frequency %
100+	0				
85	−1	85–90			
70	−2	50–69	Mild intellectual disability	9 to < 12 years	2
55	−3				
40	−4	35–49	Moderate intellectual disability	6 to < 9 years	0.4
25	−5	20–34	Severe	3 to >6 years	
10	−6	<20	Profound (»Idiocy«)	<3 years	0.04

15.2 Impairment of Judgment

Studies on the capacity to consent of patients who come in for psychiatric examination and treatment, whether voluntarily or as compulsory treatment, show significant variance (Curley et al. 2022).

There are various areas of disorders that can impair judgment; they are presented below:

1. attention, directed to the problem area or the problem, is reduced:
   - quantitatively,
   - qualitatively,

   e.g., self-attention, paying attention to illnesses, etc., attention to family with sorrows, etc. Here, educational and developmental phenomena as well as e.g., denial have an effect.
2. Availability of information:
   - Forgetting the past phase of illness, partly in schizophrenic patients,
   - Forgetting decision alternatives,
   - Lack of psychoeducational measures, lack of information about the disorder.
3. Cognitive engagement with the problem and the development of a concept:
   - Thought disorders cause the inability to engage rationally with the problem situation,
   - Refusal, defense mechanisms, denial, etc.
4. Capacity for cognitive processing of the situation or one's own symptoms—a person may, for example, only be able to deal with concrete aspects of the situation (see Table 15.1).

The efficiency of thought processes can be directed by mental operations and attention. Through suggestion, mental processing steps can apparently be overridden (Raz et al. 2006).

15.3 Diagnosis of Judgment Ability

Judgment ability is a quality of information processing to be assessed by the initial examiner—concerning insight and control ability. Do patients understand what they are consenting to, or are they incapable of consenting?

- Important for the assessment of judgment ability is recognizing a reduction in premorbid intelligence or mental retardation, for example, due to early childhood brain damage or genetic burden.
- Furthermore, a content-related thought disorder, especially a delusion that affects judgment ability in certain areas, must be recognized. If a delusion exists, judgment ability is generally impaired, as not all areas of knowledge can be freely accessed in the

judgment process (Fodor 1983). It is possible that in the area not affected by the delusional topic, "appropriate" judgments may be found—however, this has not been investigated. Additionally, if, for example, a delusion is florid and emotionally disturbing, affective-cognitive complexes determine the person's thinking.

15.3.1 Examination Procedures

Logical Tasks of Intelligence Tests
In many examination proposals, finding similarities (e.g. between banana and apple) or finding differences (e.g. between stairs and ladder) is asked. (see HAWIE intelligence test, finding similarities, Tewes 1994). However, good intelligence performance, see above, is not a proof of unimpaired judgment ability.

Explaining Proverbs
Explaining proverbs is useful for examining comprehension ability, abstraction ability, and linguistic expression ability (see chapter thinking). Several dimensions can be assessed independently:

1. Explanation of the proverb is correct—incorrect,
2. complete—incomplete (partial),
3. proverb was not explained but the person made descriptive concrete statements about the proverb (see concretism),
4. metaphorical level (of the explanation of the proverb) reached—not reached.

Interview
In the interview, the manner of deciding of the patient should be considered—for example, inquiring about a recently made decision, how the person arrived at the decision (e.g., purchase, vacation, etc.). What was the decision requirement, what kind of information was needed. In discussing the recently made decision, an attempt is made to clarify to what extent the person considered the decision alternatives and what the decision criteria were in that case—how much effort the person put into the decision (or did they decide "from the gut" or thoughtlessly, impulsively).

As mentioned above, the person must be asked to describe the matter to be decided and the decision options.

15.4 Psychopathological Symptoms of Judgment Ability

Judgment Disorder
Definition. Disorder of judgment and voluntary, conscious decision-making in complex matters.

Example

A patient can no longer assess his financial situation, i.e., overlook the consequences of expenditures and the development of income, although he was previously able to do so. ◀

Position in Psychopathology. Not in AMDP; central for dementia and schizophrenic as well as affective psychoses.

Psychopathological Interactions. A judgment disorder that did not manifest in the development and is possibly caused genetically or by early childhood brain damage is usually due to psychiatric disease factors or newly occurring neurological disease. Disorders of consciousness, attention, language comprehension, formal or content-related thinking, affectivity, or action organization may be present.

Differential Diagnostic Distinctions
1. acquired intelligence disorder, comprehension disorder, agnostic, aphasic disorders, working memory, executive disorder,
2. non-rational decision:
   - decision style: "decide from the gut"
   - impulsive decision.

Further Characterization.
It must be a conscious decision. Insight disorder due to impaired semantic processing (in relation to world knowledge and self-knowledge) and disorder of mental transformations (see intelligence tests), or disorder of control, availability, and maintenance of decision alternatives regarding the execution of the decision.

Self-/other persons's judgment. Usually little insight into a judgment disorder.

Interview for Rating. Ask the person being examined to explain the facts and decision options.

Neuropsychology/objectification. In addition to the above-mentioned presentation of the facts and options—in the interview using an example of a recent decision explain the decision requirement , describe assessment and decision criteria.

Severity. Mild: Not all insight-relevant content and decision-relevant options fully available—with fundamentally uncertain judgment ability—severe: globally neither capable of insight into the decision facts nor capable of control for rational decision regarding all possible options.

Specifications
- Partial—regarding specific areas of facts that are not accessible to rational decision due to delusion, etc.
- capacity to consent—also partial, in impaired insight in one'sillness,
- Specifically incapacity to contract

Personality Influences. Hysterical mode of decisions, where decisions are made more emotionally and less rationally . Impulsivity as a personality trait.

Conceptual Problems of the Feature. Complex feature that gains special significance through the legal framework in clinical everyday life (especially capacity to consent).

Difficulty in grading severity. Possibly, the requirement to be able to access all possible content is unrealistic?

Neuroscientific/Cognitive Neuroscientific Models
Complex task that can be disrupted neuropsychologically at various points—from the semantic processing of the facts with availability of all thought content to the execution of an appropriate decision algorithm.

Acquired Intelligence Disorder
Definition. The intelligence level is reduced as a result of an illness. Specifically: the ability to solve problems, perform mental transformations that were previously successful, is no longer possible.

Example

A patient who had successfully performed a highly complex profession as an engineer is no longer able to perform simple calculations, makes mistakes in simple logical intelligence tasks. ◀

Further Characterization: In the case of reduced intelligence, automatic and effortful mental transformations are generally impaired (but no specific disorder of modules such as the language or perception module—according to Fodor 1983). The spectrum of intelligence tasks must be examined.
The feature is not defined in the AMDP system.

Differential Diagnostic Considerations: A depressive pseudodementia must be excluded. This refers to the depressive patient's giving up on demanding thinking tasks. Furthermore, Ganser's syndrome must be distinguished, a "hysterical" pseudodementia with gross misjudgments.

Psychopathological Interactions:

- Reduction of performance in intelligence tests (without a decrease in competence).
- Interaction by further psychopathological impairments. There may be doubts that neuropsychological foundations of intellectual functions are not disturbed (such as agnostic, aphasic, apraxic, amnestic, working memory, or executive disorders) which lead to reduced performance in intelligence tests.

Neuropsychology, objectification: For the diagnosis of the reduction of intelligence, the estimation of premorbid intelligence is necessary.

Premorbid intelligence

- non-verbal intelligence tests, e.g., non-verbal part of the HAWIE-R (Tewes 1994), LPS3 (Horn 1983),
- estimation based on school education, number of completed school classes, exams, type of school, grade level
- New word reading tests; MWT-B (Lehrl 1995), word-nonword distinction,
- Lector test (Reischies et al. 2005), reading of foreign words with different pronunciation possibilities.

Specification: global reduction of intelligence—partial reduction limited to certain dimensions of intelligence

Disorders in disease perception and change assessment

Diagnostically, there are 3 levels:

1. Does the person perceive, experiences what the examiner considers a symptom, i.e., does he perceive changes in the mental processes or the body?
   - this is often not the case, especially in behavioral disorders, e.g., in aggressive behavior.
2. Does the person suffer from the perceived changes that are considered a symptom?
3. Does the explanatory concept of the perceived features, which are considered a symptom, agree with the medical-psychopathological judgment?

Anosognosia
Definition: Changes in the body and psyche, which are diagnosed by examiners as psychopathological symptoms, cannot be perceived by the person, and he cannot form a concept of the illness.

Examples

- anosognosiais particularly striking in neurology, where it was defined—for example: in hemiparesis, the patient says the hand is not paralyzed. The perception regarding the disorder is disturbed.
- Anton syndrome: There is cortical blindness, the patients experience hallucinations and claim to be able to see (often with double bookkeeping—patients let themselves be helped when walking).
- In psychopathology, anosognosia is already included in the definition of symptoms of hallucinations and delusions. ◀

Further characterization: For many, if not most, of the psychopathological features, lack of insight can occur. This represents one of the main problems of psychopathological diagnostics (and thus psychiatric therapy).

Differential diagnostic distinctions: denial, i.e., a concept of illness is achieved but defended against—in certain cases, difficult to distinguish.

Neuroscientific/cognitive neuroscientific models
Anosognosia can be explained, among other things, by the absence of mental meta-representation levels. The functionality or disturbance of self-functions cannot thus be represented in its

own mental representation—(this refers to the critical areas of mental functions for which a diagnosis is made).

Lack of feeling ill
Definition. Reduced or absent feeling of illness—the person does not suffer from the psychological symptoms that are diagnosed (and which usually lead to impairment).

Examples

- A patient with mania does not feel ill. As a patient with bipolar affective psychosis, he knows everything about his illness, which he also accepts. But currently, his condition subjectively does not meet the criteria for mania; he is in a good mood and full of drive for legitimate reasons.
- A patient with schizophrenic psychosis shows a lack of distress, although the disorder endangers the person's life or civil existence. ◀

Position in psychopathology. AMDP 97.

Related terms. anosodiaphoria.

Psychopathological interactions.
- lack of perception, experience of the disorder
- trivialization in dementia

Differential diagnostic distinctions.
- denial e.g., in shame.

Interview for rating. Question about the extent of suffering from changes in body and mind.

Neuropsychology/objectification. Other persons' judgment and behavioral observation, whether distress is recognizable.

Specifications:
- the person does not suffer from the disorder or what is diagnosed as a disorder, for example, in hallucinations with pleasant content (often e.g., also in tardive dyskinesia)

Conceptual problems of the feature:
- cultural influences, e.g., families in which every illness is denied.
- The feature of feeling ill is listed here, because it is necessary for differentiation regarding the uncooperativeness towards one's illness.

Neuroscientific/cognitive neuroscientific models
1. In positive emotions or positive content of a delusion (or hallucinations), there is no distress for the person,
2. Delusional distortion of the causes of the disorder with distorted action readiness (enemies, etc.),
3. additionally, a lack of a meta-level that could monitor the disorder of information processing.

Impaired insight in one's illness
Definition. A person cannot perceive or accept the illness dimension of his suffering, his concept of illness deviates from the medical concept of illness—despite sufficient explanation.

Examples

Despite psychoeducational measures, a patient with a delusion cannot see that the experience and behavior that led to the admission to the clinic is a psychiatric illness.

- A person with depressive symptoms due to conflicting development and dysfunctional cognitions does not see that a psychiatric disorder is present but believes that the suffering is part of his life.
- A patient with severe depression and delusion of poverty believes he is not ill but have severe, self-inflicted financial problems.
- A person impaired by compulsive actions does not see it as an illness but believes that rational arguments support the repetition of the compulsive acts.

- A patient with somatization disorder has a false concept of illness: He believes he is suffering from the seemingly present somatic syndrome and exclusively demands an internist. ◀

Position in psychopathology. AMDP 98, symptom intransigence.

Psychopathological Interactions. Delusion, Hallucination, hypochondria, somatization disorder, intellectual disability.

Differential Diagnostic Distinctions.
- simplifying but educationally useful concept of illness (as applied in behavioral therapy).

Further Characterization. False concept of illness caused by various factors—also due to social pressure, conformity pressure.

Interview for Rating. Question about the concept of suffering of the affected person self. Assess spontaneously expressed disease model.

Neuropsychology/objectification. Observe the engagement with the medical concept of illness—affective signs of a non-rational attitude.

Severity. Minor doubts about the diagnosis up to severe behavioral effects of uncooperativeness towards one's illness.

Specifications
- symptom intransigence,
- anosognosia accompanying
- optional: in case of depressive mood,
- uncooperativeness towards one's illness related to classification units of mental disorders.

Consequences:

- diagnostic compliance disturbed? A patient does not allow diagnostic examinations,
- uncooperativeness (AMDP 99), therapeutic compliance disturbed or abolished.
  Personality influences. Antisocial, narcissistic, paranoid, querulous, etc.

Conceptual Problems of the Feature:

- antipsychiatric attitudes in the zeitgeist promote uncooperativeness towards one's illness.

Neuroscientific/Cognitive Neuroscientific Models
1. Due to a lack of meta-levels that could realize a perception of the disorder, or a lack of intellectual valences, or rejection of engagement with the problem; the discrepancy with the medical diagnosis is not perceptible and therefore not further processed.
2. Incompatibility of the concept of illness with the understanding of one's own person—resulting denial—clarify:—What does the diagnosis mean for the person; is the diagnosis compatible with the person's fundamental attitudes?
   - What gain could the patient achieve with the denial of the disorder?

References

Curley A, Watson C, Kelly BD (2022) Capacity to consent to treatment in psychiatry inpatients—a systematic review. Int J Psychiatr Clin Pract 26:303–315

Fodor JA (1983) The modularity of mind. MIT Press, Cambridge

Lehrl S (1995) Mehrfachwahl-Wortschatz-Intelligentest (MWT-B), 3. edn. Hogrefe, Göttingen

Horn W (1983) Leistungsprüfsystem L-P-S, 2. edn. Hogrefe, Göttingen

Raz A, Kirsch I, Pollard J, Nitkin-Kaner Y (2006) Suggestion reduces the stroop effect. Psychol Sci 17:91–95

Reischies FM, Wertenauer F, Kühl K-P (2005) Lector—ein Untersuchungsverfahren zur Bestimmung des verbalen Bildungsniveaus. Nervenarzt 76:849–850

Tewes U (Ed) (1994) HAWIE-R. Hamburg-Wechsler Intelligenztest für Erwachsene—Revision 1991. Huber, Bern

16 Outlook

In this book, the psychopathological symptoms are described and placed in a neuroscientific context. The aim is to explicate the scientific background of the symptoms.

1. Neuroscientific Explanation
   A neuroscientific explanation of all individual symptoms is still pending—in many cases, there is still no generally accepted neuroscientific model of the symptoms—further research is needed.
   Many aspects of the neuroscience of psychopathology are still hypothetical or merely model assumptions that need further verification.
   Psychopathology has an evolutionary anthropological dimension, which has received less attention in connection with the specific symptoms to this day. For we know far too little about the psychological structures that could have formed in phylogenetic development and also have a specific individual impact on mental disorders today (Reischies 2021). Far too little is still known about the development of syndromes, the syndrome dynamics, as discussed, for example, for the panic syndrome.
2. What is a Psychopathological Symptom
   In psychopathology, attempts are made to define the smallest descriptive units of psychic dysfunction in disorders and diseases. Errors can occur in both directions: There are relevant subgroups that make a division of the symptom-features necessary, or conversely, a group of features has a common neuroscientific-psychological basis and differs only marginally, e.g., only in severity of the dysfunction.
   The main focus of classical psychopathology is on the symptoms of more severe mental illnesses, traditionally even on psychoses. Today, many more people are treated psychiatrically than at the time of the development of psychopathology, both through psychotherapy and psychopharmacotherapy. This results in a problem of the severity range that is the focus of psychopathological investigations.
3. Mental Illness
   If it is already difficult to define mental, psychic illness (Heinz 2014), then a new, even more difficult problem arises: The delineation of an intermediate suffering—that is, the definition of (1) mentally healthy, (2) intermediate mental disorder, and (3) mental illness (Helmchen et al. 2000).
   If the simple WHO demand for complete mental and physical well-being is accepted as a definition of mental health, and the problematic definition of mental illness for severe disorders, then the question remains, how can the intermediate mental disorder be defined? Is it sufficient to speak, on the one hand, of deviating from complete mental well-being

F. M. Reischies, *Psychopathology*, https://doi.org/10.1007/978-3-662-70293-2_16

and, on the other hand, of not fulfilling the definition of "mentally ill"? It seems that this conception corresponds to today's societal practice. Rarely do recognized scales or tests exist that allow for the identification of a normal range, a gray area, and a clearly pathological area (see Mild Cognitive Impairment, Reischies 1999).

Apart from definitional obstacles, there is the unresolved question of whether intermediate mental disorders are characterized by milder manifestations of symptom-features—compared to a severe psychiatric illness—or whether they are incomplete syndromes, etc. Can one assume suffering from a symptom in the intermediate range of mental disorders?

4. Many Symptoms and Terms Not Explained:
In the diagnostic criteria according to ICD and DSM, many more psychopathological features and symptoms are mentioned than are presented in this book—mostly features that are not addressed in classical psychopathology. Among them are characteristics of personality disorders. The following are some features that belong to this group:
Terms from various areas, predominantly the area of personality disorders, that were not presented:
   - Disturbed contact behavior, disturbed eye contact, physical distance,
   - emotionally cold, relationship disorder, rational detachment; intentional disorder; social withdrawal,
   - submissive, solitary, autistic features, lack of empathy, shy, seductively interacting,
   - manipulative, exploitative
   - insecure, socially retarded, avoidant, overly cautious, introverted
     conscientious, scrupulous, perfectionistic, pedantic
   - selfish, reckless, cynically, bitter, irresponsible, approving the suffering of others, egocentric, profile- neurotic, self-dramatizing
   - sensitive, irritable, easily offended, irritable weakness,
   - mild cognitive impairment
   - performance-oriented, avoiding effort, tendency to forget tasks
     arrogant, blaming others, competitive, jealous, power fantasies, awareness of rank, tactical handling of the truth
5. Psychopathological Levels
Initially, it is not even clear how those mental functions arise that are undoubtedly present in adult humans, such as consciousness. This is being intensively investigated. A self also exists as a psychological entity. However, too little is known about this. The place neurons and grid neurons provide the living being with a signal for localisation in space at all times, like in a modern navigation system ("I am here", in relation to the other locations on the map). Certainly, the self further develops in constant interaction with its socio-cultural interactions. Related terms include identity and the concept of the person, each with different emphases, about which little is also known. The self is then again a starting point for the development of diverse psychopathological experiences.
It is certain that many of these and other questions of psychopathology need to be examined more closely in order to determine further disease- and health-promoting factors and ultimately to improve the diagnosis and therapy of psychological symptoms.

References

Heinz A (2014) Der Begriff der psychischen Krankheit. Suhrkamp Verlag, Frankfurt

Helmchen H, Linden M (2000) Subthreshold disorders in psychiatry: Clinical reality, methodological artifact and the double-threshold problem. Compr Psychiatry 41:1–7

Reischies FM (1999) Leichte kognitive Störungen. In: Helmchen H, Henn F, Lauter H, Sartorius N (Eds) Psychiatrie der Gegenwart, 4. edn. Springer, Berlin, pp 225–246

Reischies FM (2021) Leid-Erleben, ein Fundament der Psychopathologie. Pabst Scientific Publishers, Lengerich

MIX
Papier aus verantwortungsvollen Quellen
Paper from responsible sources
FSC® C105338

If you have any concerns about our products,
you can contact us on
ProductSafety@springernature.com

In case Publisher is established outside the EU,
the EU authorized representative is:
Springer Nature Customer Service Center GmbH
Europaplatz 3, 69115 Heidelberg, Germany

Printed by Libri Plureos GmbH
in Hamburg, Germany